Musculoskeletal Medicine and Surgery

For Churchill Livingstone

Commissioning Editor: Michael Parkinson
Project Development Manager: Jim Killgore
Project Manager: Frances Affleck
Designer: Erik Bigland

Musculoskeletal Medicine and Surgery

J. Glynne Andrew MD FRCS

Senior Lecturer in Orthopaedic Surgery, University of Manchester Department of Orthopaedic Surgery, Hope Hospital, Salford, UK

Ariane L. Herrick MD FRCP

Senior Lecturer in Rheumatology, University of Manchester Rheumatic Diseases Centre, Hope Hospital, Salford, UK

David R. Marsh MD FRCS

Professor of Trauma and Orthopaedic Surgery, The Queens University of Belfast, Musgrave Park Hospital, Belfast, UK

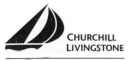
CHURCHILL
LIVINGSTONE

EDINBURGH LONDON NEW YORK PHILADELPHIA ST LOUIS SYDNEY TORONTO 2000

CHURCHILL LIVINGSTONE An imprint of Harcourt
Publishers Limited

© Harcourt Publishers Limited 2000

 is a registered trademark of Harcourt Publishers
Limited

The right of J. Glynn Andrew, Ariane L. Herrick and
David R. Marsh to be identified as authors of this work
has been asserted by them in accordance with the
Copyright, Designs and Patents Act 1988.

First published 2000

ISBN 0443 05698 6

British Library Cataloguing in Publication Data
A catalogue record for this book is available from the
British Library

Library of Congress Cataloging in Publication Data
A catalog record for this book is available from the
Library of Congress

Note
Medical knowledge is constantly changing. As new
information becomes available, changes in treatment,
procedures, equipment and the use of drugs become
necessary. The authors and the publishers have, as far as
it is possible, taken care to ensure that the information
given in this text is accurate and up-to-date. However,
readers are strongly advised to confirm that the
information, especially with regard to drug usage,
complies with the latest legislation and standard of
practice.

The
publisher's
policy is to use
**paper manufactured
from sustainable forests**

Printed in China

Preface

This book is principally intended for undergraduate medical students. These are exciting and challenging times in undergraduate medical education, reflected in major changes in the undergraduate curriculum in most medical schools. Our aim in writing this textbook was to embrace these changes, with their emphasis towards problem-based, system-orientated teaching, and to provide an integrated textbook covering what we perceived as the 'core curriculum' of musculoskeletal disease and injury.

What we mean by an 'integrated' approach to musculoskeletel problems is that the book spans the traditional territories of both rheumatology and orthopaedics. We feel this approach is justified. For many years the Universities of Manchester and Belfast have successfully taught rheumatology and orthopaedics together, and many medical schools are now adopting this approach. Its advantage (as opposed to teaching 'rheumatology' with medicine and 'orthopaedics' with surgery) is that students have the opportunity to concentrate on the musculoskeletal system, learning how to assess problems (with the emphasis on history taking and examination techniques) and how different disease processes and injuries adversely affect the integrity of this system. At an undergraduate level many of the traditional divisions between rheumatology and othopaedics are false or at least unhelpful. For example, if a patient presents with shoulder pain the important point is to have (a) the basic clinical skills to assess the problem and (b) a knowledge of the likely disease processes or injuries likely to be responsible for the patient's presenting symptoms. Thinking separately about rheumatological 'diseases' which affect the shoulder and about orthopaedic 'conditions/injuries' giving rise to

shoulder pain is not the best approach. This book attempts to break down these divisions.

The undergraduate curriculum has a large number of different priorities and we specifically set out to cover only the core curriculum, hoping that interested students will obtain more detailed descriptions elsewhere. With some subjects this was easier than for others. We had to balance the need for some structured disease/injury descriptions (albeit brief) with the philosophy of the problem-based approach. Our final decision was to have three main sections:

- An introductory section describing the approach to diagnosis and management, and incorporating a chapter on pain.
- A section outlining the main joint diseases (both inflammatory and 'degenerative') and connective tissue diseases. This covers clinical features and both rheumatological and orthopaedic management as appropriate. The final three chapters of this section adopt a regional approach, describing upper limb, foot and spinal problems. These regional chapters cover many soft tissue and spinal disorders which are common and often insufficiently covered in other texts. We deliberately chose to have a 'foot chapter' rather than a 'lower limb' chapter, because we felt foot problems warranted a chapter in their own right and important hip and knee conditions are covered in other chapters.
- A trauma section.

It has not been possible to provide an identical template for each chapter. Most chapters begin with a case history, which gives an example of the sort of problems with which the patient might present. Some chapters include more than one case history. When a chapter deals with several different conditions linked by a common theme (for example, the chapters on polyarthritis and bone disorders) we have begun with a case history, but have included shorter 'scenarios' to emphasise important clinical points. While it is not necessary to read the case history to follow the structure of the chapter, we recommend that you do, and then consider the problems described in the context of the chapter. After the case history we have included a key points box in each chapter. These are the things you must know, and are expanded upon in the chapter. The remaining structure varies but includes, where appropriate, epidemiology, pathology, history and examination, and an approach to investigation and treatment.

While much basic scientific and clinical research is currently underway, only occasionally have we referred to this, as we felt it outwith the remit of the core curriculum. However, it is a 'core fact' that in recent years our understanding of musculoskeletal disease and injury (with a major emphasis on molecular and cellular biology) has greatly increased, and new avenues of treatment are continually being explored.

We hope that this textbook will help you to achieve three objectives. Firstly, to develop good history taking and examination skills relevent to the patient with musculoskeletal disease or injury. Secondly, to understand and know about the common and important musculoskeletal conditions. Thirdly, to gain an insight into the challenges of musculoskeletal disease and injury, and into how much is achievable for our patients.

J. G. A
A. L. H
D. R. M

Acknowledgements

We are grateful to several of our colleagues from the University of Manchester for helpful comments and discussions about the manuscript. In particular we thank Professor A.J. Freemont, Dr C. Hutchinson, Professor M.I.V. Jayson and Dr P.L. Selby. In addition, we are very grateful to all those colleagues who have helped us by providing some of the illustrations for the textbook and to the staff of the Department of Medical Illustration at Hope Hospital for their help also in producing the slide collection. We would particularly like to thank Professor C.S.B. Galasko for his assistance with illustrations.

Contents

1 | Introduction to musculoskeletal medicine

There are four features of musculoskeletal medicine which make its practice particularly enjoyable:

- It is mainly about disability and the quality of life. The available medical and surgical treatments are often very effective in improving patients' function.
- Musculoskeletal disease processes comprise a complex interplay of genetic and environmental factors. Understanding of cell-biological processes is beginning to yield new treatments which may prove to be even more effective.
- Many rheumatic diseases are multisystem: diagnosis and management require a broad range of medical skills.
- There is a multidisciplinary approach to treatment, involving collaboration between physicians, surgeons and many others.

Key points

- Musculoskeletal disease impairs the quality of life by reducing the ability to move and often by causing pain.

- The severity of musculoskeletal disease varies enormously.

- There is a huge demand for relief from musculoskeletal symptoms.

- Many musculoskeletal disorders are localised but some are multisystem, e.g. rheumatoid arthritis, so a combined system approach to musculoskeletal medicine and surgery is best.

- Fractures are common, especially in the elderly.

Life is movement, movement is life

The musculoskeletal system allows us to move; this is fundamental to human existence. The various parts of the system are specialised for different kinds of movement, but patients with disorders limiting any of these will experience significant disruption of their ability to function normally in their social and work environments, and a consequent fall in their quality of life.

It is worth considering the importance of the skeletal system in evolution. The development of vertebrates after the Cambrian explosion resulted in a proliferation of life forms. The large terrestrial animals that developed have distinctive features, including the presence of a calcified endoskeleton. The other most successful terrestrial animals are insects; their size is strictly limited by their skeletal arrangement. The development of the musculoskeletal system was therefore intrinsic to the establishment of vertebrate life on land. Furthermore, the great leaps which allowed humans to establish dominance over other animals included the adoption of the upright posture and bipedal locomotion. The legacy of that change is reflected to a large extent in the patterns of musculoskeletal disease we now have to treat.

Disorders of the musculoskeletal system have affected mankind since prehistory; archaeologists have discovered fossil bones showing arthritic changes. However, musculoskeletal medicine and surgery have expanded in importance and size remarkably in the last 50 years, reflecting both the increased longevity of populations in developed countries and the increased possibilities for treatment of diseases which have relatively low mortality rates but which cause severe symptoms.

Currently, both rheumatology and orthopaedic surgery are large and expanding specialities.

The musculoskeletal system comprises not only bones, joints and ligaments, but also muscles and all their attached tendons and their tendon sheaths. In addition, some conditions affecting the nerves supplying the peripheral parts of the body are treated by orthopaedic surgeons and rheumatologists. Disorders affecting these various structures occur throughout the body, and disorders of the musculoskeletal system are very prevalent in the community. Most people will be affected by symptomatic osteoarthritis at some time of their life. It is estimated that about 25% of the workload of general practitioners arises from musculoskeletal disorders. There are also a variety of paramedical professions that collaboratively and independently provide care for the musculoskeletal system (including physiotherapists, podiatrists, osteopaths, chiropractors), further emphasising the demand for relief from musculoskeletal symptoms.

The nature of musculoskeletal disorders varies from the minor to the life-threatening. Many are localised to only a few areas of the body, but systemic conditions such as rheumatoid arthritis can affect not only the musculoskeletal system but most other body systems as well.

The severe, generalised conditions require treatment both by medical means and by surgery; there is increasing integration of such services at a hospital level in the UK and elsewhere. Close working relationships between rheumatologists and orthopaedic surgeons, including combined clinics, provide the best quality care. Furthermore, with the vast numbers of patients presenting with musculoskeletal complaints, the primary doctor in general practice or the A&E department needs to know who can be treated in that primary setting (the majority) and who needs rheumatological or orthopaedic expertise. For these reasons, many medical schools integrate the teaching of musculoskeletal medicine and surgery.

Trauma has been described as the plague of the 20th century and is the commonest cause of death in young adults in the West. The components of the musculoskeletal system are much more exposed to trauma than are other body systems, so fractures are commoner than injuries to other internal organs. A further function of the skeleton is to participate in the management of mineral stores; when bone metabolism becomes unbalanced the skeleton may become unduly susceptible to trauma. The ageing populations of many countries are now experiencing an epidemic of osteoporosis and osteoporotic fractures. Orthopaedic surgery provides a wide variety of methods to treat fractures and soft tissue injuries; success of such treatment may be life-saving or may dramatically reduce morbidity.

PROCESSES OF MUSCULOSKELETAL DISEASE

An evolving feature of most areas of medicine is the increasing understanding of the biological basis of both normal function and disease. Research in musculoskeletal medicine is extremely active and some examples of recent changes in understanding are given below.

Some musculoskeletal conditions are strongly determined by inheritance, e.g.:

- osteogenesis imperfecta, in which abnormal type I collagen renders bones brittle and very susceptible to fracture
- muscular dystrophy, in which progressive degeneration of muscle occurs from a young age.

Others are clearly environmentally induced, the most obvious example being trauma. Everyone's tibia will fracture if a car hits it hard enough.

However, the majority of musculoskeletal conditions involve a combination of environmental trigger and genetic susceptibility. For example, there is evidence of a genetic component to susceptibility for several of the rheumatic diseases. The MHC (major histocompatibility complex) contains many polymorphic loci, and some of these are associated with autoimmune diseases. There is an association, for example, between rheumatoid arthritis and HLA-DR4 (Ch. 8). However, some triggering antigen in the environment is likely also to be required to produce the disease. Reactive arthritis (Reiter's disease) occurs most commonly in patients who are positive for HLA-B27, following a triggering infection at a distant site (Ch. 8). It is also the case that those patients who are HLA-B27-positive tend to have more persistent and chronic disease than those who are HLA-B27-negative.

Our understanding of genetic susceptibility is linked to increasing knowledge of the mechanisms of disease at the level of cell biology. This opens up the possibility of developing new treatments which harness that knowledge. For example, the abnormal immune response involved in the pathogenesis of rheumatoid arthritis is extremely complex and involves the actions of cytokines such as tumour necrosis factor-alpha (TNF-alpha). In view of this, antibodies to TNF-alpha are currently being studied in the treatment of the disease. In another area, since fractures are followed by a process of healing which involves the regeneration of bone, administration of a growth factor, bone morphogenetic protein, is being tried as an adjunct in fracture treatment because of its ability to induce bone formation.

The multisystem aspects of musculoskeletal medicine

Many of the disease processes that affect the musculoskeletal system simultaneously affect other parts of the body. This is because they affect connective tissues and blood vessels at many different sites. Most of these 'multisystem' conditions are inflammatory and associated with abnormalities of the immune system. Therefore a primarily musculoskeletal condition such as rheumatoid arthritis may have manifestations elsewhere, e.g. in the lungs. A good example of a multisystem connective tissue disease is systemic lupus erythematosus (SLE) which is an inflammatory disease associated with a number of abnormalities in immune function. Patients with SLE may present with a variety of symptoms other than joint problems, including rash, tiredness, or chest pain (to name only a few).

Conversely, a primarily non-musculoskeletal disease may present first in the joints or muscles. An example is hypothyroidism, which may present with myopathy.

Therefore a broad range of general medical skills is necessary in the diagnosis of rheumatological disease. These skills are also necessary in management as many of the drugs prescribed to patients with musculoskeletal diseases are potentially toxic, and so very careful assessment of the risk–benefit ratio for each drug is always necessary for each individual patient. This assessment should take into account any other medical conditions the patient might have and any other drugs he/she is already being prescribed. Management also includes that of non-musculoskeletal manifestations of disease, as well as interrelating with all members of the musculoskeletal team as described below.

The musculoskeletal team

Orthopaedic surgery continues to progress rapidly, with an explosion of new techniques and ever more specialised skills which allow ambitious reconstructions of damaged musculoskeletal structures. Rheumatology already has powerful anti-inflammatory agents and, if molecular biology yields the answers we hope it will, more subtle interventions in musculoskeletal conditions will become possible. But the therapeutic potential of these individual medical skills is greatly amplified by the adoption of a team approach (Fig. 1.1).

Clearly there is not much an orthopaedic surgeon can do about an inflammatory condition that is causing pain in all joints and affecting soft tissues as well. Equally, there is no point in expecting a rheumatologist to cure a broken leg with tablets. But there are many situations, particularly in inflammatory arthritis, where the patient needs a combination of the two doctors' skills: medical treatment directed at inflamed tissues and surgery to certain selected musculoskeletal structures where mechanical reconstruction can give significant improvement in function.

However, the need for a team approach goes much wider than this, because of the importance of rehabilitation in recovery from musculoskeletal disease. Even full resolution of a musculoskeletal problem will always leave a legacy of muscle wasting, joint stiffness or local osteoporosis through disuse that will require guidance and encouragement if it is to be overcome. Far more

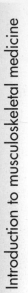

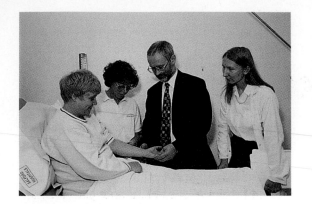

Figure 1.1 Some members of the multidisciplinary team.

help will be needed if some permanent deficit has to be accepted and lifestyle adapted accordingly. The input of specialist nurses, physiotherapists and occupational therapists can dramatically speed up the process of recovery, lead to a higher quality of end result and help reduce the stress and disruption to patients' lives caused by musculo-skeletal disease.

Taken together, these therapeutic possibilities mean that health care professionals have a great deal to offer patients with musculoskeletal disease.

2 | Taking a musculoskeletal history

Case history – trauma

A 30-year-old man was seen in the fracture clinic complaining of knee problems for a period of a fortnight. He had already been seen in the A & E department. His problems started when playing football: in a tackle he had twisted his knee. This became painful and he had to leave the field about 5 minutes after the accident because he could not bear weight normally. The knee swelled up overnight, and he noted that he could not straighten it fully, although he could bend it normally. The knee remained painful, especially on the medial side. He expected it to improve, but it failed to do so.

The doctor in the orthopaedic department told him that the story was 'typical of a torn cartilage' and admitted him forthwith with a view to arthroscopy. This confirmed a bucket handle tear of the medial meniscus, which was blocking full extension of the knee.

Case history – non-trauma

A 62-year-old man with an 8-year history of rheumatoid arthritis presented with a 2-week history of gradually increasing breathlessness and a dry cough. He was on treatment for hypertension but had no previous cardio-respiratory complaints. Six months previously he had been commenced on methotrexate because of his active joint disease. He was also on treatment with prednisolone and ibuprofen.

He was a non-smoker. He had had to give up his work as a teacher 5 years previously because of his joint problems. A widower, he lived alone in a second floor flat, but was considering selling this.

He attended his GP, who was concerned at how breathless he was and arranged hospital admission that day for further assessment and treatment. His GP explained that there were several possible causes of the breathlessness, including an infection, the rheumatoid arthritis itself, or the methotrexate treatment.

The kind of history required from a patient with musculoskeletal complaints depends crucially on whether the patient reports a traumatic incident which initiated the symptoms. If the problem is caused by a known mechanical insult, with previous good health, the history can concentrate on the details of the injury and assessment of its effects; general systemic enquiry is needed only to predict the functional consequences of the injury and to assess the risks of anaesthetics and other elements of the treatment that will be required. On the other hand, if the symptoms are of spontaneous, or at least non-traumatic, onset, then a wide-ranging medical history is required if important factors are not to be

---

Key points

- Taking a careful history is often the most important step in a diagnosis.

- Distinguish between trauma-related and non-trauma-related problems.

- For trauma, take a detailed history of the mechanism of injury.

- For non-trauma, take a full history including careful systemic enquiry.

- Assess the functional consequences of the problem in the context of the patient's life.

missed in the diagnosis of the musculoskeletal problem.

There are exceptions to this simple dichotomy – traps for the unwary. For example, a child may present with a clear history of minor trauma (as reported by a parent) at the start of an episode of a painful swollen joint. This could easily be septic arthritis of non-traumatic origin, because parents naturally look for the simplest and most familiar explanation for things like swollen joints – and children are *always* knocking themselves. Or an elderly person could present with a fractured femoral shaft after a fall – it could be an ordinary osteoporotic fracture, or it could be a pathological fracture through a bony metastasis.

However, despite the need to be on the lookout for such traps, it makes sense to have two different approaches, depending on whether the problem is post-traumatic or not. Therefore, if that aspect of the history is not already glaringly obvious, your first question needs to establish whether there is any preceding injury.

HISTORY FOLLOWING TRAUMA

The patient with multiple injuries represents a special case, dealt with in Chapter 18. Similarly, the general medical history which is needed specifically for pre-anaesthetic assessment in a patient who is heading for surgical treatment of an injury is dealt with in Chapter 5. The following is concerned with the diagnosis of the musculoskeletal consequences of a traumatic incident.

In order to understand the effects of a traumatic incident, the first thing to establish, as clearly as possible, is the *mechanism of injury* (Box 2.1). This does not just mean 'how the accident happened', it means getting a picture of what kind of force was applied to the limb. Was it a direct blow, or was it indirect violence, e.g. a twist applied to the foot causing a knee injury or a spiral fracture of the tibia? Was it a crushing injury, with likely severe soft tissue damage and a relatively minor fracture? Many classic injury patterns can quickly be found if the mechanism of injury has been understood. Ask the patient if he or she can remember exactly what happened to the limb during the accident. If the incident was a fall, ask how the patient landed

---

Box 2.1   Questions about the traumatic incident

- **When did the accident occur?**
- **How did it happen?**
- **What happened to the limb** (mechanism of injury)**?**
- **How much force was applied** (energy of injury)**?**

– onto the outstretched hand, or directly onto the elbow, point of the shoulder and so on?

Related to this, it is important to try to estimate the *energy of injury*. Many injuries have been undertreated because the large amount of energy dissipated in the tissues was not appreciated at the outset. Any road traffic accident (RTA), any fall from a height of more than 6 feet and any severe or prolonged crushing or limb entrapment usually produces a high-energy injury which must be taken very seriously. However, there are many other possible ways to get a high-energy injury and the only safe policy is to ensure you get a clear mental picture of the incident.

Having understood how the trauma occurred, the next job is to assess the consequences by eliciting the patient's symptoms. The main symptoms following musculoskeletal trauma are listed in Box 2.2.

Pain

Pain is probably the commonest and most important symptom; its assessment is so important that a whole chapter (Ch. 6) is devoted to it (the related issue of tenderness is dealt with in Ch. 3).

Box 2.2   Major symptoms after musculoskeletal trauma

- **Pain**
- **Loss of movement**
- **Symptoms of instability**
- **Swelling**

The whole raison d'être for the sense of pain is to give information about tissue damage and, in the vast majority of cases, the diagnosis can be obtained by carefully listening to the description of pain alone. This is even truer in the musculoskeletal system than in other systems where more primitive, visceral pain pathways are more dominant. Important points to ask about pain include the exact site of the pain, whether the pain radiates anywhere, the severity of the pain, the character of the pain, and when the pain developed in relation to the timing of the injury (Box 2.3). Neurogenic pain, discussed in Chapter 6, may develop some time after the initial injury.

Box 2.3   Questions about pain

- Where exactly is the pain, and does it spread anywhere?

- How severe is the pain?

- Can you describe the type of pain?

- Did the pain come on immediately after the injury?

Loss of movement

'Life is movement' and loss of movement is the next commonest complaint after pain. The problem may be loss of motor power, or there may be damage to a joint. Sometimes the problem is a reflex inhibition of muscle action due to pain, or protective muscle spasm. (Questions about loss of movement are given in Box 2.4.)

Loss of *active movement* (movement by the patient, without any help from the doctor examining) in the area of an injury may be neurological, due to peripheral nerve injury, or mechanical, due to disruption of a muscle or its tendon. In order not to miss the former possibility, always enquire about *sensory loss*; but beware – shortly after injury patients may not yet have realised that an area has become numb. They may well have noticed, however, a change in the *quality* of sensation, and if you phrase your question in those terms (asking the patient to make a comparison with the uninjured limb), you will

---

Box 2.4   Questions about loss of movement after injury

- When did the loss occur:
  — immediately after the injury
  — soon after, as swelling developed
  — much later (suggesting fibrosis)?

- Were there symptoms suggestive of joint dislocation (someone may have reduced it)?

- Can the joint be moved passively?

- Are there symptoms suggestive of associated neurological deficit?

- Does the mechanism of injury suggest muscle or tendon rupture?

- Are there other symptoms suggestive of internal derangement?

---

miss less. Suspicion of mechanical disruption of muscle or tendon will usually stem from the history of the injury, e.g. a laceration in the palm. The final distinction is a matter for skilled examination, as outlined in Chapter 3.

Loss of *passive movement* (movement by the examining doctor) of a joint following injury may be due to an acute disruption of the joint architecture, including subluxation (partial dislocation) or complete dislocation. It can also be due to excessive fluid in the joint cavity as a result of the injury (see *joint swelling* below). Lesser degrees of loss of movement range may be caused by *internal derangement* (see below); the classic example is a meniscal tear in a knee joint which causes loss of full extension. Stiffness of a joint at a later stage after injury is likely to be due to fibrosis of the joint capsule or degeneration of the articular cartilage – treatment should be aimed at preventing these. The history of the mechanism of injury, the time course of symptoms since the injury, and the presence of other symptoms related to the joint will usually allow these pathological mechanisms to be distinguished.

Instability

In addition to loss of movement, there are other joint symptoms which patients may complain of following injury, e.g. symptoms suggestive of instability, indicating ligament damage. What the patient will actually say is something like 'my knee gives way'. This symptom can also be due to damage within the joint, to the joint surface (as in an osteochondral fracture) or, in the case of the knee, to a torn meniscus. Such lesions are collectively known as internal derangements; they are also likely to cause mechanical clicking or clunking, or *locking* of the joint. Locking, in a musculoskeletal context, specifically means (in the knee) a physical block to extension (in other joints it means that the joint is jammed, a feeling that is often pronounced but fairly short-lived). If these symptoms are not volunteered, you must ask specifically for them (Box 2.5).

Box 2.5   Questions about instability

- Has the joint ever given way?
- Has the joint ever locked in one position (clarify that the joint truly locks, rather than that the patient is unwilling to move it because it is painful)?
- Have there been any clunks or clicks upon movement of the joint? Are they painful?

Swelling

Following injury to a joint, the symptom of joint swelling is likely to arise. You will need to distinguish between a swelling of the whole joint, due to fluid throughout the synovial cavity, and a more localised swelling near to, but outside, the joint. Enquire as to the speed of onset of the swelling: very rapid swelling indicates a haemarthrosis (and therefore a fracture or something ruptured within the joint), whereas a swelling taking 12 or 24 hours to appear is more likely to be due to a reactive effusion of synovial fluid (see Box 2.6).

HISTORY FOLLOWING ONSET WITHOUT TRAUMA

When there is no preceding history of trauma, a much more open-ended approach to history-taking

---

Box 2.6   Questions about joint swelling

- Has there been any swelling of the joint?
- How much swelling has there been?
- Was the whole joint swollen, or just a part of it?
- How quickly after the accident did the swelling develop?

---

is needed. A detailed history of the presenting complaint must be complemented by a wide-ranging systemic enquiry. The previous medical history, family and drug history may also give clues to the diagnosis.

History of the presenting complaint

The main symptoms (Box 2.8) are similar to those following trauma: pain, swelling, stiffness and loss of function. However, your enquiry needs a different emphasis. The main questions about joints to ask about in patients with and without trauma are compared in Boxes 2.7 to 2.9.

Pain

Pain is often the patient's most distressing complaint, and when severe it interferes with all aspects of everyday life. Pain is considered in Chapter 6.

Box 2.7   Key questions about joints after trauma

- Was the joint ever dislocated?
- Has there been swelling of the joint?
  — how big?
  — whole joint or localised?
  — how quickly after the accident?
- Has the joint ever given way? (Instability)
- Have there been clunks or clicks?
- Has the joint ever locked in one position?

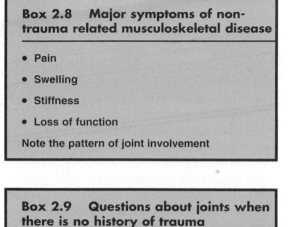

Box 2.8   Major symptoms of non-trauma related musculoskeletal disease

- Pain
- Swelling
- Stiffness
- Loss of function

Note the pattern of joint involvement

Box 2.9   Questions about joints when there is no history of trauma

- Are the joints
  — painful
  — swollen
  — stiff?
- What is the pattern of joint involvement?
- What is the time course of symptoms
  — within each day
  — since the onset?
- What are the functional consequences?

frequently complain of morning stiffness, it is usually short-lived and their symptoms are usually worse later in the day. So the duration of morning stiffness helps you to decide whether this is likely to be an inflammatory or a non-inflammatory disease.

The *pattern* of joint involvement (in both space and time) is very important:

- Is the problem monoarticular or polyarticular? For example, septic arthritis usually affects one joint, rheumatoid usually several, while osteoarthritis can do either.
- Certain diseases have characteristic distributions of joint involvement. For example, rheumatoid arthritis tends to have a symmetrical distribution with early involvement of the small joints of the hands and feet (but sparing the distal interphalangeal joints of the hand).
- The time course of the disease may be characteristic. For example, the patient with gout may have one acute attack followed by months of being symptom-free. If further attacks occur, then the interval between the second and third attacks is shorter, and as time goes on the attacks become closer and closer together. By contrast, patients with osteoarthritis often have a slow progression of their joint complaints, whereas in rheumatoid arthritis, disease progression is very variable – many patients have a relapsing remitting disease characterised by intermittent 'flares'.

Swelling

Enquire about swelling of the joints. If there has been swelling, which joints? Swelling of a joint may be due to fluid, soft tissue or bone, or a combination of these. Ask how long the swelling has been present: an acute onset of knee swelling, for example, suggests monoarthritis, whereas bony knee swelling due to osteoarthritis may have been present for years. Some effusions are painless, but usually an inflamed joint will be stiff and painful as well as swollen.

Stiffness

Ask if the patient is stiff on waking in the morning. A cardinal symptom of inflammatory joint disease, such as rheumatoid arthritis, is stiffness first thing in the morning, which tends to improve with activity. This morning stiffness may last several hours. Such patients may also stiffen up later on in the day after resting (post-inactivity *'gelling'*). Although patients with osteoarthritis also

Loss of function

Enquire as to how joint problems have restricted the patient's activities. Musculoskeletal disease is a major cause of disability. Ask the patient what he/she is unable to do because of pain or stiffness. Walking is often limited in patients with lower limb problems. Patients with inflammatory joint disease and back problems may experience severe loss of function in activities of daily living such as washing, dressing and going to the toilet.

Remember that the importance of a specific loss of function is relative to an individual's daily life and aspirations. This applies to both trauma – and non-trauma-related musculoskeletal problems. For example, a ligamentous strain will be a major handicap to a professional athlete or musician, whereas this would be considered a minor problem by many other patients.

Systemic enquiry

There are several reasons why a full history may be helpful (Box 2.10):

- Clues to the correct diagnosis may be revealed. Several diagnoses have characteristic associated features which are non-musculoskeletal. For example, in the patient presenting with a monoarthritis, a recent diarrhoeal illness would suggest a reactive arthritis. A history of psoriasis suggests psoriatic arthritis. Moreover, many diseases which are not primarily musculo-skeletal may present with musculoskeletal problems. For example, hypothyroidism may begin with a myopathy presenting with generalised aches and pains. A full systemic history should then reveal weight gain and cold intolerance. Malignancies which have metastasised to bone may present with a pathological fracture, and therefore a history of recent weight loss and breathlessness may be highly relevant.

- A patient may have internal organ involvement in what is primarily a musculoskeletal disease. For example, rheumatoid arthritis, systemic lupus erythematosus (SLE) and the vasculitides are all potentially multisystem diseases and relevant symptoms will be missed without a full assessment. Indeed, connective tissue diseases and vasculitides can present simply with pyrexia of unknown origin and other features of multisystem inflammatory disease, without specific musculoskeletal symptoms.

- Drugs used to treat several inflammatory diseases affecting the musculoskeletal system can have side-effects which may be overlooked if not specifically queried. For example, patients on methotrexate may develop cough and breathlessness due to methotrexate pneumonitis (this could have been the problem in the patient in the Case history). Therefore the development of new symptoms in a patient with joint inflammation or connective tissue disease should always prompt the question: 'Is this part of the underlying disease, or could it be drug-related?'

- Patients with musculoskeletal disease or injury may require surgery and need medical assessment before it (and the associated anaesthesia) can be undertaken. This issue is covered in more detail in Chapter 5.

In conducting your systemic enquiry, there are some aspects which are particularly relevant to the patient with musculoskeletal problems (Box 2.11).

Box 2.10   Importance of a full systemic enquiry

- Provides clues to the diagnosis of musculoskeletal disease
  — associated features, e.g. at illness onset
  — systemic disease with musculoskeletal manifestations

- Highlights multisystem effects of musculoskeletal disease, aiding diagnosis e.g. lung involvement in rheumatoid arthritis

- Can identify drug toxicity, e.g. methotrexate pneumonitis

- Part of pre-operative assessment in cases needing surgery

Box 2.11   Systemic questions particularly relevant to musculoskeletal disease

- Have you been feeling well in yourself?

- Have you felt hot or shivery?

- Have you had any rashes?

- Have you had any unusual colour changes in your skin?

- Have you had any problems with your eyes?

Also ask about cardiovascular, respiratory, gastrointestinal, genitourinary, and neurological symptoms

General

Patients with active inflammatory joint or connective tissue disease, or infection, often feel non-specifically tired. Sometimes tiredness is partly related to anaemia, which can occur as part of the inflammatory disease process or for other reasons (e.g. secondary to non-steroidal anti-inflammatory drug treatment, which can cause gastrointestinal blood loss, which can be occult).

If a patient feels feverish, think of infection.

Skin

Many rashes are associated with articular disease. These are described in the relevant chapters. Examples include the rash of psoriasis, the evanescent rash of systemic onset juvenile chronic arthritis, and the characteristic rash on the soles of the feet in Reiter's disease (termed 'keratoderma blenorrhagica').

Mottled, purplish or blue-black fingers or toes are likely to be ischaemic and this may indicate vasculitis or microcirculatory disease associated with connective tissue disease. If you think a patient has connective tissue disease, ask about *Raynaud's phenomenon* (episodic colour change of the extremities in response to cold – classically the digits turn white, then blue, then red). Raynaud's phenomenon can occur in association with a variety of connective tissue diseases, e.g. systemic sclerosis and SLE, although it is often a 'primary' phenomenon, especially when it occurs in young women.

Eyes

Many inflammatory and connective tissue diseases are associated with eye problems. For example, *iritis* can occur in association with the spondyloarthropathies. *Dry eyes* are one of the features of Sjögren's (sicca) syndrome, which can occur alone or in association with connective tissue disease. Ask also about dryness of the mouth.

Past medical history

The past medical history may be important for several reasons (Box 2.12). It may well be relevant to the presenting complaint and suggest a likely

---

> **Box 2.12 Previous medical problems**
>
> - May be relevant to diagnosis
> - May influence medical management
> - May affect decisions regarding surgery

---

diagnosis. For example, in the patient presenting with back pain:

- a history of breast carcinoma raises the possibility of spinal metastases
- a history of hysterectomy and bilateral oophorectomy puts the patient at increased risk of osteoporotic vertebral collapse in later years
- a patient with a history of psoriasis may have developed a spondyloarthropathy

Information obtained from the past medical history may alter decisions regarding medical management, including drug treatment. For example, non-steroidal anti-inflammatory drugs (NSAIDs) should be avoided if there is a recent history of peptic ulceration. An intensive physiotherapy programme for back pain may not be appropriate for a patient with ischaemic heart disease.

Past medical history may affect decisions regarding surgery. For example, a recent myocardial infarction would necessitate postponement of an elective total hip replacement.

Drug history

There are several reasons why you must take an accurate drug history (Box 2.13). The drug history may be relevant to the diagnosis. Drugs prescribed for different medical problems may cause, or predispose to, musculoskeletal disease. For example, diuretics cause a rise in serum uric acid, and therefore predispose to gout. Corticosteroids may lead to osteoporosis and therefore to fractures, as well as to a condition called avascular necrosis. Elderly patients prescribed antihypertensive treatment may develop postural hypotension and may therefore be more likely to fall and to injure themselves.

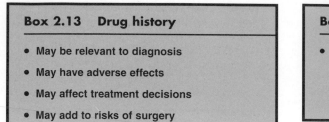

Box 2.13   Drug history

- May be relevant to diagnosis
- May have adverse effects
- May affect treatment decisions
- May add to risks of surgery

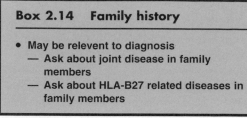

Box 2.14   Family history

- May be relevent to diagnosis
  — Ask about joint disease in family members
  — Ask about HLA-B27 related diseases in family members

All drugs, including those prescribed for musculoskeletal disease, can cause adverse effects. Unless you know which drugs the patient is taking, then abnormal clinical features may not be recognised as side-effects of drug treatment. For example, an iron deficiency anaemia may be the result of an NSAID.

The choice of treatment may depend on previous and present drug therapy. Examples include:

- *Previous therapy.* In a patient who has active rheumatoid arthritis not controlled on current drug treatment, you must check which treatments have already been tried before suggesting a change in treatment. You should also ask why any previously prescribed drugs were discontinued. Was this due to lack of effect (in which case perhaps a higher dose could be tried) or because of adverse drug effects?
- *Present therapy.* Always be aware of the possibility of drug interaction. For example, if a patient is on anticoagulant therapy, NSAIDs are best avoided if possible, as they might induce gastrointestinal bleeding, which could be catastrophic.

A patient's drug treatment may increase the risks of surgery. For example, a patient on immunosuppressive drug treatment may be at increased risk of postoperative infection.

Family history

A family history of musculoskeletal disease should always be sought, as this may be relevant to diagnosis (Box 2.14). Many inflammatory joint/connective tissue diseases are partly genetically determined. This means that there is an increased incidence of the disease in first-degree relatives. In a patient with inflammatory joint disease, always ask specifically about a family history of inflammatory bowel disease and psoriasis (as well as of spondyloarthopathies such as ankylosing spondylitis; see Ch. 8). These can all be associated with the tissue type. HLA-B27 (see Ch. 8).

Rarely musculoskeletal diseases have a Mendelian form of inheritance. One example is osteogenesis imperfecta (autosomal dominant or autosomal recessive), which is associated with inherited abnormalities of collagen and is characterised by brittle bones. Another example is haemophilia (sex-linked). Although haemophilia is not primarily a musculoskeletal disease, patients may present with recurrent haemarthroses and are at high risk of developing secondary osteoarthritis in those joints.

Another important point to bear in mind is that patients who develop musculoskeletal symptoms may be especially worried about these if they have a close relative (e.g. mother, sister) with severe joint disease.

Social history

In patients with musculoskeletal problems, both with and without a history of trauma, the social history is particularly important. Without it, you will not be able to appreciate the impact on the patient's life of the disability produced by the condition. Nor will you be in a position to make realistic treatment plans that will bring about worthwhile improvement.

Important questions include the following:

- *What sort of housing do you have, and is there anyone else at home*? Are the bedroom, bathroom and toilet upstairs? Is there a bath or a shower, and can the patient manage this? Is there anyone else at home who can help? Remember that disability may increase temporarily after surgery.

- *What job do you do?* This may be important for several reasons. A proportion of musculoskeletal problems may be work-related, e.g. certain back problems and some upper limb disorders. Also, the ability of a patient who has developed a musculoskeletal problem to return to work will depend on the nature of the work as well as the diagnosis. For example, a patient who has developed an inflammatory arthritis may be able to return to light duties, but not to heavy labouring. Joint problems may make travelling to work difficult.
- *Do you smoke, and how much alcohol do you drink?*

Smoking is a risk factor for osteoporosis.

Alcohol is a risk factor for gout and for injuries.

You should also be aware that patients with musculoskeletal disease (e.g. severe inflammatory arthritis) may have poor body image as a result of their deformities, and difficulties with sexual relationships. These factors have a major influence on psychosocial well-being.

Box 2.15   Social history

Ask particularly about

- **housing and support at home**
- **occupation and the workplace**
- **smoking habit and alcohol consumption**

3 | Examination of the musculoskeletal system

Case history – trauma

A 25-year-old man driving a car was involved in a road traffic accident. He was brought by ambulance to the A & E department. The ambulanceman reported that the front of the car had been considerably crushed. The patient was able to explain that his right knee was rammed violently against the dashboard and that he now had severe pain in the right knee and hip. The assessment of the A & E trauma team was that the injuries were confined to the right lower limb, and the orthopaedic surgeon was called to see the patient before any X-rays were taken.

Visual inspection revealed that the right lower limb was short compared with the left and lay in a flexed and internally rotated posture. There was bruising over the patella and a large swelling above and to the sides of this bone, in the distribution of the synovial cavity of the knee. Palpation of the swelling suggested it consisted of a large volume of fluid, which was presumed to be blood because of the speed with which it appeared. The front of the knee was extremely tender to the touch. Attempted movement of both the knee and the hip produced considerable pain with very little mobility present. As the surgeon examined the leg below the knee, the patient realised that he could not feel the surgeon's touch and he was unable to move the ankle, although there was no sign of local damage there.

Together with the history of the mechanism of injury, the findings suggested that there had been an intra-articular fracture in the knee and a dislocation of the hip produced by the driving backwards of the femur. Furthermore, it seemed that there had been injury to the sciatic nerve where it ran behind the hip joint. The surgeon sent the patient for X-rays to define the details of the bony injuries and began making arrangements to take him urgently to theatre for reduction of the hip dislocation.

Case history – non-trauma

A 70-year-old female patient was brought by ambulance to the A & E department. Her home help had found her unwell at home, tired and unable to rise from her chair. Very little history was available, but she was known to have long-standing rheumatoid arthritis and normally walked around the house with two sticks. The home help had given her medication to the ambulanceman – prednisolone 7.5 mg daily, ranitidine 300 mg daily and calcium supplements.

On examination she was drowsy. She had a temperature of 37.8°C. Her heart rate was 100/min, and her blood pressure 130/80 mmHg. There were coarse crepitations at both lung bases. With respect to the musculoskeletal system, she had signs of destructive rheumatoid arthritis with deformities of her hands (ulnar deviation at the metacarpophalangeal joints, Z-thumbs), with limited passive movements of the wrists, elbows (with fixed flexion deformities), shoulders and neck. However, there was no evidence of active synovitis of any of these joints, suggesting to the rheumatologist who was called to see her that her rheumatoid arthritis was inactive. However, in the lower limbs she was very tender over the left knee, which was warm and swollen. This knee also had a surgical scar, suggesting that it was prosthetic. She cried out when the doctor attempted to flex the knee. The right knee was not significantly swollen, and flexed to 90°. The left ankle was also warm, swollen and tender, with pain elicited on slight movements of the ankle and subtalar joints. While right ankle and subtalar movements were also limited, there was no swelling. There was metatarsophalangeal subluxation bilaterally.

The working diagnosis was septic arthritis of the left ankle and prosthetic left knee, and bronchopneumonia, against a background of treatment with prednisolone and joint destruction due to rheumatoid arthritis. Pus was aspirated from the left ankle. The on-call orthopaedic surgeon arranged for urgent surgical lavage of the left knee. Prior to her transfer to the ward, blood was taken for blood cultures, full blood count, ESR and biochemical profile.

Key points

- Regional and systemic examinations are often just as important as local examination of the site of maximum symptoms.

- To be focused and fruitful, examination needs to be guided by the history and informed by a knowledge of musculoskeletal pathology.

- In order to record and communicate findings, it is necessary to learn professional terminology and conventions of description, e.g. of the ranges of joint movement.

- You can only learn examination technique by practising it on patients.

- A useful routine to approach any joint is *look, feel and move*.

- Certain issues are particularly important in certain joints, such as stability in the knee or range of movement at the hip. You need to practise specific routines for assessing these.

The two case histories demonstrate how a careful clinical examination is crucial in making the correct diagnosis. This chapter is arranged as follows:

- Some introductory comments, followed by a very basic description of bone, joints and peripheral nerves.
- A brief section outlining the importance of the systemic as well as the musculoskeletal examination.
- General points of musculoskeletal assessment and description. This will introduce many of the concepts which are then put to the test in the examination of the individual joints.
- A regional atlas of examination techniques. Different joints are used as exemplars of key points in examination technique. For example, assessment of joint swelling and joint stability are highlighted in the section on the knee, but the same basic principles are relevant to other joints/regions. Boxes throughout the text emphasise that the basic approach to the examination of any joint/region has the same common elements.

As you begin to examine a patient with a musculoskeletal problem, you need to have taken a good history and to have some knowledge about the patterns of musculoskeletal disease, so that you already have a theory about what could be wrong and what you may find. Without this, your examination will be poorly directed and you will miss things – the eye cannot see what the mind does not know. For example, if a patient's principal complaint is of pain in the leg and foot, your examination may miss the point if you do not know that the differential diagnosis includes radicular pain from lumbar spinal disease.

Furthermore, your examination will be unrewarding without the patient's cooperation. You should have established rapport in the course of taking the history, checked that the patient is happy to be examined by you, knowing that you are a student, and arranged for a chaperone to be present if the patient is of the opposite sex. The patient should be comfortable and warm, not on public view, and the relevant parts of his or her anatomy should be adequately exposed right at the beginning of the examination. *You should have established whether any parts you intend to examine are painful to touch.*

When examining the limbs, you will make full use of the fortuitous fact that patients often have a normal limb with which to compare the abnormal one, by examining each feature on the normal side first. If your examination is to be a useful contribution to the patient's care, you need to know not only what to look for, but also how to communicate your findings. This requires knowledge of the terminology and conventions used by your fellow professionals to describe things: the functional anatomical descriptors of the bones and joints, the musculotendinous units which move them, and the peripheral nervous network which controls that movement.

Bone may be cancellous or cortical. The former is found in small rounded bones and at the expanded ends of long bones near the joints. It is designed to absorb impacts, if necessary by sustaining small fractures of its constituent trabeculae – like the crumple zone at the front of a car – which can heal quickly. Cortical bone forms very strong, stiff tubes which provide the long lever arms that comprise our limbs. The topography of a long bone is described in relation to the growth plate – *physis* – or the scar where it used to be in adults (see Fig. 3.1). The prefixes *dia-* and *epi-* (as in diaphysis and epiphysis) come from the Greek meaning 'between' and 'beyond', respectively. Between these two zones is the metaphysis, *meta* meaning 'transitional'.

Joints are like the hinges of a door. In one sense they allow movement, while in another sense they prevent it: they normally only allow movement in certain directions. Most are synovial, i.e. they have gliding cartilage surfaces lubricated and nourished by synovial fluid (the fluid produced by the synovium, which lines the joint cavity). Other types of articulations are found, such as the intervertebral discs, which function quite differently. However, all joints are guarded by ligaments which constrain movement between the adjacent bones. In a simple hinge joint (Fig. 3.2), the main ones are the collateral ligaments, which prevent movement at right angles to the correct plane of joint movement. Smooth joint movement depends on the articular cartilage, and the health of this tissue depends on nourishment by the synovial fluid. Disturbance of this mechanism constitutes a large part of the subject matter of musculoskeletal medicine, and the complicated interplay of mechanical forces and cellular reactions which underlie it is fascinating. In some joints – principally the knee – the congruence of the opposing surfaces, which is essential for stability and the even distribution of pressure, is partly achieved by the presence of separate cartilaginous spacers, or menisci, within the joint, and these may also play a significant role in causing symptoms. Further discussion of the structure of synovial joints is given in Chapter 22 on joint injuries.

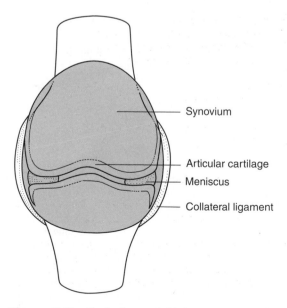

Figure 3.2 Typical synovial joint structure.

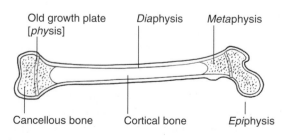
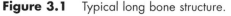

Old growth plate [*phy*sis]   *Diaphysis*   *Metaphysis*

Cancellous bone   Cortical bone   *Epi*physis

Figure 3.1 Typical long bone structure.

The neuromuscular system. Although some passive stability to the various linkages within the skeleton is provided by the ligaments around joints, the system is not stable without active postural control by the neuromuscular system. Energy-efficient locomotion and skilful manipulation of the world about us are also the products of a feedback control system of great elegance and, normally, reliability. Proprioception (literally, 'sense of oneself') and a fine tactile sense through the skin provide the basis for the central nervous system to perform this remarkable integration; deficits in the control system produce dramatic effects on body posture and control.

Figure 3.3 shows, in a gross simplification, the nerve fibres involved in motor control (the gamma motor neurones, whereby the CNS can control the sensitivity of the muscle spindles, are not shown). These are all large, myelinated, fast fibres. However, peripheral nerves also transmit the many smaller fibres which subserve the sense of pain. Our understanding of their function is even less complete than that of motor control, yet they are crucial to musculoskeletal medicine.

Musculotendinous units. Being able to move around and manipulate things in the environment depends also on the mechanical transmission of force generated by muscles to the bones, often going round corners in the process. The functional anatomy of the tendons, their guiding sheaths and the specialised structures whereby they, or muscle fibres, insert into bone (entheses) is important in diagnosing many symptoms which patients develop in response to the strains of everyday life or following traumatic incidents.

As with the history, it is important to make a full systemic examination in patients presenting with musculoskeletal problems without a clear traumatic aetiology and in trauma patients who may have other injuries or require surgery. Narrowing the focus somewhat, it is then a good idea to observe the integrated function of the affected region: standing and walking for the spine and lower limb; grasping and manipulating for the upper limb. If you are faced with a patient who has a widespread rheumatological problem, observe and record the pattern of involvement of joints and muscles between the limbs. Then you can proceed to specific examination of the relevant joints, bones, muscles and tendons, nerves and skin. A description of the techniques and terminology used is given here in two sections: (1) a discussion of general principles, and (2) an atlas of specific examination techniques for different regions.

SYSTEMIC EXAMINATION

The injured patient (especially if multiple injuries have occurred) may be unwell with signs of shock (see Ch. 18), and may require resuscitation prior to any surgery.

In the non-traumatic case, systemic examination is required for the same reasons as a full history (see Ch. 2). You may:

- Find clues to the diagnosis. For example, a small patch of psoriasis may point to a diagnosis of psoriatic spondyloarthropathy.
- Find evidence of internal organ involvement. Basal crepitations in a patient with rheumatoid arthritis could be due to pulmonary fibrosis, which can be a feature of rheumatoid arthritis.
- Suspect drug toxicity. For example, a purpuric rash (which the patient would probably draw to your attention) might be due to drug-induced thrombocytopenia (this can occur with gold and other antirheumatic drugs) (Fig. 3.4).

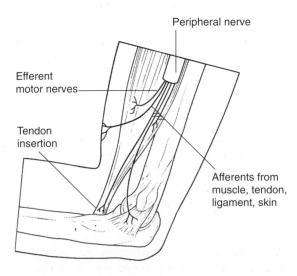

Peripheral nerve

Efferent motor nerves

Tendon insertion

Afferents from muscle, tendon, ligament, skin

Figure 3.3   Neuromuscular control elements.

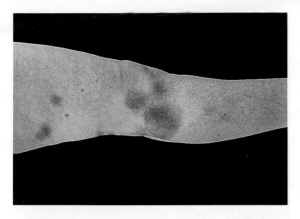

Figure 3.4 Purpuric rash in a patient with drug-induced thrombocytopenia.

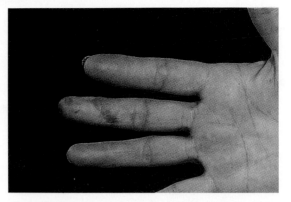

Figure 3.5 Digital cyanosis in a patient with Raynaud's phenomenon secondary to systemic sclerosis.

- Alter decisions regarding treatment, including surgery. If an elderly patient is in a degree of cardiac failure you would hesitate to prescribe a non-steroidal anti-inflammatory drug (these can cause fluid retention and therefore exacerbate cardiac problems) and the patient would be at increased risk from an anaesthetic and from surgery.

Specific points about what to look for on systemic examination are made in the relevant chapters but some general points can be made.

General

Always check the temperature. A high temperature suggests infection, but can occur with connective tissue disease including vasculitis (inflammation of the blood vessels) or sometimes with malignancy. Also look for pallor, weight loss and lymphadenopathy, all of which may indicate chronic inflammatory or malignant disease.

Mucous membranes, skin and nails

A tremendous amount of information can be obtained from these. Look for mouth ulcers, skin rashes and areas of skin discoloration. Many different forms of rash occur in the different rheumatic diseases and some are disease-specific. Rashes also occur as side-effects of several of the antirheumatic drugs. An area of erythema may be due to underlying infection, whereas cyanosed

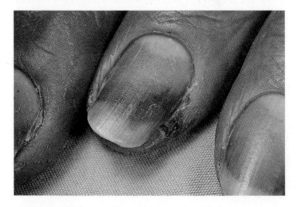

Figure 3.6 Splinter haemorrhages.

extremities can be found in certain connective tissue disorders (Fig. 3.5). Cyanosis occurring after limb trauma is suggestive of vascular involvement.

Multiple splinter haemorrhages (Fig. 3.6) may occur in vasculitis as well as in bacterial endocarditis. They should always prompt a search for more serious clinical features of systemic disease. Typical nail changes occur in psoriasis, with nail pitting and onycholysis (separation of the nail plate from the nail bed).

Eyes

A number of rheumatic diseases are associated with eye involvement. While this may not be clinically apparent, requiring specialist

Examination of the musculoskeletal system

investigation (e.g. detection of chronic anterior uveitis in juvenile chronic arthritis by slit-lamp examination), some problems are obvious (e.g. the painful red eye of acute anterior uveitis associated with the B27-related spondyloarthropathies, or scleritis associated with rheumatoid arthritis).

GENERAL POINTS OF MUSCULOSKELETAL ASSESSMENT AND DESCRIPTION

In learning the art of musculoskeletal examination, it is useful to have in your mind the framework *look – feel – move*. This sequence was distilled from very wide experience by the great orthopaedic teacher Alan Apley. As you approach any joint, ask yourself: what do I need to *visually inspect*; what do I need to *palpate*; what do I need to *move*?

There are several specific features to look for when examining a patient with musculoskeletal disease. A quick check list is given in Box 3.1.

Joints

The pattern of involvement in rheumatological cases

In the patient with joint disease, the pattern and site of joint involvement can be important diagnostically. For example, the metatarsophalangeal joint of the great toe is often affected in gout, and therefore acute swelling of this joint in a middle-aged or elderly patient is suggestive of gout. However, beware because this joint is also often affected by osteoarthritis. In a young woman with polyarthritis, arthritis of the small joints of the hands or feet is suggestive of rheumatoid arthritis or systemic lupus erythematosus, whereas large joint, lower limb involvement with restricted spinal movement is suggestive of a spondyloarthropathy.

Deformity

Learn to recognise and describe common deformities of a limb or a single long bone. The same words are used to describe deformities within one long bone or between bones connected by a joint in the same limb, based on the anatomical planes (Fig. 3.7).

Varus and valgus. These are angulations in the

Box 3.1 Points to look for when assessing the musculoskeletal system

The pattern of joint involvement for each joint:

- deformity (*look*)
- the overlying skin (*look*, and *feel* for temperature)
- joint swelling (*look* and *feel*)
- tenderness (*feel*)
- range of movement (*move* and at the same time *feel* for crepitus; ask whether the patient experiences pain on movement, and watch their face for signs of pain)
- stability (*move* and *feel*)

Also, always assess whether the combination of signs suggests joint inflammation; i.e. swelling, tenderness and pain on motion.

For the affected region:

- muscle bulk (*look*, *feel* and ask the patient to *move* against resistance)
- sensibility (*feel*)
- blood supply (*look* for colour change and then *feel* for temperature and pulses)
- lumps (*look* and *feel*)

Note: remember it is also important to look beyond the musculoskeletal system, especially when there is no history of trauma or when surgery is indicated.

---

coronal plane. In varus, the distal segment is inclined towards the midline; in valgus the distal segment is angulated laterally (Fig. 16.1). Thus genu valgum is knock-knee, and tibia vara is an outward bow of the tibia (Fig. 3.8).

Procurvatum and recurvatum. These are angulations in the sagittal plane. In procurvatum, the apex of the deformity protrudes anteriorly; in recurvatum it points posteriorly. Genu recurvatum is a hyperextended knee; a long bone shaft fracture may heal with a procurvatum deformity.

Internal and external rotation. These are angulations in the transverse plane. The direction given is that of the distal segment with respect to

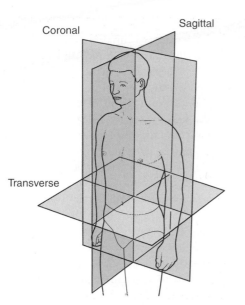

Figure 3.7   The three anatomical planes.

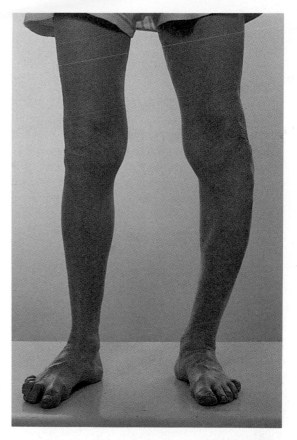

Figure 3.8   Tibia vara in Paget's disease (the distal tibia is inclined towards the midline). Courtesy of Dr T. O'Neill.

the proximal. With an externally rotated tibia, the foot points outwards.

Real and apparent shortening.   This distinction is important in the lower limb, where tilt of the pelvis combined with adduction of one hip can result in legs which lie parallel with apparently different lengths, although the bones are actually the same length.

The main spinal deformities (scoliosis and kyphosis) are described in more detail in Chapter 14 on paediatric orthopaedics.

The overlying skin

In addition to signs of current inflammation, the skin bears evidence of past history. Look for *sinuses* – points where infected material has found its way to the surface – and note whether they are actively draining. Check for *scars* (traumatic and surgical). A search for skin pustules is essential in a patient who is scheduled for surgery, particularly operations involving implantation of prostheses or other metalwork. *Vasomotor instability* may be indicated by abnormal erythema, purple colour or pallor. In chronic painful conditions, or following nerve injury, this may be associated with *trophic change* – shiny, tight, hairless skin and spindling of

---

Box 3.2   Check list of things to examine about joints

- Deformity
- Swelling
  — effusion
  — synovitis
- Tenderness
- Inflammation (temperature)
- Range of movement
  — active
  — passive
- Pain on movement
- Stability

digits. Previous soft tissue injury may leave an area of *induration* – also a sign of previous deep vein thrombosis in the legs.

Joint swelling

It is crucial to be able to distinguish between a joint effusion (which may be blood, pus or synovial fluid), synovial thickening and other swollen structures around joints. This is especially important in the exposed, superficial joints, the knee and elbow. A swollen joint may be inflamed. Features of acute and chronic joint inflammation are described below under 'signs of inflammation'.

Tenderness

Tenderness may be localised or diffuse. It is one of the cardinal signs of inflammation (see below). Localising an area of tenderness may indicate the likely cause of a patient's problems. For example, tenderness at the knee joint line may indicate a tear in the meniscus. Patients with the condition fibromyalgia (see Ch. 6) have tenderness at a number of specific sites.

Range of movement

Know which movements are important for each joint and what is the convention for describing them. Examine passive or active movements as convenient (often active for upper limb, passive for lower), but both if there is doubt about the integrity of the motor system moving the joint. Assess how much of the limitation is due to pain and how much to mechanical block (watch the face). A mechanical block to joint movement is often described as a fixed deformity in the opposite direction; for example, a loss of extension at the hip is classically described as *fixed flexion*. When assessing movement, feel for *crepitus* (a crunching or grating which may be felt over a moving joint). Coarse crepitus is sometimes audible – it commonly occurs with joint damage, e.g. in osteoarthritis.

Joint stability

Know what stabilisers are important for each joint and how to stress-test them. Look out for subluxation and dislocation.

Signs of inflammation

The cardinal signs of inflammation are redness, warmth, swelling and pain. Not all elements may be present. Classically, an inflamed joint is swollen, tender and painful on movement. In an acute monoarthritis (Ch. 7) of a superficial joint such as the knee, there may also be redness, the joint may be hot, and the tenderness and pain on movement may be extreme. In patients with more chronic (but active) inflammation, such as the patient with rheumatoid arthritis, joints are unlikely to be red, but other signs of joint inflammation are present (albeit less intense than in an acute monarthritis). Classically in patients with active inflammatory joint disease such as rheumatoid arthritis, the joint feels 'boggy' due to the hypertrophied synovium. Inflammation of the synovium is termed synovitis. Remember that synovial swelling affects tendon sheaths as well as synovial joints.

Affected region

Muscles

Look for wasting: it can be a consequence of disuse (especially quadriceps) or denervation (e.g. the thenar eminence in median nerve compression). If it is helpful to chart muscle power, use the MRC scale (M0–5, Box 3.3). Muscle tenderness may indicate myositis.

Sensibility

Much can be learned from mapping out an area of altered sensibility and comparing it with

---

Box 3.3   MRC motor scale

0 – no contraction

1 – flicker or trace of contraction

2 – active movement, with gravity eliminated

3 – active movement against gravity but not resistance

4 – active movement against gravity and resistance but not full power

5 – normal power

Box 3.4   MRC sensory scale

0 – absence of sensibility

1 – deep cutaneous pain sensibility

2 – superficial cutaneous pain and some tactile sensibility

3 – tactile sensibility plus some two-point discrimination

4 – normal sensibility

---

segmental dermatomes and peripheral nerve territories. Describing the degree of alteration in sensibility is more difficult; the MRC sensory scale (S0–4, Box 3.4) is available, but it was really designed for the specific purpose of monitoring recovery from peripheral nerve injury. The important thing is to distinguish protective sensibility from tactile sensory acuity: the former will prevent skin damage from occurring but both are needed in the hand for normal function. It is also important to distinguish ordinary tenderness from painful hypersensitivity or allodynia (see Ch. 6).

Blood supply

Check the main pulses. In lower limb conditions, check in the groin, the popliteal fossa and behind the medial malleolus. Arterial disease causes pain in the legs and so enters into the differential diagnosis of lower limb pain. Furthermore, its presence may affect decisions about the advisability of surgery. In the upper limb, diminished pulses may indicate thoracic outlet compression, which could also be affecting nerves and causing pain. Venous disease should also be noted, since phlebitic or post-phlebitic soft tissue heals poorly after surgery. Patients with connective tissue disorders (e.g. systemic sclerosis) may have microcirculatory disease, in which case they may have signs of digital ischaemia but normal major pulses.

Lumps

Abnormal swellings are a common presenting complaint. Their analysis depends on diagnosis of what they consist of and where they arise from – questions which are mainly answered by physical examination, although imaging techniques and aspiration or biopsy are often used for confirmation. It is essential to be able to distinguish cystic from solid swellings by eliciting *fluctuation*. The composition of solid swellings can be deduced from their *hardness*, ranging from bony lumps to lipomata. The deep *attachment* of a swelling, elicited by attempting to move it, often allows you to deduce the layer (subcutaneous, intramuscular) in which it lies and the deep structures to which it is related. If the lump is in the region of a joint, then ask yourself whether it could be in the synovial cavity. If not, it could still be a *ganglion*, arising from the joint (these may have a history of variations in size), but it could also be one of the anatomically recognised bursae which commonly give problems, especially around the knee and elbow.

A number of rheumatic diseases are associated with superficial swellings, e.g. rheumatoid modules, gouty tophi and tendon xanthomas.

REGIONAL ATLAS OF EXAMINATION TECHNIQUES

You cannot fully investigate every bone and every joint in the examination of each patient. Decide which you are going to concentrate on, given the history and what you have observed so far. If you remember to think about and observe the integrated function of the affected region first, your subsequent examination of individual structures will be much more rewarding.

Depending on the likely pathology, your examination may be focused on a particular type of abnormality; some of these are best described in certain joints or regions where they are classically taught (see Table 3.1).

In the regional atlas which follows, these 'exemplars' of types of abnormality will usually be described first in each regional section because they are the most important for you to learn and apply. They are not necessarily the things examined first when you are faced with a patient. The best person to develop an order in which you apply tests to a particular joint or region is you, as

Table 3.1
Types of joint abnormality and exemplar regions

Type of abnormality	Exemplar joint or region
Joint stiffness	Hip
Joint swelling	Knee
Localised tenderness	Knee
Loss of external stabilisers and internal derangement of a joint	Knee
Joint deformity	Knee + foot
Problems with soft tissue structures around a joint	Shoulder
Sensibility	Hand
Synovitis	Hand
Tendon rupture	Hand
Neurological deficit	Spine

a result of observing senior colleagues and your own practice. Most people find that a basic framework of *look–feel–move* is helpful. However, as a medical student it is best to have a structured approach to the examination of each joint or region (which you may modify when you have more experience), and each regional section includes a subsection with a box outlining the key features to be included in the examination. In addition to 'exemplar' points and the box outlining the structured approach, for each region we include subsections which are of particular importance, e.g. range of motion in the section on the knee.

Finally, always remember to consider the possibility that symptoms do not necessarily originate from the site where they are felt – a classic example is that pain in the knee may arise from the hip. Therefore, examine other musculoskeletal sites or for internal organ involvement, as appropriate.

LOWER LIMB

Examination of the lower limb comprises an assessment of gait and any limb length discrepancy that might be present, followed by examination of the hip, knee, ankle and foot.

Gait

Examination of gait will allow you to observe the integrated function of the lower limbs. Careful observation allows the recognition of several characteristic patterns caused by specific deficits.

Antalgic limp

A painful lesion anywhere in one lower limb causes the patient to try to reduce the amount of time spent taking weight on that limb – the *stance phase* of the gait cycle. The gait cycle is therefore asymmetrical in time, with shorter steps taken on the painful limb.

Trendelenburg gait

This gait results from weakness of the hip abductors, most commonly due to shortening of these muscles because of abnormal proximal position of the greater trochanter where they are inserted. Because the abductors are weak, when the weight is taken on the affected limb, the opposite side of the pelvis dips down. *Trendelenburg's test* (Fig. 3.9) is performed by asking the patient to stand on one leg and observing the occurrence of this pelvic dip, which may take a few seconds to occur. When Trendelenburg-positive patients walk, they keep their balance, in spite of the pelvic dip, by leaning their upper body over the weak hip, to shift their centre of gravity. This is most apparent when the patient walks towards you; their shoulders make exaggerated side-to-side movements as this manoeuvre is performed.

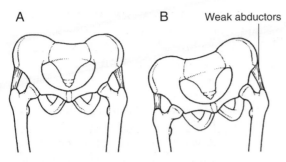

Figure 3.9 Trendelenburg's test.
A. Symmetrical bilateral stance. **B.** Pelvic tilt when weight taken on affected leg (with other knee bent).

Limp of limb length discrepancy

This may also give rise to a pelvic tilt, with lateral movement of the shoulders as in a Trendelenburg gait. Since the abductors are likely to be normal, however, the patient may keep a horizontal pelvis and dip vertically up and down, flexing the knee in the longer limb to clear the ground during the *swing phase* of gait. Try walking on the edge of a pavement, with one foot in the gutter, to understand the choice such a patient has to make, and how tiring it is.

Drop foot

Inability to dorsiflex the ankle (due to a peroneal nerve lesion) renders the patient at risk of tripping over the toes during the swing phase. To avoid this, patients adopt a high-stepping gait on that side, flicking the foot forward at the end of the swing phase. Sometimes such a patient will also swing that leg outwards to help clear the ground and bring the foot in sharply at the end of swing phase. The stance phase usually begins with *heel strike*, but in a patient with a drop foot, heel strike is replaced by slapping the whole foot on the ground simultaneously.

Equinus contracture

Although patients with drop foot are unable to dorsiflex their ankle actively, the passive movement is usually retained. In patients with equinus contracture, passive dorsiflexion is also lost; this means they cannot get their heel to the ground during stance phase. Again they have a

difficult choice: adapt the gait to that of a limb length discrepancy or try to get the heel down and force the knee into hyperextension (this is sometimes called '*back-kneeing*'); both patterns are seen.

Fixed hip flexion

Patients with stiff hips are often unable to extend them – they have a fixed flexion. This disturbs the flow of normal gait because, at the end of each stance phase, the hip normally extends as the opposite leg swings forward to plant the foot at the beginning of the next step. Inability to do this means that the pelvis is halted suddenly in its forward progress and the opposite leg has to terminate its swing prematurely. The stop–start forward motion of the pelvis makes walking uneven and very tiring.

Limb length equality

As described above, inequality in the lengths of lower limbs has a drastic effect on gait. It is also bad for the lumbar spine, producing a scoliosis, and leads almost inevitably to low back pain. Checking for limb length discrepancy is a fundamental step in most cases of lower limb assessment, since there are so many ways in which one limb can suffer shortening (Box 3.5).

Just as limb length discrepancy can lead to tilting of the pelvis during standing or walking, the reverse can also happen. The pelvis may be

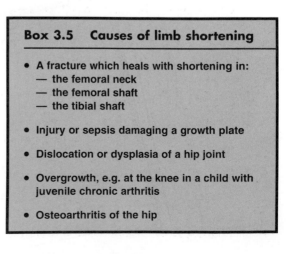

Box 3.5   Causes of limb shortening

- A fracture which heals with shortening in:
  — the femoral neck
  — the femoral shaft
  — the tibial shaft

- Injury or sepsis damaging a growth plate

- Dislocation or dysplasia of a hip joint

- Overgrowth, e.g. at the knee in a child with juvenile chronic arthritis

- Osteoarthritis of the hip

tilted due to a fixed curvature of the spine or, more commonly, because there is an *adduction contracture* of one hip joint, so that the only way the patient can retain parallel legs (a prerequisite for walking!) is to lift up the pelvis on the affected side (Fig. 3.10). The effect of this is to produce *apparent shortening* of that limb. This must be distinguished from the *real shortening* that results from damage to the bones.

The key step in making this distinction is to look for tilting of the pelvis. With the patient lying straight on the examination couch (supine), feel for the anterior superior iliac spines; this takes practice and may be difficult in overweight patients. They are most easily felt with the thumbs, sliding up to them from below. Once these are located, it is not difficult to judge whether they are lying at right angles to the patient's long axis, and to adjust the patient's posture until they are. After you have done this, look at the patient's heels – real leg length discrepancy is then directly observable.

If, because of fixed hip adduction or for any other reason, you cannot get the pelvis to lie square, another technique is to measure real lengths directly with a tape measure from the anterior superior iliac spine to the medial malleolus (Fig. 3.11A). Apparent lengths can be measured from the xiphisternum or umbilicus to each medial malleolus, with the pelvis lying in its habitual tilted position (Fig. 3.11B).

Another approach is to examine the patient standing: observe whether the heels are both on the ground and, kneeling behind the patient, feel the iliac crests with the flat of the index fingers on each side. Pelvic tilt is readily appreciated in this way. Most orthopaedic and rheumatological clinics are equipped with 'standing blocks' – blocks of wood of various (marked) thicknesses, which can be placed under the heel of the short limb until both you and the patient feel that the pelvis is level. The advantage of this is that it leads directly to the prescription of the correct size of heel-raise from the surgical appliances department. The inter-relationship between scoliosis and limb length discrepancy is shown in Figure 3.12.

Hip (exemplar for joint stiffness)

Joint stiffness

The hip is a deep, stable joint. Therefore, stability and ligament integrity are rarely the issue (except in babies; see Ch. 14); what is important is the *range*

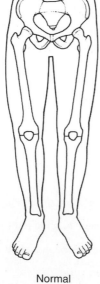
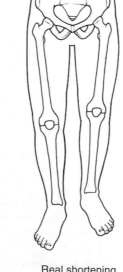
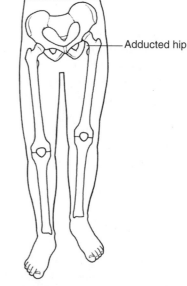

Adducted hip

Normal   Real shortening   Apparent shortening

Figure 3.10   Lower limb shortening: normal, real and apparent.

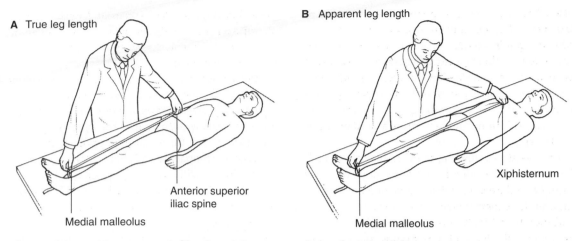

A True leg length

B Apparent leg length

Xiphisternum

Anterior superior
iliac spine

Medial malleolus

Medial malleolus

Figure 3.11 Measurement of leg length (measure right leg first, then left).

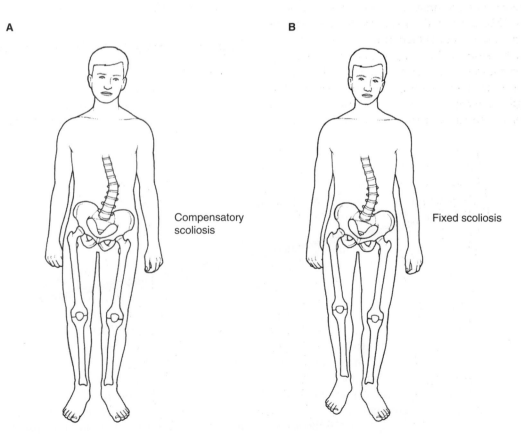

A

B

Compensatory
scoliosis

Fixed scoliosis

Figure 3.12 Interrelationship between scoliosis and limb length inequality.
A. A true leg length discrepancy has resulted in a compensatory scoliosis.
B. A fixed scoliosis has resulted in an apparent limb length discrepancy.

of motion. Theoretically, a complete description of the range of motion of a joint includes, for all the possible degrees of freedom of that joint, both the *active range,* that which the patient is able to produce by muscle action, and the *passive range* achievable by the examiner. In practice, one is selective, and the active range is less commonly tested for the hip. The commonest indication for measuring the range of motion in the hip is probably the evaluation of osteoarthritis, which causes stiffness both by degeneration of the joint cartilage and by the associated scarring contraction of the joint capsule.

The range of movement in the hip can be analysed in three planes: sagittal, coronal and transverse. The movements in the sagittal plane are flexion and extension; in the coronal plane, abduction and adduction; in the transverse plane, internal and external rotation. As the hip joint capsule contracts, it pulls the joint into flexion and adduction; this combination produces the typical fixed deformity of advanced osteoarthritis. Rotation is lost at an early stage. Assessment therefore boils down to testing for fixed flexion (loss of extension in less severe cases) and fixed adduction (loss of abduction) and loss of internal and external rotation.

The key point of technique is to avoid being fooled by rotation of the pelvis. As in the comparison of leg lengths, remember that the human body has little choice but to contort itself in such a way that both legs are more or less parallel and point to the ground. So, as we have already seen, fixed adduction does not lead to scissoring of the legs; instead the pelvis tilts. If a patient has flexion deformities of the hips, it will not be the legs that point forwards – they will be vertical and it will be the pelvis that rotates.

Testing for fixed flexion and for fixed adduction. Controlling the pelvis when testing for fixed flexion is the essence of the Thomas test (Fig. 3.13). By flexing the opposite hip (the one thought to be normal), the lumbar lordosis is eliminated; this is confirmed by placing one hand under the lumbar spine and feeling it squashed. If the tested hip has a fixed flexion, this manoeuvre will cause that thigh to lift. An analogous manoeuvre is required to demonstrate or exclude fixed

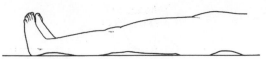

A   Resting position: legs flat, lumbar lordosis present

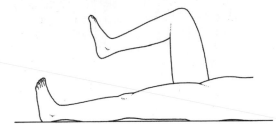

B   No fixed flexion: no lift when lordosis eliminated by flexing normal hip

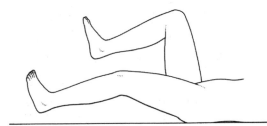

C   Fixed flexion: tested leg lifts when lordosis eliminated

Figure 3.13   Thomas test.

adduction (Fig. 3.14). Again the pelvis is locked into a standard anatomical position by manipulating the other hip, this time in the coronal plane, by abducting it to its limit and rendering the pelvis horizontal.

Testing internal and external rotation. This is not beset by the problem of pelvic mobility, since the pelvis does not so easily rotate in the transverse plane, being broad and flat. The problem here is that rotation can be tested with the hip either flexed or extended, and one needs to standardise. Rotation-in-flexion is easier to measure since, with the knee flexed as well, the tibia can be used as a pointer. However, most clinicians report rotation-in-extension, since that is the functionally important movement when standing and walking. The best indicator of femoral rotation is then the patella which, despite being rounded, has the

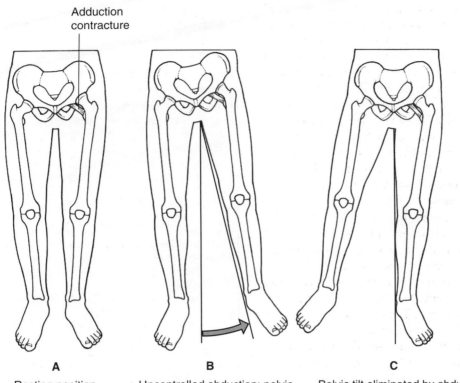

A
Resting position
legs parallel

B
Uncontrolled abduction: pelvic
tilt gives spurious abduction

C
Pelvic tilt eliminated by abducting
other hip: fixed adduction apparent

Figure 3.14 Testing for fixed abduction.

virtue of sitting firmly in the trochlear groove of the distal femur and faithfully reproduces the latter's rotation.

Reporting of range of movement. The most rigorous measurement is pointless unless the results are reported in a standard format that will be understood by others. Figure 3.15 shows the accepted conventions for recording ranges of movement at the hip. An economical way to record the findings in, for example, a patient with a normal right hip but a stiff left hip showing 20° fixed flexion, 15° fixed adduction and 10° of fixed internal rotation would be as shown in Table 3.2. Sometimes an even more economical notation is adopted which would record the abnormalities as:

- flexion   20–90
- adduction   15–25
- IR   10–30

Structured approach to examination of the hip
We have concentrated on the assessment of joint stiffness, but there are other aspects of hip examination in the patient presenting with problems thought to be arising in and around the hip (Box 3.6). Several conditions can give rise to symptoms around the hip and it is important to check for these, especially if hip movements appear normal and are pain free (Box 3.7). Some of these are local soft tissue disorders within the region of the hip, while others arise from elsewhere. Common causes of pain in the region of the hip are:

- trochanteric bursitis – the greater trochanter will be tender on palpation
- ischiogluteal bursitis – pain is aggravated by sitting
- adductor enthesopathy – pain and tenderness are localised over the adductor insertion

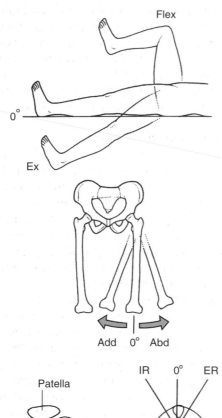

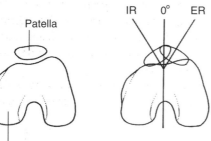

Figure 3.15 Conventions for reporting range of movement at the hip. Note: for internal and external rotation, imagine that the patient is lying supine on the couch and you are at the end (looking towards the patient's head). The cross-section is then through the left knee.

Table 3.2
Recording range of movement

	Flex	Ext	Add	Abd	IR	ER
Left	90	−20	25	−15	30	−10
Right	120	10	30	30	30	30

- meralgia paraesthetica – an entrapment neuropathy of the lateral cutaneous nerve of the thigh, causing symptoms in the anterolateral thigh.

Box 3.6   Structured approach to examination of the hip region

Patient supine on couch
- **Check** the position of the pelvis and measure limb length if inequality is suspected
- *Look* for any soft tissue abnormality, scars, or obvious deformity
- *Feel* for any areas of local tenderness (e.g. trochanteric bursitis)
- *Feel* and *move* to examine the range of hip movements, and note whether these are painful:
  — flexion and extension (test specifically for a fixed deformity)
  — abduction and adduction (test specifically for a fixed deformity)
  — internal and external rotation
- Perform any neurological examination as clinically indicated. This should include assessment of muscle power

Patient standing
- *Look* from behind for a pelvic tilt. Perform Trendelenburg's test if abductor weakness is suspected
- *Look* at the patient walking to assess gait

Remember that pain felt in the hip may not arise from the hip joint.

Box 3.7   Other conditions giving rise to symptoms around the hip

- *'Local' soft tissue conditions*:
  — trochanteric bursitis
  — ischiogluteal bursitis
  — adductor enthesiopathy or strain
  — meralgia paraesthetica

- *Musculoskeletal disorder at another site*, e.g. lumbar disc pathology (especially high lumbar)

- *Symptoms arising from other structures*, e.g. femoral hernia

Possible extrinsic causes of hip symptoms
Remember to examine the lumbar spine (especially high lumbar) – spinal disorders can give rise to pain in the hip. Disease of non-musculoskeletal structures can also cause pain in the hip, e.g. a femoral hernia.

Knee (exemplar for joint swelling, for localised tenderness, for testing for stability and for deformity)

The knee differs from the hip in several ways:

- it is near the surface, so swelling and inflammation are much more apparent, both to the patient and to the examiner
- it relies on ligaments and muscles, rather than bone geometry, for stability
- it has internal soft tissue structures, the menisci, which share some of the load across the joint
- it moves principally in one plane.

Because of these features, there are two aspects of joint evaluation which are particularly fruitful to learn about in relation to the knee: joint swelling and joint stability.

Before dealing with these, one crucial indicator of trouble in the knee joint must always be looked for first – *quadriceps wasting*. The quadriceps muscle at the front of the thigh is essential for stability and active movement of the joint, but reflex inhibition of its activation is one of the first effects of almost any painful knee condition. It then becomes wasted at an incredible speed and the extra instability which this causes is often a big contributor to the symptoms by the time the patient is first seen. By the same token, building the muscle back up again by active exercise is an essential component of treatment.

Simple inspection will usually reveal quads wasting, provided the patient has been adequately exposed. You cannot examine a knee by asking the patient to roll up his/her trouser leg. Insist on having trousers removed – with a chaperone present if necessary – then compare the two thigh muscles. Quantify the degree of wasting with a tape measure. First measure a fixed distance above the top edge of the patella (say 10 cm) on both legs,

and mark the skin with a pen. Then measure the circumference of each thigh, ensuring that the tape is perfectly at right angles to the long axis, with the same edge of the tape alongside the mark for both measurements. Express the degree of wasting as the difference between the two circumferences: 'the left knee shows 3 cm of quads wasting'.

Swellings around the knee

Is it within or outside the joint? Significant swelling within the synovial cavity of the knee appears horseshoe-shaped, the central defect being caused by the patella. Although the patella does have fluid behind it, being rigid it does not bulge as much as the softer regions of the cavity. The opposite configuration is found in prepatellar bursitis, a cystic swelling in front of the kneecap with nothing around it (Fig. 3.16).

If you find a swollen synovial cavity, the next thing to decide is whether it is composed of hypertrophied synovium or whether it is normal synovium which is distended by fluid within the joint. Hypertrophied synovium has a 'doughy' consistency which is, with practice, distinguishable from liquid. You cannot learn this from reading – get your hands on as many swollen joints as possible.

Examinating for a knee effusion. Fluid is detected by palpation and its essential property –

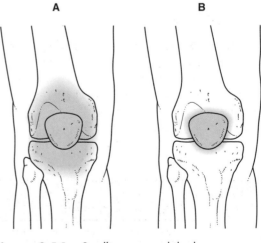

Figure 3.16   Swellings around the knee. **A.** Pattern of joint effusion. **B.** Pattern of prepatellar bursitis.

fluctuation – is no different in the knee joint from anywhere else. There are several techniques for demonstrating fluctuation of fluid in the knee joint:

- A large effusion, producing a clear horseshoe-shaped swelling, can be demonstrated to be fluid by pressing or tapping with one hand at one side of the joint and detecting the transmitted mechanical disturbance on the other side with the other hand.

- A moderate effusion can be diagnosed by looking for the 'patellar tap'. The patella is pushed gently posteriorly by the fingertips, which detect a distinct tap when the patella hits the front of the femur. This will not work if the effusion is too large (the patella will never hit the femur) or too small (the patella will be resting on the femur to start with). A good way of demonstrating the patellar tap is shown in Figure 3.17. The synovial fluid is compressed into the middle of the joint space, behind the patella, by exerting pressure downwards and towards the knee with the right and left hands. Maintaining this pressure, the examiner can 'tap' the patella downwards on to the femur with the index finger.

- A small effusion is best detected by swishing the fluid from one arm of the horseshoe to the other. Sweep the flat of the hand upwards from the joint line on the lateral side, flushing the effusion into the medial half of the joint. Then sweep it back again by a similar movement on the medial side, while looking intently at the lateral surface of the joint. If there is an eggcupful or so of fluid, you will see it progress down the lateral aspect in a wave.

Remember also to examine behind the knee. A popliteal cyst (Baker's cyst) is a common finding, especially in a patient with knee problems (e.g. osteoarthritis or rheumatoid arthritis.).

Having established that the synovial cavity contains fluid, you need to determine what kind of fluid it is – blood, synovial fluid or pus. Although the history may often give a strong indication of this, it is often necessary to perform a needle aspiration to be certain (Fig. 3.18).

The distinction between blood and synovial fluid is important after trauma to the knee: blood

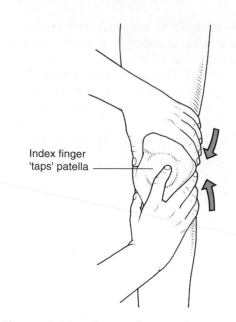

Index finger 'taps' patella

Figure 3.17   The patellar tap. The examiner's hands exert pressure downwards and towards the knee joint, forcing any fluid behind the patella. The patella is then 'tapped' with the index finger.

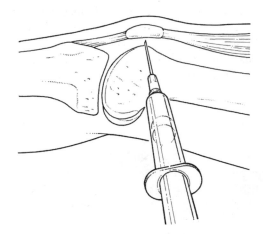

Figure 3.18   Aspiration of the knee joint. This can be via either a medial or a lateral approach. A 'no touch' technique must be used.

implies that some intra-articular structure has actually ruptured. A further diagnostic clue is that a fracture will usually produce obvious fat globules (bone marrow is rich in fat) floating on the surface of the blood. If the swelling occurred within minutes of an injury it will probably be blood; if it came up overnight, it will probably be synovial fluid.

The distinction between synovial fluid and pus is important in diagnosing monoarthritis (see Ch. 7) and in cases of polyarthritis where sepsis can occur on top of inflammatory synovitis. Pus is more likely to be associated with the classic signs of inflammation, which should always be looked for, comparing with the other side:

- the overlying skin may show erythema
- the joint may be felt to be warm when stroked with the back of the hand
- the joint may have recently become much more painful, especially on movement.

Localised tenderness

Identifying sites of local tenderness may be important diagnostically, and this is well demonstrated in the knee. Tracking down the cause of a knee effusion starts with a search for areas of tenderness by gentle palpation. Inflammatory synovitis is likely to cause diffuse tenderness, but many traumatic lesions produce tenderness with characteristic localisation. The crucial step is to locate the *joint line* – the easily palpable edge of the tibial plateau – and to relate the site of maximal tenderness to it (Fig. 3.19).

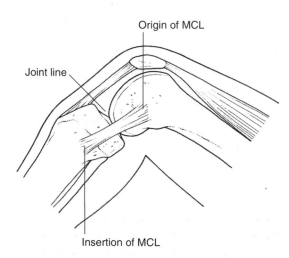

Figure 3.19 Localised tenderness around the knee. MCL, medial collateral ligament.

The commonest example of this is in a patient with effusion and pain on the medial side of the knee following a sporting injury. Tenderness on the joint line, especially when associated with loss of full passive extension, suggests a meniscus lesion. Osteoarthritis is another common cause of joint line tenderness in the knee, especially in older patients. Tenderness above or below the joint line suggests a medial ligament injury due to a valgus stress and you can expect to find pain and possibly laxity on stress testing.

Testing knee joint stability

Although stability of the knee joint depends heavily on quadriceps and hamstring muscle control, it also requires the integrity of two pairs of ligaments. The medial and lateral collateral ligaments provide stability in the coronal plane – resistance to valgus and varus angulation. The cruciate ligaments provide stability in the sagittal plane – resistance to forward and backward subluxation of the tibia on the femur. In addition to their structural integrity, normal function of these ligaments depends on their resting at the correct length; this may be disturbed by loss of bone under the articulating surfaces or by damage to the spacers of the knee joint (the menisci). Abnormalities in this anatomy will cause the patient to complain of a sensation of the knee 'giving way', and the aim of examination is to provide an explanation for this symptom.

Collateral ligament stability. The basic strategy is to apply a valgus stress to test the medial collateral ligament (MCL) and a varus stress to test the lateral collateral ligament (LCL) (Figs 3.20 and 3.21). In each case the degree of both angulation and pain produced is compared with the other side. The trap is that, with the knee fully extended, both the cruciate ligaments are tight and function as a 'middle collateral ligament', preventing coronal angulation even if one of the true collaterals is ruptured. Therefore, this test needs to be done with the knee slightly flexed, between 10° and 20°. This requires practice: if the knee is too flexed, the application of valgus or varus stress to the tibia simply rotates the limb.

As well as noting that there is an increase in opening of the knee joint compared to the other

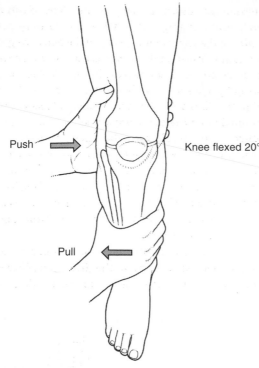

Push · Knee flexed 20°

Pull

Figure 3.20 Testing medial collateral stability. Push medially with the proximal hand on the femoral condyle, and pull with the distal hand at the ankle.

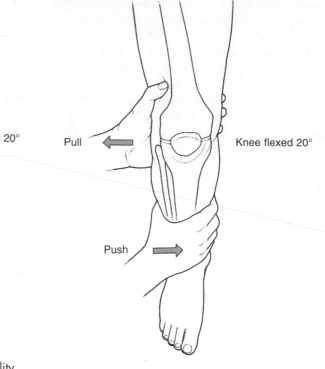

Pull · Knee flexed 20°

Push

Figure 3.21 Testing lateral collateral stability. Pull with the proximal hand on the (medial) femoral condyle, and push with the distal hand at the ankle.

side, note whether the opening comes to an abrupt stop (the ligament is stretched but at least partly intact) or appears to be unconstrained except by muscle action (the ligament is completely ruptured). This is important for treatment. In addition, ask the patient to try to tell you exactly where it hurts when you apply the stress and feel for tenderness. You can often localise the damage to one or other insertion (tibial or femoral) of the ligament in this way.

Cruciate ligament instability. The strategy of this test is to try to move the tibia in the sagittal plane while holding the femur still. This can be done with knee extended (Lachman's test) or flexed to 90° (anterior drawer test). Many orthopaedic surgeons prefer the former, but you need big hands to grasp the two bones and the latter method is easier. Figure 3.22 shows how to perform the test, and Figure 3.23 shows the theory behind it.

Feel the degree to which the tibia moves forwards, compared with the opposite leg, when you pull on it. If it moves more than in the opposite knee, the anterior cruciate ligament (ACL) must be disrupted. However, as the diagram shows, you must check before you apply any force whether the tibia is resting in a posteriorly subluxed position, indicating a ruptured posterior cruciate ligament (PCL). If it is, there will be excessive anterior movement, but only to restore the tibia to its correct location; the ACL is intact.

Rotatory instability. Many people show abnormal sagittal laxity without having any symptoms. It seems that the real problems following cruciate rupture arise when the tibia can rotate on the femur. This is detected by the pivot shift test. It is difficult to perform and is part of postgraduate training.

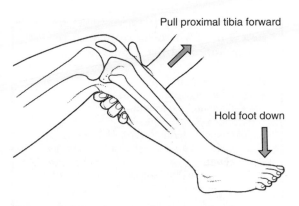

Pull proximal tibia forward

Hold foot down

Figure 3.22 Anterior drawer test for the anterior cruciate ligament (knee at 90°). NB – don't sit on a rheumatoid foot!

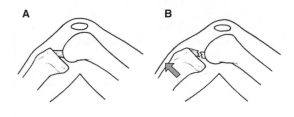

A B

C D

Figure 3.23 Principles of the anterior drawer test. **A.** Normal resting position. **B.** True anterior drawer: ruptured ACL. **C.** Posterior subluxation: ruptured PCL. **D.** False anterior drawer. Excessive anterior movement can result from rupture of either cruciate ligament. The important point is the starting position.

Joint deformity

The final feature for which we use the knee as an exemplar is joint deformity. Knee deformities are common, and can exacerbate problems at the knee. In addition to the need for stability to be provided by soft tissues, another consequence of the simple geometry of the articulating surfaces at the knee is that the ability of the cartilage to stand up to a

lifetime of stress is very dependent on the *mechanical axis* (Fig. 3.24). A line drawn from the centre of the femoral head (where the body weight enters the lower limb) to the centre of the ankle joint (where the load passes through to the foot) normally passes through the centre of the knee joint. If it does not, then there is unequal loading of the medial and lateral compartments of the knee, which can accelerate the development of osteoarthritis. The angle between the mechanical axis and the anatomic axis of the femoral shaft is normally between 5° and 7° (greater in females), because of the offset created by the femoral neck. In the tibia, the anatomic and mechanical axes more or less coincide.

When examining the knee, you should look at the mechanical axis from the front. Significant abnormalities are apparent as *genu valgum* (knock-

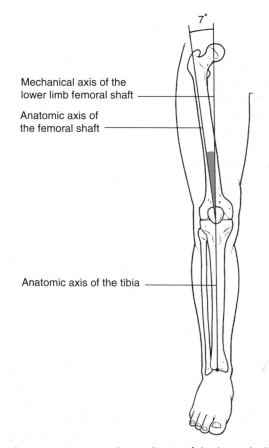

7°

Mechanical axis of the lower limb femoral shaft

Anatomic axis of the femoral shaft

Anatomic axis of the tibia

Figure 3.24 Mechanical axis of the lower limb.

knee) or *genu varum* (bow legs), either may be unilateral or bilateral. Precise measurements require long X-rays which have the hips and ankles on one film.

Other deformities of the knee have been referred to earlier in this chapter: fixed flexion deformity (common in inflammatory arthritis) and genu recurvatum (common in patients with hypermobility).

Range of movement

When testing for instability, we are dealing with abnormal movement. Measuring and documenting the range of normal movement is much simpler than in the hip. The convention is that full extension is recorded as 0° and the flexion range is given in degrees from that point. Check carefully that the passive extension really is full – loss of just a few degrees can be a tell-tale sign of an important lesion, such as a torn meniscus. Pick the two legs up by the heels while standing at the end of the examination couch; as the two knees lie side by side, slight differences in their height, indicating a slight loss of extension (fixed flexion), will be apparent. Normal knees can flex to around 140°; less than 120° makes it difficult to rise from a chair.

The knee is one lower limb joint where it is important to check the active range, at least to check that full extension can be produced by quadriceps action. The reason is that the extensor apparatus – the quadriceps muscle and tendon, the patella and the patellar tendon inserting into the tibial tubercle – can all be disrupted by injury. A discrepancy between the active and passive ranges is described as an *extensor lag*.

When assessing movement at the knee always feel for crepitus, by placing a hand over the knee as it flexes.

Structured approach to examination of the knee

This is outlined in Box 3.8. The knee is frequently a source of symptoms, causes including trauma, osteoarthritis and inflammatory arthritis.

Possible extrinsic causes of knee symptoms

Examine the lumbar spine and the hip, both of which can give rise to knee pain.

Box 3.8   Structured approach to examination of the knee

Patient supine on couch
- *Look* for any scars, rashes, erythema, swelling, muscle wasting or obvious deformity
- *Feel* the skin temperature and for any areas of local tenderness (especially along the joint line).
- *Feel* any swelling, and decide whether this is:
  — synovial
  — fluid (patellar tap)
  — bone
  — a combination of the above
  (remember to feel behind the knee)
- *Feel* and *move* to examine the range of knee flexion, feeling for crepitus during movement of the knee. Note whether movement is painful
- *Feel* and *move* to test for instability of:
  — collateral ligaments
  — cruciate ligaments
- Perform any neurological examination as clinically indicated. This should include assessment of muscle power

Patient standing
- *Look* for deformity (from in front of the patient and from the side)
- *Look* at the patient walking to assess gait

Remember that pain felt in the knee may not arise from the knee, and particularly may arise from the *hip*.

Ankle and hindfoot

The ankle and subtalar joints allow the transmission of body weight through the tibia and foot through all stages of the gait cycle, even if the ground is uneven. In order to do this comfortably, they have to be sufficiently supple and the main point of examination is to look for limitation of their range of movement. (As the ankle and hindfoot are usually examined with the forefoot, we shall describe the basic approach to their examination together, in the next section.)

The ankle joint

Ankle movement is described as plantarflexion

and dorsiflexion (Fig. 3.25): this is less ambiguous than flexion and extension. A loss of dorsiflexion is particularly important, and fixed plantarflexion (i.e. the ankle cannot even get up to the neutral position) is graced with the name of *equinus*, since it mimics the posture of the horse. Loss of ankle movement may be due to osteo- or inflammatory arthritis, but can also be a consequence of immobilisation (e.g. after cast treatment of a tibial fracture) when it is due to fibrosis of the capsule and other soft tissues around the joint. As well as recording the passive range, it is important to note whether the same range can be achieved actively, since loss of active dorsiflexion is relatively common as a result of deep peroneal nerve injury (*drop foot*).

The subtalar joint

The subtalar joint provides inversion and eversion of the hindfoot. In order to estimate the range, stand at the foot of the bed, holding the heel in one hand while supporting the calf with the other (Fig. 3.26). Swing the calcaneum from side to side and compare the two sides. It is difficult to measure the exact amount of inversion – eversion; most people report 'slight', 'moderate' or 'severe' limitation.

The midtarsal joints

Figure 3.27 demonstrates the assessment of midtarsal movements. This time it is the heel which is stabilised by one hand (as opposed to the calf when testing subtalar movements), the other hand holding the foot just proximal to the metatarsophalangeal (MTP) joints. Care must be taken not to compress the MTP joints, which are often tender in patients with inflammatory

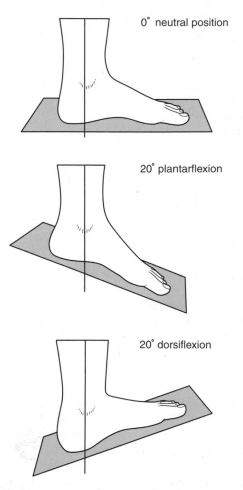

0° neutral position

20° plantarflexion

20° dorsiflexion

Figure 3.25 Measurement of ankle movements.

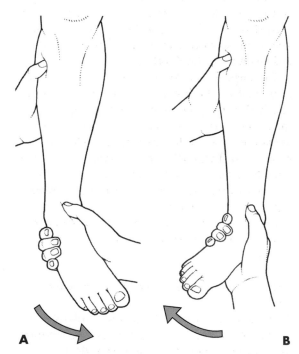

A   **B**

Figure 3.26 Testing subtalar movement. The left hand stabilises the calf; the right hand holds the hindfoot and 'rocks' it into inversion (**A**) and eversion (**B**).

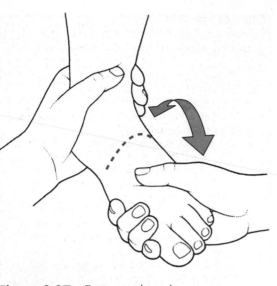

Figure 3.27   Testing midtarsal movement. The heel is stabilised with one hand and the forefoot is plantarflexed and dorsiflexed with the other.

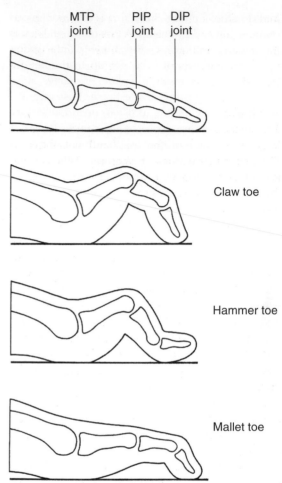

Figure 3.28   Forefoot deformities.

arthritis (see below). Midtarsal movements are principally plantarflexion and dorsiflexion. Midfoot movements (tarsometatarsal joints) also contribute to inversion and eversion.

Forefoot (exemplar for deformity)

Forefoot problems are extremely common. Many patients have forefoot deformities of either the hallux or the other toes (Fig. 3.28).

The metatarsal heads and the pads of the toes take a lot of weight during normal walking: all the acceleratory forces pass through them to the ground. Unless the load is evenly shared between them all, the overlying skin is subjected to excessive stress and it responds by thickening and forming *callosities*. Inspection of the plantar skin for these is the logical way to start examination of the forefoot. Often, pressure over callosities is painful, whether it is caused by walking or by the examining doctor. In rheumatoid arthritis, for example, the MTP joints become hyperextended/subluxed and the metatarsal heads become prominent in the sole of the foot. In this position the toes are unable to contribute much to weight-

bearing and the skin over the prominent metatarsal heads is often very thickened and tender. Tenderness over the MTP joints can be an early sign of rheumatoid arthritis.

Callosities can also occur on the dorsal surface, due to pressure against the shoe; this is a clue that there is deformity of the toes due to fixed postures of one or more of the toe joints. Leaving aside the hallux, three main patterns of toe deformity occur, all of which have their counterparts in the hand. *Claw toe* is like the ulnar palsy pattern of claw hand – the MTP joint is hyperextended and both interphalangeal joints are flexed. *Hammer toe* is like the boutonnière deformity in the fingers – the proximal interphalangeal (PIP) joint is flexed.

Mallet toe is like mallet finger, the distal interphalangeal (DIP) joint is flexed. In mallet toe, the callosity and tenderness are likely to be on the tip of the toe, which is taking weight vertically instead of on the toe pad.

The hallux

The big toe deserves separate description: it bears a large proportion of the load and is subject to different abnormalities of anatomy. Whereas the lesser toes develop deformities in the sagittal plane, the hallux is most prone to a deformity in the coronal plane – *hallux valgus*. This means abduction of its MTP joint, which leads to an uncovering of the metatarsal head on the medial aspect. This prominence, often supplemented by thickening of the bone (formation of an *exostosis*) and formation of a bursa, due to the excess pressure which results on the medial side, is what constitutes a *bunion*. In severe degrees of hallux valgus, the big toe is also pronated, i.e. rotated so weight is taken on its medial aspect. In such cases, the big toe is able to take very little weight and the extra strain is thrown on to the lesser toe MTP joints.

Two other aspects of the hallux need to be examined. The first is inflammation: the hallux MTP joint is the commonest site for gout. Redness, swelling, exquisite tenderness and pain on movement are the signs. The second is limitation of movement of the MTP joint due to osteoarthritis, known as *hallux rigidus*.

Structured approach to examination of the ankle and foot

This is outlined in Box 3.9. The ankles and feet are commonly affected by either local problems or systemic inflammatory disease. Remember to assess for Achilles tendon problems and for plantar fasciitis, both of which are common causes of pain. The Allen test for Achilles tendon rupture is described in Chapter 23. Also assess the blood supply – vascular insufficiency may cause or contribute to foot problems.

Possible extrinsic causes of ankle and foot symptoms

Remember that pain in the ankle and foot may arise from the lumbar spine (radicular pain).

Box 3.9   Structured approach to examination of the ankle and foot

Patient supine on couch
- *Look* for any scars, swelling, colour change, deformity or callosities
- *Feel* the skin temperature and for any areas of local tenderness
- *Feel* any swelling, and decide whether this is:
  — synovial (in which case determine whether it is diffuse, suggesting joint inflammation, or more localised, suggesting tenosynovitis)
  — bone
  — oedema (which may reflect cardiac or other important general medical problems)
  (Remember, if appropriate, to palpate the Achilles tendon, looking for tenderness and swelling, or over the plantar fascia insertion into the calcaneus.)
- *Feel* and *move* (noting whether movement is painful) to examine the range of:
  — ankle dorsiflexion and plantarflexion
  — subtalar inversion and eversion
  — midtarsal movements
  — movements at the MTP and IP joints
- Perform any neurological examination as clinically indicated. This should include asessment of muscle power
- *Feel* for the posterior tibial and dorsalis pedis pulses (especially if you suspect arterial insufficiency)

Patient standing
- *Look* at the appearance of the foot, looking for deformity such as pes planus or hindfoot pronation
- *Look* while the patient stands on tiptoe (this is difficult and painful if there is Achilles tendinitis, and very difficult on the affected foot if the Achilles tendon is ruptured)
- *Look* at the patient walking to assess gait

Remember that pain felt in the ankle and foot may arise elsewhere.

Neurological examination in the lower limb

The commonest reason for neurological testing in the lower limb (in connection with musculoskeletal examination) is to look for abnormalities of the nerve root supply. Nerve root values (for muscles and reflexes) are given in the section on the spine (p. 61). However, it must be recognised that as well as testing such neurology when assessing patients with overtly spinal problems, it is vital to address this in patients with problems which seem, at first sight, to arise purely within the limb. This is because so many complaints of limb pain or dysfunction eventually turn out to arise from spinal pathology.

However, peripheral nerve lesions also occur, although they are less common in the lower than in the upper limb. The motor weaknesses resulting from lesions of the various nerves of the lower limb are shown in Table 3.3. Peripheral nerve examination is particularly important after lower limb injury, such as a tibial fracture when, for example, a deep peroneal nerve lesion can lead to a drop foot. The nerve lesion can either be a direct consequence of the injury or develop later as a consequence of compartment syndrome (see Ch. 19).

Table 3.3
Motor weakness resulting from lesions of various nerves of the lower limb

Peripheral nerve	Muscle group affected
Femoral	Knee extensors
Obturator	Hip adductors
Sciatic	Knee flexors/hamstrings
Posterior tibial	Ankle and toe plantarflexors
Deep peroneal	Ankle and toe dorsiflexors
Superficial peroneal	Ankle evertors

Box 3.10 Neurological examination of the limbs

Look
- Wasting.
- Deformity which might arise due to neurological problems, (e.g. pes cavus, ulnar claw hand

Feel and *move*
- Tone – assess this at all of the major joints of the limb in turn, examining passive motion. Consider different types of change in tone, e.g. flaccid, spastic, cogwheel
- Power – again, assess all of the major muscle groups

Reflexes – examine the major reflex arcs
- Biceps (C5, C6)
- Supinator (C5, C6)
- Triceps (C6, C7)
- Knee (L3, L4)
- Ankle (S1)

Sensation
- Touch
- Pain
- Vibration
- Proprioception
- (Allodynia)

Consider both *dermatomal* pattern of loss and pattern of loss of *major peripheral nerves*

Coordination (finger–nose test for upper limb; heel–shin test for lower limb) – this reveals something of combined sensory and motor function, but is also affected by cerebellar disorders

Provocation tests – local pressure over superficial peripheral nerve, e.g., median nerve at wrist, ulnar nerve at medial epicondyle or common peroneal nerve at fibular neck. For the test to be positive, the local pressure should reproduce the symptoms of which the patient complains

Points to note
- The most common level of spondylosis and disc protrusion in the neck is C5/6 (C6 nerve root); this leads to symptoms radiating down the radial border of the forearm to the radial side of the hand, and commonly affects the supinator jerk
- The commonest levels affected in the lumbar spine are L4/5 and L5/S1. L4/5 *disc protrusions* most commonly affect the L5 nerve root (weak toe extensors, especially extensor hallucis longus); L5/S1 most commonly affect the S1 nerve root (decreased ankle jerk). Study the dermatome chart (Fig. 3.55) to see the likely areas of change of sensation

However, testing muscle power in the acutely injured patient is difficult because of pain worsened by movement, so it is important to know the sensory supply of the main peripheral nerves as well. Thus motor examination of a patient with common peroneal nerve damage after a knee injury may be difficult. However, such a patient is likely to have an area of numbness between the first and second toes (deep peroneal nerve) or on the dorsum of the other toes and the foot (superficial peroneal nerve), which will give the diagnosis.

A structured approach to neurological examination of the limbs is outlined in Box 3.10. Upper limb peripheral nerve problems are discussed in the next section and in Chapter 15.

UPPER LIMB

Start by observing the integrated function of the upper limbs; in other words examine the patient's ability to reach out and do things. The upper limb is often described as the *hand–arm unit*. This conveys the division of labour between the shoulder, elbow and wrist, which have the job of orienting the hand in space, and the hand itself, which is adapted to exploring, grasping and manipulating objects.

The large representation of the hand in the cerebral cortex is the basis of what is described as *active touch*. This phrase encapsulates the close integration of sensory and motor function: the hand does not merely feel, it explores. Manipulation of objects requires more than just muscle contraction; sensory feedback from the skin is essential for control. As a consequence, neurological examination is very important in the upper limb.

Ask your patient to pick up a paper clip from a table surface and observe what happens (Fig. 3.29A). The patient with a stiff, painful shoulder or elbow will have to move the whole body in order to get the hand in the appropriate position. The patient with a stiff wrist, or a loss of foream rotation, will have to contort the upper arm into an ungainly posture. See if there is enough mobility in the thumb and index finger to form a *precision grip*. Loss of sensory acuity in the median nerve territory will lead to obvious clumsiness once the clip has been reached.

Ask your patient to grip and squeeze your index and middle fingers as hard as possible – both hands simultaneously. This allows an easy comparison, between the two sides, of *power grip* (Fig. 3.29B). If this is painful for the patient, find out where: it could be the hand itself (e.g. in polyarthritis), in the wrist (e.g. with a carpal injury) or at the elbow (in medial or lateral epicondylitis).

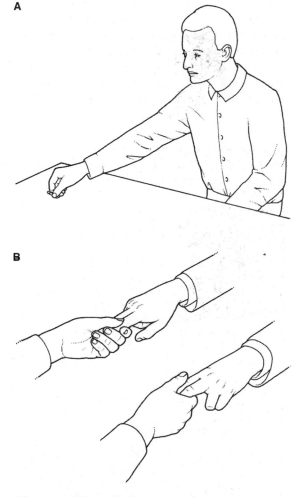

Figure 3.29 Whole upper limb screening tests. **A.** The patient picks up a paper clip. **B.** The patient (seated beside the examiner) grips and squeezes the index and middle fingers of the examiner (both hands simultaneously).

As with the lower limb section, we have concentrated on areas of examination that exemplify particular problems which can be assessed by careful clinical examination. These areas are also very relevant clinically. Thus, in this upper limb section, we emphasise assessment of soft tissue problems in the shoulder region, and assessment of sensibility, synovitis, and tendon rupture in the hand.

Shoulder

The discussion below is exemplar for problems with soft shoulder examination around a joint. The essence of shoulder examination is the range (and comfort) of active movement. Its bony and ligamentous geometry is designed for maximum freedom and therefore its stability depends on muscles and their tendons (Fig. 3.30). In particular, the passage of the rotator cuff tendons (principally supraspinatus) over the top of the humeral head and under the acromion is very important for holding the glenohumeral joint stable in all positions. It is also prone to damage because of this unusual arrangement of a soft tissue structure sandwiched between two bones across which considerable forces need to be transmitted. Evaluating the state of health of these bone/soft

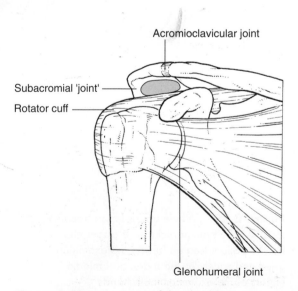

Figure 3.30   Anatomy of the shoulder.

Acromioclavicular joint

Subacromial 'joint'

Rotator cuff

Glenohumeral joint

tissue articulations is the main objective of examination of the shoulder.

A quick evaluation of the shoulder, based on the most important functional requirements, is very easy (Fig. 3.31). Simply ask the patient to:

- put their hands behind the head – this tests abduction and external rotation
- put their hands into the small of the back – this tests adduction, extension and internal rotation
- lift their arms out like an aeroplane and then point to the ceiling – this tests abduction, and allows identification of a painful arc of abduction

Watch the patient's face for signs of discomfort and observe differences between the two sides. This approach, which emphasises the role of the shoulder in controlling the position of the hand in space, is enough by itself if you are simply checking that all is well with the shoulder – say after an accident or in polyarthritis – and will alert you to look in more detail if necessary.

For a more detailed evaluation, stand behind the patient, who should also be standing, or sitting on a chair whose back does not obstruct any shoulder movement. If the patient complains of shoulder pain, the first thing is to ask them to point to the site of the pain. The patient suffering from subacromial pain will tend to place the whole palm over the deltoid region or over the biceps: the pain is diffuse. If the acromioclavicular joint (which is prone to osteoarthritis) is the seat of the pain, they will probably point with one finger straight at it (Fig. 3.32).

Testing abduction

The movement which is most revealing in analysing the shoulder is abduction (Fig. 3.33). This is not necessarily the most important movement for the patient's function, but it gives good information about the articulating structures described above. If you simply ask the patient to abduct their arm as far and as high as possible, what you will see is actually a combination of abduction at the glenohumeral joint and rotation of the scapula on the chest wall (the latter is often referred to as the

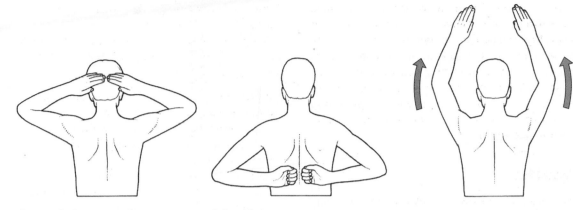

Figure 3.31 'Quick' assessment of shoulder movements.

scapulothoracic 'joint'). This combined movement, which is what the patient would actually use for function, is best described as *elevation* (Fig. 3.34). In order to analyse it into its component parts, and thereby assess the glenohumeral joint itself, repeat the exercise with the palm of your hand pressing down on the acromion, standing behind the patient, and hence fixing the scapula. Now the elevation achieved by the arm represents pure abduction. Note that 'shoulder' movements also include movement at the acromioclavicular and sternoclavicular joints.

Limitation of glenohumeral abduction can be due to capsular stiffness of the joint, and will be associated with limitation of other movements as

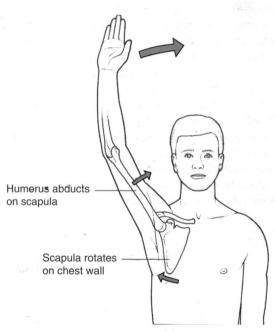

Humerus abducts on scapula

Scapula rotates on chest wall

Figure 3.33 Shoulder abduction: full elevation.

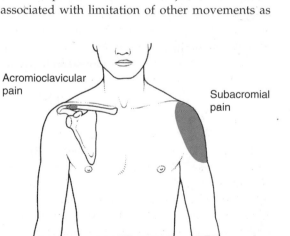

Acromioclavicular pain

Subacromial pain

Figure 3.32 Acromioclavicular (well localised) and subacromial pain (diffuse, often over deltoid and biceps).

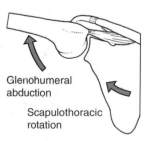
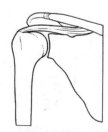

Glenohumeral abduction

Scapulothoracic rotation

Figure 3.34 Components of shoulder elevation.

described below. However, it is more commonly due to problems with the rotator cuff in the subacromial space (Fig. 3.30). Two major problems which can occur here are (1) rupture of the rotator cuff, and (2) impingement on the cuff by the bony structures which lie above it; there are two specific tests to detect these. In addition, a painful arc of shoulder abduction is most commonly caused by either a supraspinatus tendinitis or a subacromial bursitis (with or without impingement); these are described in Chapter 15.

Testing for a rotator cuff tear. This relies on the fact that the powerful deltoid muscle is only able to abduct the shoulder once the humerus has already moved towards the horizontal position. When the humerus is vertical, the line of pull of the deltoid fibres merely slides the humeral head upwards, parallel to the glenoid surface (Fig. 3.35). Therefore initiation of abduction can only be achieved by supraspinatus, the main component of the rotator cuff. Simply ask the patient to stand with the arm hanging vertically and to abduct the arm while gently restraining the elbow with the palm of your hand. Feel whether any abducting force can be generated in this position. If it can not, then the rotator cuff is probably ruptured (this can be confirmed with an MRI scan, arthrogram or arthroscopy) but the patient will probably be able to maintain abduction, if you lift the arm into the horizontal, by the action of deltoid.

Testing for subacromial pain. The test for subacromial impingement is to look for a painful arc during active abduction. This means that the

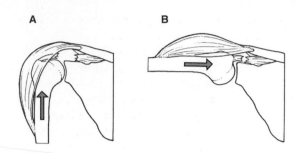

Figure 3.35   Rotator cuff tear. The deltoid cannot initiate abduction but can maintain it.

earliest and latest parts of the arc of abduction are comfortable, but the middle is painful. This happens because the bony narrowing selectively injures the fattest section of the supraspinatus tendon (Fig. 3.36). Only when this section (which has become inflamed by the repeated trauma) is in the narrow isthmus is the pain felt. The narrowest part is often under the acromioclavicular joint, which can develop osteophytes if there is degenerative change. It is best to stand in front of the patient while testing for a painful arc, since it is important to be looking at the face for signs of discomfort. Note that impingement can occur as a result of inflammation in the subacromial area (subacromial bursitis or supraspinatus tendinitis, in which case symptoms will settle as the inflammation subsides), or as a result of bony mechanical obstruction (e.g. due to an osteophyte arising either from the acromioclavicular joint or from the tip of the acromium (Fig. 15.2, p. 232), in which case symptoms are more likely to be

No impingement   Impingement   No impingement

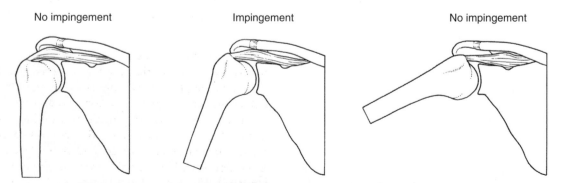

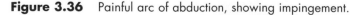

Figure 3.36   Painful arc of abduction, showing impingement.

persistent. However, in practice there is often a contribution from both elements.

Testing for acromioclavicular pain. As has already been stated, acromioclavicular pain is usually more localised than subacromial pain, although they may coexist (e.g. acromioclavicular joint osteophytes causing subacromial impingement). To test specifically for pain arising from the acromioclavicular joint, flex and adduct the shoulder by gently moving the flexed elbow across in front of the chest. This stresses the acromioclavicular joint and worsens the pain localised to it. Patients with acromioclavicular pain also experience pain at the extremes of shoulder abduction, and are also tender over the acromioclavicular joint. Feel for your own acromioclavicular joint – a slight depression between the end of the clavicle and the acromion: it can be difficult to feel in overweight patients.

Testing the shoulder movements

Having assessed abduction in some detail, to complete the assessment of range of movement at the shoulder joint, observe the following, by standing behind the patient and comparing the two sides:

- forward flexion – 'swing your arm high up in front of you' (Fig. 3.37)

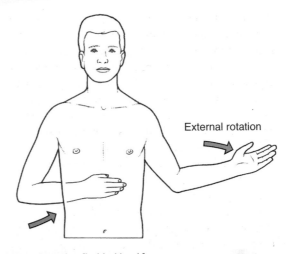

External rotation

Internal rotation [behind back]

Figure 3.38   Internal and external rotation of the shoulder.

- extension – 'swing your hand as far behind you as you can'
- external rotation – hold the flexed elbow into the side, use the forearm as a pointer (Fig. 3.38)
- internal rotation – as for external rotation (Fig. 3.38). Also, can the hand reach the small of the back (i.e. 90°)? See how high up the spine the thumbs can reach (Fig. 3.31).

Shoulder stability. Following injuries to the shoulder joint, especially those involving dislocation (see Ch. 22), a persistent instability due to capsular damage can remain. There will be limitation of the range of movement, accompanied by apprehension on the part of the patient. This should lead to an assessment of stability (covered at postgraduate level).

Contour of the shoulder

Simple inspection of the shoulder from the front may reveal important information. Wasting of the deltoid leads to a 'squared off' contour; dislocation of the acromioclavicular joint gives a step at the lateral end of the clavicle; anterior dislocation of the shoulder gives a fullness in front of the glenoid. Inspection from behind will show wasting of the supraspinatus as a hollow above the spine of the scapula.

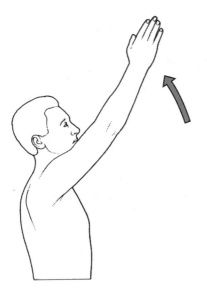

Figure 3.37   Shoulder flexion.

Structured approach to examination of the shoulder

Most of the relevant points have been already covered; these are summarised in Box 3.11. While the shoulder is a frequent site of soft tissue problems, it is also often involved in inflammatory arthritis, e.g. rheumatoid arthritis or pseudogout.

Possible extrinsic causes of shoulder symptoms

The shoulder and the cervical spine should always be examined together, since pain arising from the neck may cause symptoms in the shoulder, and vice versa. Also, patients often have both neck and shoulder problems. Pain from internal organs may be referred to the shoulder, e.g. pain arising from the pleura. Because of the innervation of the diaphragm, subdiaphragmatic pain, e.g. pain from a subphrenic abscess, may be felt in the shoulder. Remember, therefore, that shoulder pain does not always reflect a shoulder problem.

Elbow

The elbow, together with the shoulder, plays a vital role in the positioning of the hand in space. Soft tissue problems are common, mainly enthesopathies and bursitis (Ch. 15). Elbow problems, e.g. injuries, can lead to ulnar nerve damage, the consequences of which are noted mainly in the hand. The elbow is commonly affected in patients with inflammatory joint disease, e.g. rheumatoid arthritis.

The movements which occur at the elbow are flexion and extension (the normal range is from 0° to 150°) (Fig. 3.39) and pronation and supination (Fig. 3.40). Pronation and supination occur at the superior and inferior radioulnar joints.

Structured approach to examination of the elbow

This is summarised in Box 3.12. Particular points to look out for are swelling of the elbow joint itself (synovial swelling is often most easily seen and felt over the head of the radius with the elbow flexed at 90° or in the soft tissues. Common 'lumps' to be found around the elbow are a swollen olecranon

---

> **Box 3.11   Structured approach to examination of the shoulder**
>
> The patient should be standing, or seated without obstruction to shoulder movements.
>
> - *Look* for muscle wasting, swelling, skin changes (look from both in front and from behind)
>
> - *Look* at the active range of movements, and whether these produce pain
>
> - *Feel* for skin temperature
>
> - *Feel* for any areas of local tenderness of:
>   — the sternoclavicular joint
>   — the acromioclavicular joint
>   — the anterior joint capsule
>
> - *Feel* and *move* to examine the range of passive shoulder movements. Feel for crepitus and note whether the following movements are painful:
>   — flexion
>   — abduction
>   — external and internal rotation
>
> - Perform any neurological examination as clinically indicated. This should include assessment of muscle power
>
> Remember that pain felt at the shoulder may not arise from the shoulder.

bursa (Fig. 3.41), rheumatoid nodules (Fig. 8.14), and sometimes gouty tophi.

Fixed flexion deformities are common in patients with inflammatory arthritis, whereas hyperextension (beyond −10°) is seen in patients with hypermobility. Look for areas of tenderness, especially over the medial and lateral epicondyles. Specific testing for lateral epicondylitis (tennis elbow) and medial epicondylitis (golfer's elbow) is described in Chapter 15.

When assessing range of movement, look at active and then passive range. Pronation and supination are best assessed with the elbow flexed at 90° (Fig. 3.40). Remember to feel for crepitus as the joint is moved.

As with movement around any joint, a full examination is incomplete without assessing muscle power and performing the relevant neurological examination.

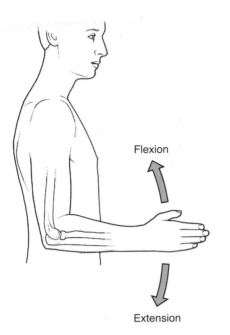

Figure 3.39 Flexion and extension at the elbow.

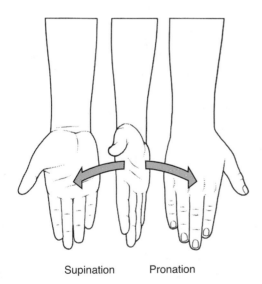

Supination   Pronation

Figure 3.40 Supination and pronation at the elbow.

Possible extrinsic causes of elbow symptoms
Pain around the elbow is usually well localised. However, pain felt in the elbow may be radicular, referred from the neck, and shoulder pain may

> **Box 3.12 Structured approach to examination of the elbow**
>
> The patient should be standing, or seated without obstruction to elbow movements.
>
> - **Look for muscle wasting, deformity, swelling, skin changes**
> - **Look at the active range of movements, and whether these produce pain**
> - **Feel for skin temperature**
> - **Feel any areas of swelling to define their nature**
> - **Feel for any areas of local tenderness, especially**
>   - **over the lateral epicondyle**
>   - **over the medial epicondyle**
> - **Feel and move to examine the range of passive elbow movements. Feel for crepitus and note whether the following movements are painful:**
>   - **flexion/extension**
>   - **pronation/supination**
> - **Perform any neurological examination as clinically indicated. This should include assessment of muscle power**
>
> **Remember that pain felt in the elbow may not arise from the elbow.**

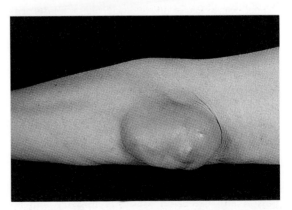

Figure 3.41 Swelling primarily due to fluid in the olecranon bursa. This patient had rheumatoid arthritis and there were rheumatoid nodules within the swelling.

radiate to the elbow. Therefore, a complete assessment of the upper limb and neck is necessary.

Wrist

The wrist is usually examined with the hand, as together they act as a single functional unit. Therefore, we shall describe the basic approach to the examination of the hand and wrist together, in the next section. However, some points about the wrist can be usefully made separately.

The wrist is commonly affected by inflammatory arthritis, expecially rheumatoid arthritis. Wrist deformity can occur in rheumatoid arthritis, most typically dorsal subluxation of the ulnar head, which is described in the next section. Look also for any areas of swelling. These may result from synovitis of the wrist itself or from synovitis of the finger extensor tendon sheaths (extensor tenosynovitis, when there is boggy swelling over the dorsum of the wrist) or of the finger flexor tendon sheaths (flexor tensynovitis, when the swelling is apparent on the palmar aspect of the wrist). Flexor tenosynovitis is one of the conditions which can be associated with median nerve compression, which results in characteristic symptoms and signs described in Chapter 15. Tenosynovitis around the wrist is also common in patients without inflammatory joint disease, when it may occur as a result of overuse (see Ch. 15).

Feel for areas of local tenderness. Tenderness may reflect injury to an underlying structure or active inflammation. Synovial swelling is not always tender. In a patient with rheumatoid arthritis, inflammatory swelling may not be tender when chronic, although it is usually tender in active disease.

The movements at the wrist (radiocarpal joint and intercarpal joints) are dorsiflexion (extension) and palmar flexion (flexion) (Fig. 3.42), and radial and ulnar deviation (Fig. 3.43). Figure 3.42 demonstrates a simple method of assessing wrist flexion and extension – any asymmetry will be quickly identifed. However, this method is not suitable in the patient with elbow problems, e.g. rheumatoid arthritis. With such patients, the examiner should support the forearm and ask the patient to flex/extend the wrist, examining first

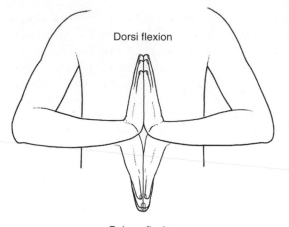

Figure 3.42   Dorsiflexion (extension) and palmar flexion (flexion) of the wrists.

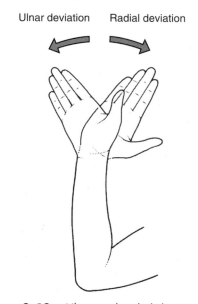

Figure 3.43   Ulnar and radial deviation at the wrists.

active and then passive movements. Movements at the inferior radioulnar joint contribute to pronation and supination.

Hand (exemplar for sensibility, tendon rupture and synovitis)

Because hand mobility is so important, as emphasised below, we describe this first, before going on to sensibility, synovitis and tendon rupture, problems which are so well exemplified in the hand. Another important feature of the hand is its susceptibility to injury and infections. These must be diagnosed accurately and early, as untreated infection can have a devastating effect on hand function.

Nomenclature. Effective communication about findings in the hand is dependent on using the accepted terminology to describe landmarks and directions. The words 'medial' and 'lateral', for instance, are ambiguous because of the ability to pronate and supinate the hand into opposite attitudes. The words 'radial' and 'ulnar' are used instead, since they are consistent. Since there are many little joints, with rather long names, abbreviations are necessary – e.g. PIP, proximal interphalangeal joint. Figure 3.44 shows the most commonly used points of reference, seen in palmar and lateral views. It is worth learning this language: it is both quick and precise.

Since the functions of the hand are manipulation and exploration, its most important attributes are *mobility* and *sensibility*; a stiff, insensate hand is useless. When treating disorders and injuries of the hand, regaining motion of the fingers is particularly important – and often difficult. Joint mobility and motor power are much more intimately blended in the hand than in larger joints elsewhere.

Examining hand mobility (Box 3.13)

Start by measuring the active range of movement. If this is deficient, measure the passive range to elucidate the cause. If the passive range is normal, the cause is loss of muscle or tendon function. If the passive range is restricted, the cause can be stiff joints or tight intrinsic muscles (e.g. interossei; this can follow injuries such as ulnar nerve transection). Sometimes persistently tight intrinsic muscles lead to joint contractures, and the two are difficult to distinguish. Ask the patient to make a fist, then a straight hand (as if about to deliver a karate blow). This will highlight where any problem lies. For instance, if a patient with a stiff PIP joint of the little finger tries to make a fist, the little finger will stick out relatively straight. If the examiner tries to coax this finger into full flexion along with the rest, all that will be achieved is

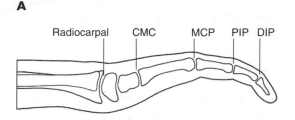

A

Radiocarpal   CMC   MCP   PIP DIP

Radius & ulna   Carpus   Metacarpal   Proximal, middle, distal phalanges

Joints

Carpometacarpal [CMC]
Metacarpophalangeal [MCP]
Proximal interphalangeal [PIP]
Distal interphalangeal [DIP]

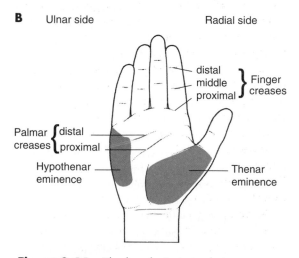

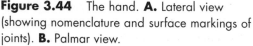

B   Ulnar side   Radial side

distal
middle   } Finger
proximal creases

Palmar { distal
creases { proximal

Hypothenar
eminence

Thenar
eminence

Figure 3.44   The hand. **A.** Lateral view (showing nomenclature and surface markings of joints). **B.** Palmar view.

discomfort for the patient. By contrast, if a patient with a cut extensor tendon tries to straighten the hand, the affected finger will droop, but the examiner will be able to lift it into line with the others.

Finger flexion. There are two ways to report the range of finger flexion which is the most important movement, since it underlies the production of a power grip. The first is to report the composite movement, in the form of pulp deficit. This is the distance between the finger pulp and the proximal

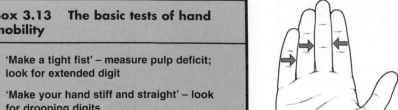

> ### Box 3.13   The basic tests of hand mobility
>
> - 'Make a tight fist' – measure pulp deficit; look for extended digit
> - 'Make your hand stiff and straight' – look for drooping digits
> - 'Make a pinch' – thumb and index pulps opposed?
> - 'Open your hand as wide as you can' – estimate span across thumb web

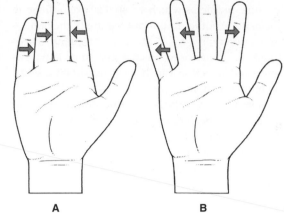

A   B

Figure 3.45   Finger adduction (**A**) and abduction (**B**).

palmar crease in maximum flexion – it should be zero. This method is suitable for charting the progress of a generally stiff hand following injury or in inflammatory arthritis. The second is to focus on the joint principally affected and report its range in the conventional way, taking full extension as 0°, as in the elbow or knee; this is appropriate for one or two joints which are stiff as a result of bony or soft tissue injury, or Dupuytren's contracture. When observing finger flexion, look out for 'triggering' — an apparent block to flexion or extension which is suddenly overcome with a jump. This is due to abnormal swelling of the flexor tendons within their fibrous sheath at the level of the MCP joint. It is worth asking the patient with hand problems about this. There may be a palpable tendon nodule or constriction of the flexor tendon sheath.

Finger extension. In testing finger extension, watch out for a trap, best described in relation to radial nerve palsy or drop wrist, where all long extensors are paralysed. The trap is that the intrinsic muscles of the fingers (lumbricals and interossei, which are mainly ulnar-innervated) are able to extend the interphalangeal joints because of their insertion into the extensor tendon over the proximal phalanx. To the unwary, this can look like active extension produced by the radial nerve. Look for active extension of the MCP joints.

Finger adduction and abduction. Testing of these is shown in Figure 3.45. This test is often performed as a test of ulnar nerve function, as the interossei are innervated by this nerve.

Movements of the thumb. The thumb has to be considered separately, since its plane of movement is at right angles to the fingers; formal description of its range of movement requires clarity about this. Abduction of the thumb is tested by holding the hand with the palm facing upwards; then ask the patient to point their thumb towards the ceiling – this is important in assessing median nerve motor function. *Adduction* is difficult to test formally, but is a major component of power grip. *Extension* of the thumb is what you do in a thumbs-up sign; it may be compromised by rupture of the long thumb extensor tendons or by radial nerve palsy. Osteoarthritis of the thumb CMC joint (a common site for osteoarthritis in the hand) may result in a generalised reduction of thumb mobility in all directions, but the main feature will be pain, well-localised to that joint. It is difficult and pointless to put numbers of degrees on these ranges of movements – the question is whether the degree of stiffness or pain is functionally important to the patient.

So the important questions are:

- Can the thumb contribute usefully to:
  — power grip (Fig. 3.46A)
  — precision pinch grip (Fig. 3.46B)
  — lateral or key pinch grip (Fig. 3.46C)?
- Can the patient produce a good span, as when lifting a beer glass without a handle?

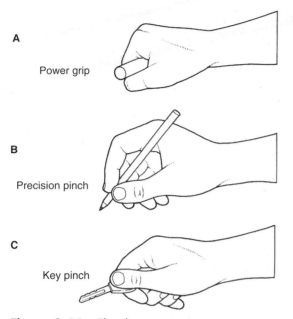

A Power grip

B Precision pinch

C Key pinch

Figure 3.46 Thumb movements.

Various pathologies may interfere with any of these functions, but loss of any will lead to functional limitation. They are thus good tests of thumb function.

Examining hand sensibility (Box 3.14)

This is a challenging exercise, because you have to rely on the patient's report of what they are feeling. This can be a problem in the first few hours after an injury which has damaged a nerve, since the patient may take some time to realise that sensibility has disappeared from part of the skin. This problem has resulted in many cases of peripheral nerve injury being missed in casualty departments. So it is not a good idea to simply stroke the skin and ask: 'Can you feel this?'. The best strategy is to stroke the skin of the relevant nerve territory of both hands simultaneously and ask whether they feel the same. If there is a denervated area, the patient will probably reply that they can feel something, but it does not feel normal. The golden rule is that this reply, in the context of a penetrating wound which could possibly have involved the nerve, means that the wound *must* be surgically explored.

> **Box 3.14   The basic tests of hand sensibility**
>
> - Simultaneously stroke the skin of the affected region and the corresponding region on the normal hand and ask: '*Do these two feel the same?*'
>
> - Map out the area of abnormal sensation

Nerve compression is much more common than nerve trauma. However, impairment of sensibility is again best demonstrated by comparing the affected with the normal side, if there is one. Putting numbers on hypoaesthesia is a complicated business involving tests of threshold and discrimination, which are useless unless expertly performed and have no part in routine clinical examination.

Having demonstrated qualitatively that there is impairment of sensibility, the next step is to map it out so as to diagnose which peripheral nerve (or cervical nerve root) is involved. Find some nearby normal skin and stroke your finger towards the affected area, asking the patient to tell you when the feeling changes; at that point mark the skin with a pen. Do this from several directions and you will easily construct a map of the denervated area, which you can match up with your anatomical knowledge. Figure 3.47 shows the territories of the major peripheral nerves, but remember that more distal injuries can damage individual digital nerves and these must be tested where appropriate. The territories of nerve roots (dermatomes) are shown in the section on the cervical spine (p. 61).

Many patients with localised nerve compression will have positive provocation tests. Thus local pressure over the median nerve, by passive flexion of the wrist to the maximum allowed (Phalen's test), by tapping over the median nerve proximal to the transverse carpal ligament (Tinel's test) or by local pressure with the examiner's thumb just proximal to the wrist, may mimic the patient's symptoms (Ch. 15). Such local pressure may also be positive with ulnar nerve problems at the elbow and the wrist.

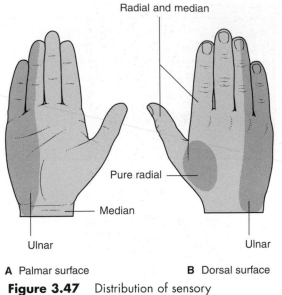

A Palmar surface   **B** Dorsal surface

Figure 3.47 Distribution of sensory abnormalities with ulnar and median nerve lesions.

Tendon problems, including ruptures

Tendons in the hand can be involved in rheumatoid arthritis; this is described later. The condition of *trigger finger* was described earlier in the section on mobility. Tendons are also frequently cut, e.g. by DIY enthusiasts, people preparing vegetables and those who enjoy fighting in pubs. The classic injuries are a cut in the palm, dividing the flexor tendons over the proximal phalanx, or a cut across the flexor surface of the wrist. Tendon lacerations are frequently accompanied by peripheral nerve injuries, which must always be carefully checked for, as described above.

Flexor tendon injuries. The cut in the palm is quite tricky to assess, because either or both of the two flexors to each finger (superficial and deep) may be divided, so they must be examined separately. The deep tendon, flexor digitorum profundus (FDP), inserts into the distal phalanx and is the only muscle–tendon unit capable of flexing the DIP joint. Flexor digitorum superficialis (FDS) inserts into the middle phalanx and is capable of flexing the PIP joint; however, FDP can do this too, since it also crosses that joint. To remove the effect of FDP, we make use of the anatomical fact that all the FDP tendons arise from a common muscle–tendon junction at wrist level;

by holding the other fingers fully extended, we prevent the action of the one belonging to the finger under examination (Fig. 3.48). Flexion of the PIP joint by FDS is then easy to see.

A complete division of FDP will result in abnormal posture of the fingers (the injured finger(s) lying in too much extension). But partial divisions and FDS injuries are often not so obvious. Do not rely on being able to see a cut in a tendon by inspecting a wound. Often the fingers were in a different posture at the time of injury and the damaged portion may have moved away from the level of the skin cut since then. If the cut is deep enough to have reached the tendon, the wound must be explored.

Extensor tendon injuries. These also need careful thought. The thumb and index have two extensors each. The single tendons to the other fingers have cross-connections on the dorsum of the hand which can reduce the degree of drooping of the affected finger. Even the single extensor tendons are complicated, because they each have two points of insertion: into the middle and distal phalanges. Thus cuts at different levels produce different effects. Again, doubt must lead to surgical exploration. Extensor tendon insertions can be avulsed without an open cut, producing a mallet finger or a boutonnière deformity. These are considered in the next section.

Abnormal hand postures due to tendon problems. The complex arrangement of flexor, extensor and intrinsic tendons means that there are are several possible patterns of derangement. It is worth knowing the classic ones and understanding how they arise.

Extensor tendon injury has different effects depending on the level at which continuity is lost (Fig. 3.49). At the distal end of the finger, the effect will confined to the DIP joint and a *mallet finger* will result. At the PIP joint level, the central slip of the extensor apparatus can be cut without injury to the lateral slips which pass to the DIP joint. This produces a boutonnière (button-hole) deformity. The same pattern is sometimes seen in rheumatoid arthritis, which can also produce a more complex derangement of extensor function, a *swan neck* deformity. This is the complete opposite of boutonnière and the explanation for it is not clear.

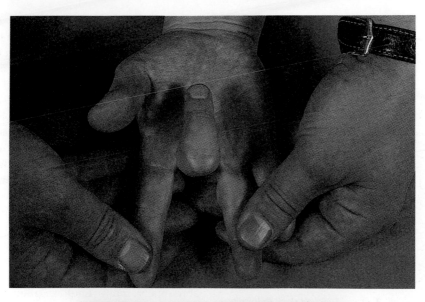

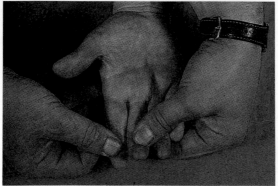

Figure 3.48 Examination of flexor digitorum superficialis (top) and profundus (bottom).

It is very disabling since it makes a power grip impossible.

Remember, once you have recognised a deformity pattern, to establish whether it is *passively correctable* – in other words, has the deformity become fixed, because of joint contracture? This has an important implication for surgical treatment: if passive correction is possible, surgery should be directed at the faulty soft tissues; if the deformity is fixed, then the bones and joints themselves will have to be addressed.

The hand in inflammatory arthritis

Remember to check for diagnostic clues: rheuma-toid nodules, vasculitic lesions, psoriatic pitting of the nails, and the typical deformities which develop, particularly in rheumatoid arthritis. The distribution of joint involvement is important diagnostically. In rheumatoid arthritis (Box 3.15), the MCP, PIP and wrist joints are affected, whereas the DIP joint is spared. Inflammatory DIP changes suggest psoriatic arthritis. In osteoarthritis (generally considered a non-inflammatory disease) the distal and proximal IP joints, and the carpometacarpal joint of the thumb are most frequently affected, but the swelling is bony and usually non-tender, distinguishing this from inflammatory arthritis.

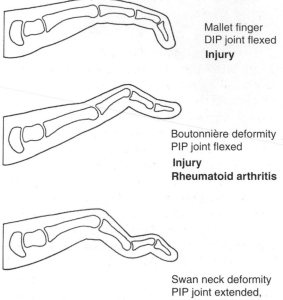

Mallet finger
DIP joint flexed
Injury

Boutonnière deformity
PIP joint flexed
Injury
Rheumatoid arthritis

Swan neck deformity
PIP joint extended,
MCP and DIP joints
flexed
Rheumatoid arthritis

Figure 3.49 Finger deformities.

Box 3.15   Hand involvement in rheumatoid arthritis

- Bulging synovium
  — from MCP and proximal IP joints
  — on the dorsum of the wrist (around extensor tendons)
  — in the palmar aspect of the wrist (around flexor tendons)

- Wasting of the dorsal interossei

- Ulnar deviation of MCP joints

- Swan neck and boutonnière deformities

- Z-deformity of thumb

- Dorsal subluxation of the ulnar head

- Vasculitic lesions on fingertips

- Median nerve compression

- Extensor tendon rupture

- Palmar erythema

Synovitis. Since the essence of inflammatory arthritis is synovitis, it is important to look for its presence when examining the hand; it is found both in joints and around tendons. Synovitis may already be obvious on inspection; e.g. in rheumatoid arthritis, the MCP and PIP joints are characteristically swollen (Fig. 3.50), in sharp contrast to the wasted dorsal interossei. As in the knee, synovitis is recognised, and distinguished from synovial fluid, by its doughy feel. As mentioned in the section on the wrist, extensor tendon synovitis is often very obvious on the back of the wrist and hand; it may be segmented into portions proximal and distal to the extensor retinaculum. Flexor synovitis is best appreciated by palpating the palm with both thumbs, then asking the patient to flex the fingers and feeling the abnormally bulky tendons gliding. As well as detecting the presence of hypertrophied synovium, try to estimate its state of inflammation by noting the degree of tenderness and pain on motion. The individual joints should be palpated individually. However, before beginning your palpation, as with any joint ask the patient about whether there is pain in that area – some patients with active rheumatoid arthritis have very tender hands. Therefore, it is important to show consideration.

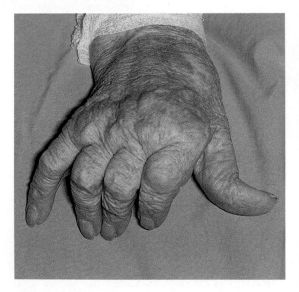

Figure 3.50 Rheumatoid hand.

Deformities. Characteristic deformities of the hand and wrist occur in rheumatoid arthritis. The whole hand may be supinated on the distal radius; this is what makes the distal end of the ulna prominent although it can usually easily be reduced (piano key sign). The wrist is often radially deviated, forming a zig-zag pattern with the ulnar deviation commonly shown by the MCP joints of the fingers. More advanced change at the MCP joints leads to their subluxation or even complete dislocation, which grossly interferes with flexion. The IP joints can adopt various patterns, swan neck or boutonnière as described above. The thumb may collapse into a zig-zag pattern.

Functional assessment. The functional consequences of widespread hand involvement in rheumatoid arthritis are the key to planning treatment. With so many joints and other structures involved, it is impossible to put everything right surgically, so a selective approach, based on functional assessment, is necessary. This is a skilled job and is best done by a hand therapist who may be a specially trained physiotherapist or occupational therapist. However, you should know the underlying principles:

- Pain-free stability of the more proximal joints is important to allow the application of grip. In practice, this means the wrist joint (for power grip) and the thumb CMC and MCP joints (for precision grip). If the erosion of these joints is severe, arthrodesis may be required. Wrist splints are often helpful.
- Finger flexion, the basis of grip, may be threatened by three things, which must be distinguished:
  — mobility of finger MCP and IP joints may be lost, necessitating surgery directed at the joints themselves
  — intrinsic muscle tightness
  — flexor tendon power may be threatened by tenosynovitis sticking the tendons to their sheaths, necessitating synovectomy.
- Sensation is needed for control of grip, particularly precision grip. The median nerve, which supplies this, can be compressed by synovitis in the carpal tunnel. If the history and sensory testing suggest this, a very simple operation to decompress the nerve may have great benefit.

The hand after injury (Box 3.16)

Swelling of the hand is almost always present after any hand injury, mostly on the dorsal surface where the skin is loose, even if the injury is on the palmar surface. It is important to note and immediately treat by elevating the limb and encouraging early active finger movement if at all possible (Fig. 3.51). Otherwise the oedema fluid will precipitate fibrin which will clog up the extensor tendons and lead to permanent loss of finger flexion: 'oedema is the mother of fibrosis'.

Notice the posture of the fingers at rest and after the patient has tried to flex and extend. Note any lacerations which could possibly have damaged underlying tendons or nerves. From these preliminaries you should pick up clues which guide formal testing of the tendons and nerves as described above.

Look for within-bone deformity which would indicate a fracture, or between-bone deformity which suggests dislocation of a joint. It is particularly important to look for *rotational deformity* of the fingers, which can occur with metacarpal or phalangeal fractures (Fig. 3.52). If left uncorrected, this leads to great loss of function, due to the fingers crossing over each other during flexion. It is best appreciated by viewing the fingertips and nails end-on.

Box 3.16   The hand after injury

- Note swelling – especially dorsal
- Note posture – signs of tendon injury
- Look for deformity – fractures and dislocations
- Site of a laceration – what deep structures could have been cut?
- Test flexor tendons – deep and superficial
- Test extensor tendons
- Test sensibility and map out loss

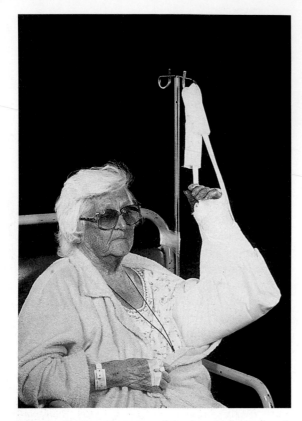

Figure 3.51 Elevation of the hand after a hand injury.

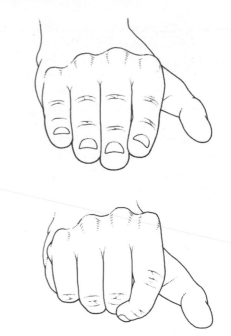

Figure 3.52 Malrotation of index finger. Visible by inspecting nail ends in extension; fingers cross in flexion. As always, it is important to compare with the other hand.

Sepsis in the hand

As in other musculoskeletal infections, sepsis in the hand may be:

- a rapidly spreading, cellulitic process – usually streptococcal
- a localised abscess – usually staphylococcal
- septic arthritis – which can be due to any organism.

The cardinal signs of inflammation are present in all cases to varying degree: pain, redness and heat, swelling, and loss of function.

The patient will soon tell you where the throbbing pain is concentrated; gently establish whether it is worsened by movement of joints or tendons. Observe the distribution of erythema; its epicentre is often obvious and almost always the seat of the infection (Fig. 3.53). Note the degree of oedema on the dorsum of the hand, which is rapid and dramatic (as after injury), and decide whether the infection is actually spreading through the oedema, as it can do at a great rate. Look for ascending lymphangitis (longitudinal red streaks on the forearm) and regional lymphadenopathy.

There are many anatomical spaces where pus can collect in the hand. Each gives a characteristic clinical picture. The common ones are:

- *paronychia* – a collection of pus in the nail bed at the proximal edge of a fingernail; it has a characteristic horseshoe shape
- *pulp space infection* – an exquisitely tender, tense swelling in a fingertip
- *tendon sheath infection* – causes pain all along the finger when the flexor tendon is moved by flexing any joint in that digit
- *septic arthritis* – gives a more localised pain at the affected joint when it is moved.

A history of human bite injury (usually acquired by punching someone in the teeth) invites specific inspection of the MCP joints which are likely to have been innoculated with anaerobes.

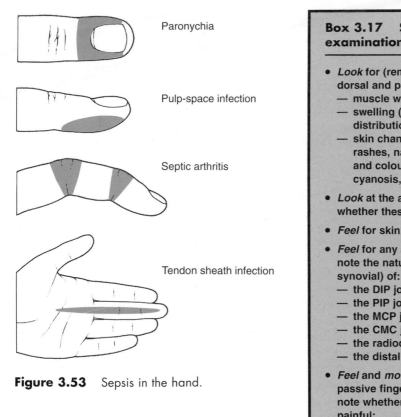

Paronychia

Pulp-space infection

Septic arthritis

Tendon sheath infection

Figure 3.53 Sepsis in the hand.

Structured approach to examination of the hand and wrist

Most of the important points have already been covered, but as with all joints it is important to structure your examination – otherwise you will miss things (Box 3.17). As well as being a common site for injury and infection, and being often involved in inflammatory arthritis, many other musculosleletal conditions are associated with clinical signs in the hands. Therefore, the hand can give many important diagnostic clues. For example, in a patient with Raynaud's phenomenon, telangiectasiae and/or calcinosis are suggestive of limited cutaneous systemic sclerosis (Fig. 9.9, p. 143). We have already stressed the importance of a detailed neurological examination. Also, remember to consider the possibility of vascular insufficiency in patients with hand problems. In patients with connective tissue diseases, circulatory problems often involve the microvasculature, and so digital ischaemia can occur even with normal arterial pulses.

Box 3.17   Structured approach to examination of the hand and wrist

- *Look* for (remembering to examine both dorsal and palmar surfaces):
  — muscle wasting
  — swelling (noting the site and distribution)
  — skin changes, including scars/wounds, rashes, nail changes, vasculitic lesions and colour changes (erythema, cyanosis, palmar erythema)
- *Look* at the active range of movements, and whether these produce pain
- *Feel* for skin temperature
- *Feel* for any areas of local tenderness, and note the nature of any swelling (bony or synovial) of:
  — the DIP joints
  — the PIP joints, and IP joint of the thumb
  — the MCP joints
  — the CMC joint of the thumb
  — the radiocarpal joint
  — the distal radioulnar joint
- *Feel* and *move* to examine the range of passive finger and wrist movements, and note whether the following movements are painful:
  — finger flexion
  — finger extension
  — finger abduction and adduction
  — thumb abduction, adduction, opposition and flexion
  — wrist dorsiflexion and palmar flexion
  — wrist radial and ulnar deviation
  — pronation and supination (inferior radioulnar joint)
- *Feel* the pulses and the skin temperature (and *look* at the skin colour) to assess the blood supply
- Perform any neurological examination as clinically indicated. This should include an assessment of muscle power, sensation, reflexes and provocation tests

Remember that pain felt in the hand and the wrist may arise elsewhere.

Possible extrinsic causes of hand and wrist symptoms

Examine the neck, upper arm and elbow – symptoms felt in the hand may have their origin

Examination of the musculoskeletal system

more proximally. Upper limb peripheral nerve problems and cervical root problems often cause problems in the hands.

SPINE

Clues to spinal pathology are often gained simply by watching how the patient moves around: walking into the consulting room, sitting or rising from a chair, climbing onto the examination couch and so on. A patient who has an inflexible or painful spinal column will move in a characteristically stiff way that is apparent even when they are fully clothed. However, a thorough formal assessment of the spine requires the patient to be undressed down to their underclothes.

Some conditions, especially inflammatory ones such as ankylosing spondylitis, affect the whole spinal column. However, in the majority of cases, one is concentrating either on the neck and corresponding upper limb neurology, or on the thoracic and lumbar spine (including the sacroiliac joints) and lower limb neurology. In both cervical and lumbar spine problems, a crucial element in analysing patients' pain is to distinguish between *referred* pain and *radicular* pain. The importance of neurological examination must be emphasised in the assessment of patients with spinal problems; thus we chose examination of the spine to demonstrate how musculoskeletal and neurological examination (here described under 'examination of distal parts') go hand in hand.

Neck

The two important features of neck (cervical spine) examination are identification of local signs and neurological examination of distal parts. The distal parts affected are most commonly the upper limbs, as a result of root compression due to disc protrusion or foraminal stenosis, in turn due to cervical spondylosis (Ch. 17). However, all distal parts (trunk and lower limbs) may be affected if there is cord compression at cervical spine level. It should be recalled that upper motor neurone signs (weakness, spasticity, hyperreflexia) are distinguishable from lower motor neurone signs (weakness, flaccidity, hyporeflexia). Extensor

plantar responses suggest an upper motor neurone lesion. Cord compression is more frequently associated with widespread sensory impairment than is more peripheral nerve compression.

When examining and treating neck disorders, it is important to be aware of the devastating results of cervical instability – a cautious approach is required. In chronic spinal conditions many patients complain of a degree of pain which does not appear to bear a good relationship with the objective evidence of underlying pathology (e.g. as demonstrated on MR scans). It is important to recognise such patients, as they often respond poorly to surgical treatments but may be helped by more conservative measures, including psychological support.

Local examination

Look. Initial inspection may show that the patient has abnormal movement of the head or neck, or abnormal posture; for example, patients with anylosing spondylitis may have loss of the normal cervical lordosis (Fig. 8.12, p. 119). In acute injuries, the neck and shoulders should be inspected for bruising and deformity; the pharynx should also be inspected, as upper cervical fractures often result in visible bruise or haematoma in the posterior pharyngeal wall.

Feel. Initial palpation localises tenderness, which may be located over the vertebral bodies or over the paraspinal muscles. Such paraspinal muscle tenderness may be associated with spasm. In the short term, spasm can be caused by injury or resultant instability, and should be regarded as a possible warning sign of underlying damage. In more chronic conditions, spasm is often a reflection of the pain experienced from the underlying disease. The spinous processes should be palpated for the presence of steps or gaps. In particular, after an acute trauma the whole of the spine should be palpated (after rolling the patient on to the side using a suitably safe technique) for gaps and boggy swellings, in order to assess the presence of a spinal fracture. This is an important adjunct to X-rays in this circumstance, as not all fractures are initially detectable on X-ray, and not all X-rays taken in emergency situations are technically satisfactory.

Tenderness at certain specific points around the neck and shoulder are characteristic of fibromyalgia, which is being increasingly recognised in patients presenting with neck and other pains (Ch. 6). Therefore, tenderness at these sites (occiput, low cervical, origin of supraspinatus and over the trapezius), together with a characteristic pattern of symptoms, is suggestive of fibromyalgia and should prompt a search for the other well recognised trigger points.

Move. Cervical movements should be assessed in three planes: flexion (normally the chin can touch the chest) and extension (normally the eyes can look straight upwards); rotation to each side (normally it is possible to bring the chin so it is directly over the shoulder); and lateral flexion to each side (it is just possible to touch the shoulder with the ear) (Fig. 3.54). Restrictions of these ranges should be noted. These may be due to actual joint stiffness, inhibition by pain or muscle spasm. Therefore assess both active and passive movements.

Distal examination

This should include neurological assessment of both upper and lower limbs. For this it is essential to have the patient undressed. Points for inspection include wasting of muscles and fasciculation. Palpation or movement reveals the tone of the limb with presence of spasticity or flaccidity. Assessment of strength should include all major muscle groups (Box 3.18), although it is often difficult and unnecessary to identify most individual muscles. The testing of strength is notoriously subjective, but the MRC rating scale (Box 3.3, p. 22) is at least widely known and used. Tendon reflexes should be examined for the standard five reflexes:

* biceps (mainly C5, C6)
* supinator (C5, C6)
* triceps (C6, C7)
* knee (L3,4)
* ankle (S1).

The plantar responses must be assessed. Sensation should be studied using touch (as a crude screening test) or fine and sharp touch and vibration (if significant sensory disturbance is suspected). It is essential to know the dermatomes

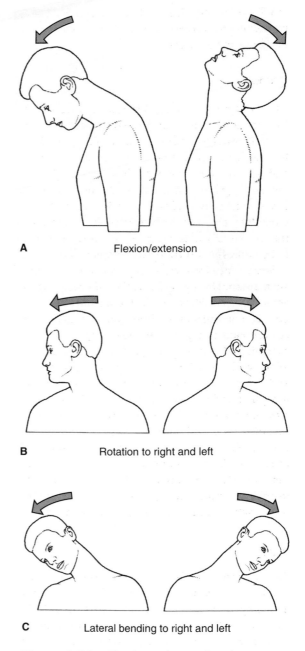

A Flexion/extension

B Rotation to right and left

C Lateral bending to right and left

Figure 3.54 The three planes of neck movement.

to make sense of this examination (Fig. 3.56). Non-dermatomal loss may be explained by a local lesion of a peripheral nerve (Fig. 3.56), peripheral neuropathy, or a central lesion.

Box 3.18   Muscle groups to test

- Shoulder flexors (C5,6), abductors (C5,6), extensors (C6,7)

- Elbow flexors (biceps, brachialis: (C5–7); extensors (triceps: C6–8)

- Wrist extensors (C7,8), flexors (C6–8)

- Fingers long flexors (C8,T1), long extensors (C7,8), intrinsics (C8,T1)

- Hip flexors (iliopsoas: L2,3), abductors (glutei: L5, S1)

- Knee extensors (quadriceps: L2–4), flexors (hamstrings: L5,S1)

- Ankle extensors (tibialis anterior: L4,5), flexors (gastrosoleus: S1,2)

- Toes long flexors (S2,3) and extensors (L5), intrinsics (S2,3).

Note root values are an approximate guide only

Box 3.19   Structured approach to examination of the neck

- *Look* for any abnormal posture or skin changes

- *Look* at the active range of movements, and whether these produce pain

- *Feel* for any areas of local tenderness

- *Feel* and *move* to examine the range of passive movements:
  — flexion and extension
  — rotation to the right and left
  — lateral bending to the right and left

- Assess the neurological state of the upper and lower limbs

- *Feel* the pulses and the skin temperature (and *look* at the skin colour) to assess the blood supply

Remember that pain felt in the neck may arise elsewhere

Structured approach to examination of the neck

Most points have already been covered and are summarised in Box 3.19. Patients who have a cervical rib may develop a thoracic outlet syndrome, when compression of the lower trunk of the brachial plexus and the subclavian vessels can occur. Therefore, if this is suspected, assess the peripheral vasculature of the upper limb as well as its neurology.

Possible extrinsic causes of neck symptoms

Pain in the neck may be due to an upper respiratory problem. Pain arising in the shoulder may be felt primarily in the neck (and vice versa). Anginal pain may be referred to the jaw.

Thoracic spine

The thoracic spine is much less mobile that the cervical and lumbar spines, and movements are often assessed along with those of the lumbar spine. Because of the anatomy of the thoracic vertebral bodies, these permit more rotation than in the lumbar spine. The thoracic spine is frequently the site of problems in patients with osteoporosis, and many elderly patients and patients attending the rheumatology clinic have osteoporotic vertebral collapse, resulting in accentuation of the thoracic kyphosis. The thoracic spine may be affected in conditions which involve the whole skeleton, such as ankylosing spondylitis.

The main elements of a thoracic spine examination are as follows:

- *Look* for any deformity, e.g. an abnormal kyphosis, or scoliosis. A deviation of the spine laterally is described as scoliosis, discussed earlier in association with limb length discrepancy and below in the lumbar spine section. The scoliosis is usually described by the side of the convexity. Figure 3.55 demonstrates a patient with a scoliosis convex to the left.

- *Feel* for areas of local tenderness. Patients with acute vertebral collapse are usually very tender over the affected vertebral body.

- *Assess movement.* Rotation is assessed by stabilising the pelvis (this is most easily done by placing your hands on the iliac crests to ensure that the pelvis does not rotate), then asking the

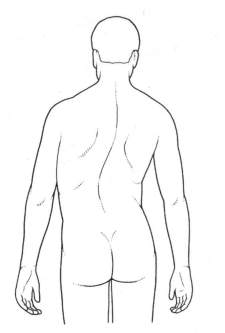

Figure 3.55 Thoracic scoliosis, convex to the left.

patient to twist to the right and to the left. Movement at the costovertebral joints can be assessed by measuring the chest expansion; this should be at least 5 cm, but is often markedly reduced in patients with ankylosing spondylitis.

Lumbar spine and sacroiliac joints

Local examination

Look. You should perform an initial inspection with the patient standing. Inspect from behind and from the side. The spine is normally straight in the sagittal plane, but has cervical and lumbar lordosis and a thoracic kyphosis. The cervical or lumbar lordosis is frequently lost due to painful conditions in the respective area. You may see a scoliosis. This used to be called kyphoscoliosis, but it is now clear that the principal problem in such spines is abnormal rotation, often due to excessive lordosis. Scoliosis may be fixed in which case it is still apparent when the patient bends forward, or mobile, in which case it will disappear on bending. As discussed earler, the condition may be caused by limb length discrepancy. A mild scoliosis or tilt

may occur with severe unilateral back pain, particularly disc protrusion.

Feel and move. Palpate for areas of tenderness. The movements occurring at the lumbar spine are flexion and extension, and lateral flexion (Fig. 3.57). Flexion may be examined using Schober's test (Fig. 3.58). The position of the dimples over the posterior iliac spines are noted or marked. A tape measure is used to mark positions in the midline 5 cm below these two points and 10 cm above (i.e. 15 cm apart). The positions should normally extend to a distance of at least 20 cm apart on full forward bending in normal patients. This is usually described as Schober 20/15. Loss of lumbar flexion may occur due to 'degenerative' disease or acutely painful conditions. Gross stiffness arises in conditions such as ankylosing spondylitis (with associated 'bamboo spine', Ch. 8), when movement is characteristically reduced in all planes. Watch the patient during movement. The spine may not move with a regular rhythm between being upright and flexed. Sudden catches or wriggles may be present during the motion; this is often thought to result from some degree of structural spinal instability, such as in spondylolysis (p. 252).

In examining the lumbar spine, you should also look for the presence of steps or gaps between vertebrae. This may be a sign of spondylolisthesis (slip of one vertebra forwards on the vertebra below it). In the common form, the slip occurs at the level below that where the step in the spinal processes is felt. Thus the commonest site of this condition in young adults is at L5–S1; if this occurs the step is felt between the L4 and 5 spinal processes.

The sacroiliac joints. These should be examined for local tenderness, which occurs in sacroiliitis which is common in the spondyloarthropathies. However, eliciting sacroiliac tenderness is difficult, due to the position of the joints. The sacroiliac joints may be stressed by asking the patient to lie on their side and then counter-rotating the chest and pelvis. This results in a torsional force at the sacroiliac joint. Sacroiliac pain is a typical cause of referred pain down the back of the leg, often as far as the knee. Contrast this with radicular pain, where nerve root entrapment may result in pain from the back as far as the foot.

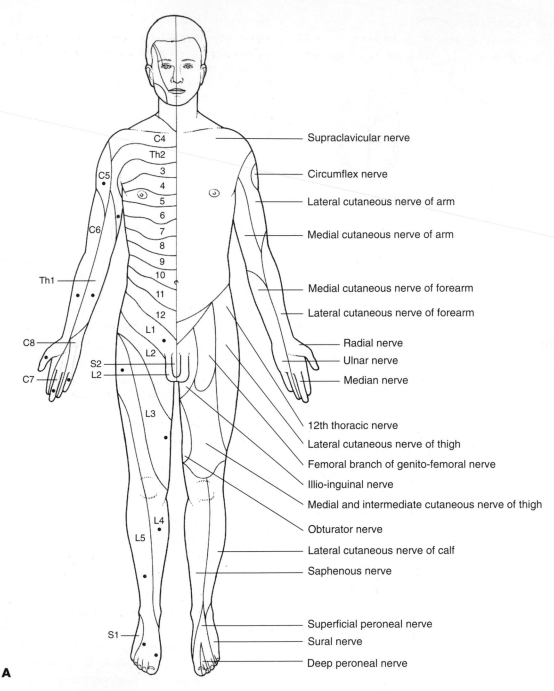

A

Figure 3.56 Segmental and peripheral nerve innervation. **A.** Anterior view. **B.** Posterior view.

Distal examination

Nerve root entrapment is an important part of lumbar spinal disease. There are two important tests which you need to know: the straight leg raising test and the femoral stretch test.

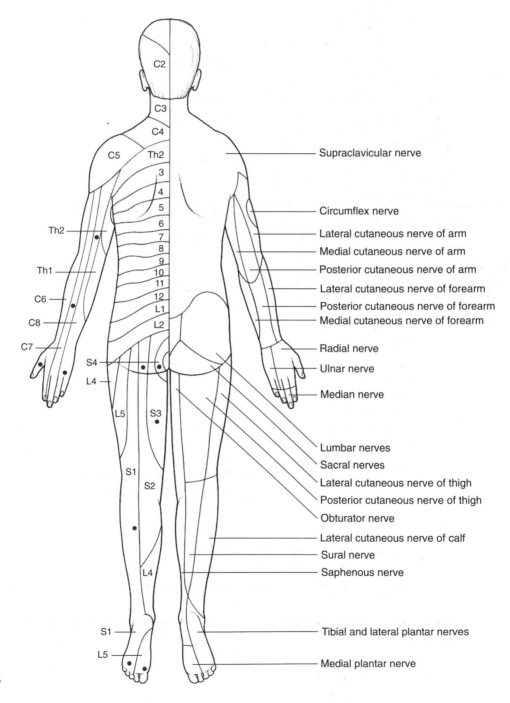

Supraclavicular nerve

Circumflex nerve

Lateral cutaneous nerve of arm

Medial cutaneous nerve of arm

Posterior cutaneous nerve of arm

Lateral cutaneous nerve of forearm

Posterior cutaneous nerve of forearm

Medial cutaneous nerve of forearm

Radial nerve

Ulnar nerve

Median nerve

Lumbar nerves

Sacral nerves

Lateral cutaneous nerve of thigh

Posterior cutaneous nerve of thigh

Obturator nerve

Lateral cutaneous nerve of calf

Sural nerve

Saphenous nerve

Tibial and lateral plantar nerves

Medial plantar nerve

C2, C3, C4, C5, Th2, 3, 4, 5, 6, 7, 8, 9, 10, 11, 12, L1, L2, Th2, Th1, C6, C8, C7, S4, L4, L5, S3, S1, S2, L4, S1, L5

B

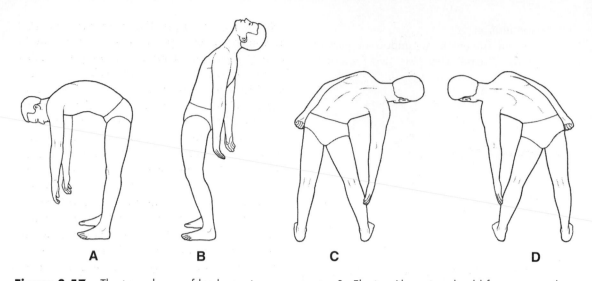

Figure 3.57   The two planes of lumbar spine movements. **A.** Flexion (the spine should form a smooth curve). **B.** Extension. **C, D.** Lateral flexion (to the right, to the left).

Straight leg raising (SLR) test. To check this, examine the patient lying supine. Check that the hips and knees are not painful by ensuring that there is a normal range of flexion without pain. Then passively raise the legs in turn as high as possible; normal patients can reach 90° (more or less, depending on age and flexibility) (Fig. 3.59). Marked reduction in the ability to straight leg raise is often caused by nerve root tension in the lower

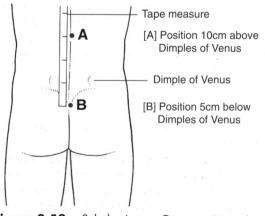

Tape measure

[A] Position 10cm above Dimples of Venus

Dimple of Venus

[B] Position 5cm below Dimples of Venus

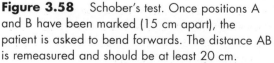

Figure 3.58   Schober's test. Once positions A and B have been marked (15 cm apart), the patient is asked to bend forwards. The distance AB is remeasured and should be at least 20 cm.

lumbar spinal roots. Occasionally, raising one leg will cause pain radiating down the other leg (cross leg pain). The pain on straight leg raise may be increased by passive dorsiflexion of the foot. The best sign of nerve root tension is a markedly asymmetric straight leg raise; the side with the reduced straight leg raise is usually the side with the nerve root entrapment.

The femoral nerve stretch test. This employs the same idea as SLR – what is being looked for is nerve root tension. Ask the patient to lie on their side (affected side uppermost). With the knee straight, gently extend the hip as far as it will go. Then flex the knee; a positive result is pain felt in the anterior thigh. This is a nerve tension test for the upper lumbar roots (Fig. 3.60).

Distal neurology. At this stage it is important to test distal neurology, including tendon reflexes, power and sensation. The principles are the same as for the cervical spine, and the muscle groups to test are outlined in Box 3.18. Limb dermatomes and peripheral nerve innervations are shown in Figure 3.56. It is essential to remember to examine the most distal nerve roots (S2–4). These may be affected by various proximal conditions, including compression of the spinal cord. However, they are particularly vulnerable to compression at the cauda equina, the leash of nerve roots which

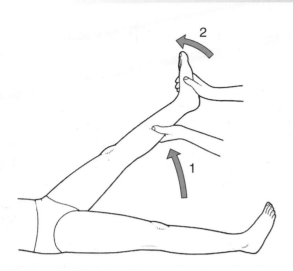

Figure 3.59 Straight leg raising test. After the limb has been raised to the position which produces pain (1), dorsiflexion at the ankle (2) exacerbates that pain.

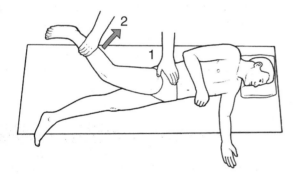

Figure 3.60 Femoral nerve stretch test. Extend the hip as far as possible (1) and flex the knee (2).

occupies the spinal canal below the termination of the cord at L1. Central compression of the cauda equina, typically by a central disc protrusion, results in loss of sphincter function (both urinary and anal) and perineal numbness. The loss of sphincter function may result in incontinence or retention; such retention is usually pain-free, while voiding under these circumstances may be associated with a loss of the normal sensation of micturition. Loss of sphincter function from this cause is often permanent; it is vital to check for perineal sensation and anal tone in patients with severe back problems.

Spinal patients, in particular, require a holistic assessment. Some spinal patients may exhibit degrees of pain which appear inappropriate to the level of organic disease found. Such patients can be difficult to assess; the natural tendency is to overinvestigate in order to 'exclude' an organic basis to their pain. This is often not the best approach, and safe assessment of such patients requires particular skill as well as a sympathetic and humane approach. Several tests are suggestive of spinal pain which will prove to be non-organic. In the lumbar spine, these include the ability to sit up on a couch with the knees straight, but an inability to straight leg raise when laid flat to more than a few degrees. Also, very superficial tenderness (e.g. pinching the skin) may yield protestations of pain, as may trunk rotation by rotating the pelvis (without rotation of the lumbar spine). Finally, axial loading of the spine by pressing downwards on the head should not normally lead to lumbar pain. These 'inappropriate signs' (of Waddell) are indicators that lumbar spinal pain may prove to be non-organic. However, they do not prove that the patient is a malingerer, or that medical science cannot help.

Structured approach to examination of the lumbar spine

Most points have already been covered and are summarised in Box 3.20. A number of different pathologies can affect the lumbar spine, including metastatic disease. Therefore, all patients must have a full clinical assessment.

Possible extrinsic causes of lumbar spine symptoms

Low back pain may arise from intra-abdominal or pelvic pathology. Always consider these possibilities, especially if there is no obvious abnormality on lumbar spine examination. Claudication may mimic radicular pain, and so the peripheral pulses should be checked. Remember to examine the abdomen – abdominal aortic aneurysms may cause back pain

---

Box 3.20   Structured approach to examination of the lumbar spine and sacroiliac joints

Patient standing

- *Look* for any abnormal posture (both from behind and from the side) or skin changes. If scoliosis is present look also with the patient flexed forward

- *Look* and *feel* for any steps of gaps between vertebrae

- *Look* at the active range of movements, and whether these produce pain:
  — flexion and extension
  — lateral bending to the right and to the left

- *Look* at the patient walking

Patient supine

- *Move* the limb and *look* for signs of nerve root tension:
  — straight leg raising test
  — femoral nerve stretch (with the patient on their side)

- Assess the neurological state of the lower limbs

- *Feel* the pulses and the skin temperature (and *look* at the skin colour) to assess the blood supply

Patient lying prone

- *Feel* for any areas of local tenderness, including over the sacroiliac joints; then stress the sacroiliac joints.

Remember that problems experienced in the region of the lumbar spine may arise elsewhere.

The temperomandibular joint

This deserves mention, albeit briefly, because it is commonly involved in inflammatory arthritis, especially in rheumatoid arthritis. Patients with temperomandibular problems complain of pain on mouth opening and closing, e.g. when chewing.

Children with juvenile chronic arthritis may have temperomandibular joint involvement. Because this occurs during growth it can lead to micrognathia (hypoplasia of the jaw, with chin recession). This is most obvious on looking from the side.

When temperomandibular joint involvement is suspected, look for any swelling and feel for tenderness. Watch the patient during mouth opening and jaw movements – is there pain on motion, or any asymmetry of movement?

4 | Principles of investigation of musculoskeletal disease

Case history — trauma

A 60-year-old woman was admitted after sustaining a fracture of her right humerus with a minor fall. Two years previously she had undergone a mastectomy for carcinoma of the breast. She was in a great deal of pain on admission from both her humerus, which had been painful for several weeks, and her left thigh. On admission, her X-rays showed evidence of bone destruction in the mid-humerus (the site of the fracture), but X-rays of the femora looked normal. A plasma biochemical profile checked prior to surgery showed that she was hypercalcaemic. This was treated with intravenous fluids. The humerus was treated with an intramedullary nail.

Further investigations were carried out during the same admission. A technetium-99 bone scan showed multiple areas of increased uptake. As well as in the humerus, these were in the left femur (subtrochanteric region), the ribs and the lumbar spine. Subsequent review of X-rays of the femur showed just discernible changes around the lesser trochanter; the femur was fixed prophylactically with a nail. After this she was able to walk almost normally and reported that her pain was much improved. Before discharge, radiotherapy was carried out (a single dose) to the right femur, humerus and lumbar spine. Her serum calcium was kept under review by the oncologists.

Case history — non-trauma

A 62-year-old woman presented to her GP with a 6-month history of back pain. While the GP felt this was most likely to be due to lumbar spondylosis (he knew that she already had cervical spondylosis from a cervical spine X-ray taken 2 years previously), she looked a little tired and he requested a full blood count and erythrocyte sedimentation rate (ESR). To his surprise she was anaemic with a haemoglobin of 101 g/L and the ESR was 70 mm/h. She was referred for further investigation. Serum globulin level was high, serum electrophoresis showed a paraprotein and testing for Bence–Jones' proteinuria was positive. X-ray of the lumbar spine was suggestive of osteoporosis, but there were no areas of vertebral collapse. She was referred to

---

Key points

- Investigations may be crucial in making the diagnosis. More often, however, they are used to support a suspected diagnosis.

- A careful history and examination guide investigations.

- A full blood count, ESR and plasma biochemical profile are useful 'screening tests'. If any of these is abnormal, ask why.

- Rational management of fractures would be impossible without X-rays.

- Investigations are used to monitor activity and severity of certain diseases (e.g. rheumatoid arthritis) and to identify adverse drug effects at an early stage.

- There have been several recent major advances in the methods of imaging the musculoskeletal system, e.g. computed tomography (CT) and magnetic resonance imaging (MRI).

Principles of investigation of musculoskeletal disease

a haematologist. Bone marrow showed diffuse infiltration with plasma cells, confirming the diagnosis of myeloma.

Investigations are used to support a diagnosis already suspected from the history and examination, or to monitor disease activity and severity. They are also used in 'safety monitoring' of certain drugs. In rheumatic disease, investigations are seldom, in themselves, 'diagnostic' although occasionally they can be. For example, the finding of Gram-positive organisms in synovial fluid aspirated from a hot swollen knee is diagnostic of septic arthritis. In orthopaedics, however, the diagnosis is often made on the basis of X-rays; this is especially true for fractures. Recently, dramatic advances have been made in imaging methods for the musculoskeletal system. These have substantially improved our understanding and management of some conditions.

The aim of this chapter is to outline the main types of investigation which are useful in the assessment of patients with musculoskeletal disease (Box 4.1). It should be remembered that *investigations are never a substitute for a meticulous clinical history and examination.* Indeed, investigations should always be considered in light of the clinical features presented by the patient. If the two sets of information do not appear to fit together, judgement is required to decide on the relative weights to give to the different pieces of information. An excellent example is magnetic resonance imaging (MRI) of the spine. Most adult patients with backache have identifiable lesions on MRI – but then so do many control patients without symptoms. Thus, this investigation should be regarded as confirming clinically, suspected pathology in this situation; if it is used blindly as a fishing expedition for data, confusion and inappropriate treatment will result.

BLOOD TESTS

Haematology

A full blood count often gives important information and should be performed in most patients presenting with musculoskeletal problems. Patients with inflammatory disease

---

Box 4.1   Main investigations in patients with musculoskeletal disease

Blood tests
- Haematology
  - full blood count
  - ESR/plasma viscosity
- Biochemistry
  - urea and electrolytes
  - liver function tests
  - urate
  - bone biochemistry
  - immunoglobulins
  - muscle enzymes
  - C-reactive protein
- Immunology
  - rheumatoid factor
  - antinuclear factor
- HLA-typing

Urine tests
- Dipstix (protein, blood)
- Microscopy (red blood cells, casts)
- Biochemistry:
  - 24 h protein
  - Bence–Jones' protein
  - creatinine clearance

Synovial fluid analysis
- Microscopy
- Culture

Radiology/nuclear medicine
- Plain X-rays
- Ultrasound
- Bone scan/white cell scan
- Computed tomography (CT)
- Magnetic resonance (MR) imaging
- Measurement of bone density

Arthroscopy

Pathology
- Synovial biopsy
- Bone biopsy
- Muscle biopsy

Electrophysiology
- Electromyography
- Nerve conduction studies

---

often have a normochromic normocytic anaemia ('anaemia of chronic disease'), although sometimes the anaemia is hypochromic and microcytic and therefore difficult to differentiate from iron deficiency. If there is any doubt, the patient must be investigated for blood loss. Occult blood loss can occur secondary to the use of non-steroidal anti-inflammatory drugs (NSAIDs). In iron deficiency, typically the serum ferritin and iron are low, and the iron binding capacity high, whereas in the anaemia of chronic inflammatory disease the serum iron is again low, but the ferritin is normal (or high) and the iron binding capacity normal (or low) (Table 4.1). However, the picture can be confused by the fact that ferritin is an acute-phase reactant, rising with inflammation, and so may be 'falsely' elevated in the patient with rheumatoid arthritis and concomitant iron deficiency. A haemolytic anaemia may occur in systemic lupus erythematosus (SLE).

A raised white cell count is suggestive of infection. Patients with SLE may have a low white blood count (in particular the lymphocyte count is low), and the platelet count and haemoglobin may also be low. The platelet count may be elevated in a patient with active inflammatory disease. The haemoglobin, white cell or platelet count may fall with bone marrow suppression, which can occur with several of the drugs used to treat severe inflammatory disease.

The erythrocyte sedimentation rate (ESR) is a non-specific test, but it rises in inflammatory disease (including infections) and malignancy. A raised ESR requires explanation, although it should be noted that there is a rise in ESR with ageing. Patients with non-inflammatory disease such as osteoarthritis and soft tissue rheumatism should not have an elevated ESR. The ESR is classed as one of the measures of the 'acute-phase response', which occurs in patients with

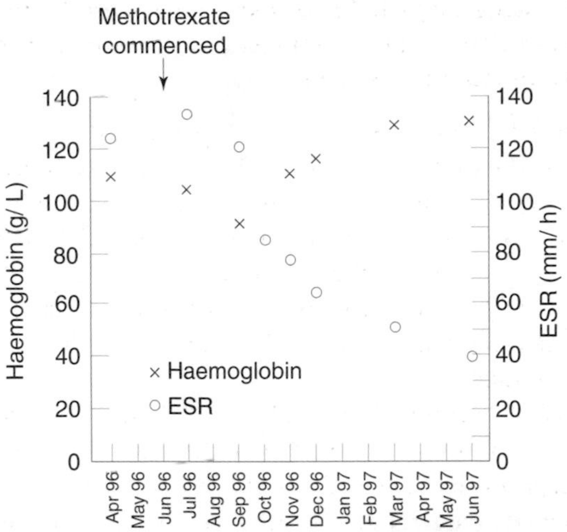

Figure 4.1 Rise in haemoglobin and fall in ESR in a patient with rheumatoid arthritis as a 'flare-up' of disease settled (after commencing methotrexate).

inflammation, and can be used as a marker of disease activity in patients with, for example, rheumatoid arthritis. As a patient's inflammatory disease becomes less active, typically the ESR falls and the haemoglobin rises (Fig. 4.1). Other markers of the acute-phase response are the plasma viscosity and the C-reactive protein.

Biochemistry

As with a full blood count, a blood biochemical profile, including bone biochemistry, is a useful screening test in patients presenting with musculoskeletal disease, especially in the context of non-specific or multisystem disease. This should be normal in patients with osteoarthritis or soft tissue rheumatism.

Derangements in renal or liver function may occur as a result of organ involvement in multisystem inflammatory disease, or as a side-effect of drug treatment. For example, treatment with methotrexate may cause hepatotoxicity. Patients with inflammatory disease often have a raised globulin level, due to a polyclonal rise in immunoglobulins: IgG, IgA and IgM may all be elevated. This is a reflection of the acute-phase response. However, if a patient has raised

Table 4.1
Typical blood count results for anaemia of chronic disease and iron deficiency

Condition	Ferritin	Serum iron	Total iron binding capacity
Anaemia of chronic disease	N or ⇑	⇓	N or ⇓
Iron deficiency	⇓	⇓	⇑
N = normal			

globulins and a raised ESR, it is worthwhile checking the serum protein electrophoresis in order not to miss a monoclonal gammopathy or 'paraproteinaemia' (increased amounts of a single immunoglobulin in the blood). This may be due to myeloma.

Calcium and alkaline phosphatase levels may be abnormal in patients with malignancy or metabolic bone disease (Ch. 11). The blood urate level should be checked if gout is suspected. Muscle enzymes, including creatine kinase, may be raised in patients with inflammatory or other forms of myopathy, indicating that muscle damage has occurred.

Immunology

The rheumatologist makes frequent use of the immunology laboratory as there are several immunological tests which contribute to the diagnosis and monitoring of rheumatogical disorders. A number of rheumatic diseases are associated with circulating autoantibodies, and detection of these antibodies forms the basis of many of these tests.

It is important to understand what is meant by the 'sensitivity' and 'specificity' of these immuno-logical tests, because some are sensitive, but not very specific, whereas others are highly specific, but not very sensitive. This concept is important in interpreting the results of a particular test.

If a test is sensitive for a particular disease then most of the individuals with that disease will have a positive test, but it is possible that individuals with other diseases may also have a positive test. If a test is specific for a particular disease then usually a proportion of affected individuals will have a positive test (this proportion may only be a minority), but it is highly unlikely that anyone without that disease would have a positive test.

If a patient presents with clinical features suggestive of a generalised rheumatic disease then a blood sample should be sent for rheumatoid factor and antinuclear antibodies.

Rheumatoid factor

Rheumatoid factor can be regarded as an IgM antibody directed against an IgG antibody. It is present in the serum of 75–80% of patients with

rheumatoid arthritis at some stage in their illness. Rheumatoid factor is not a specific test: it can be found in patients with other diseases, including other autoimmune diseases, infections, and also in the elderly ('false-positive' rheumatoid factor). Therefore:

- a patient can have rheumatoid arthritis but be rheumatoid factor-negative
- the finding of rheumatoid factor in a patient's blood does not mean the patient has rheumatoid arthritis.

Rheumatoid factor can be measured in a number of ways, e.g. by the sheep cell agglutination test (SCAT). It is useful to have some understanding of the principles underlying this test (Fig. 4.2) in order to interpret its result, which is usually given as a titre (e.g. 1:64). The serum under test is added at increasing dilutions to the sheep red blood cells coated with immunoglobulin. The result is the highest dilution at which the sheep cells agglutinate. A titre of 1:32 or greater is generally regarded as positive (this depends on the particular laboratory). This means that even when the patient's serum is diluted 32 times, it still causes agglutination. Some patients with rheumatoid arthritis have very high titres, e.g. 1:2048. The higher the titre, the less likely it is that the result is a false-positive. Conversely, a result of 1:<16 is negative.

The highest titres of rheumatoid factor tend to be found in patients with severe rheumatoid arthritis, often with erosive disease and internal organ involvement (Ch. 8).

Antinuclear antibodies

Antinuclear antibodies are found in several rheumatic diseases. Most patients with SLE have antinuclear antibodies, but these may also be found in patients with rheumatoid arthritis, juvenile chronic arthritis, systemic sclerosis, mixed connec-tive tissue disease and a number of other auto-immune diseases. Therefore, testing for antinuclear antibodies is a sensitive, but not specific, test.

Antinuclear antibodies are usually detected by an immunofluorescent technique (Fig. 4.3). The patient's serum, in increasing dilutions, is incubated with a substrate tissue, such as mouse

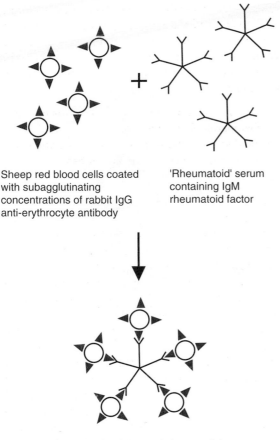

Sheep red blood cells coated with subagglutinating concentrations of rabbit IgG anti-erythrocyte antibody

'Rheumatoid' serum containing IgM rheumatoid factor

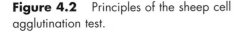

Agglutination [clumped sheep cells]

Figure 4.2 Principles of the sheep cell agglutination test.

liver or kidney or an epithelial cell line termed 'HEp-2'. The section is then washed, fluorescein-labelled anti-human immunoglobulin is added, and it is viewed under ultraviolet light. The result is the highest dilution at which the section fluoresces (Fig. 4.4). As with rheumatoid factor, the result is reported as a titre, and the higher the titre, the more positive the test. For example, a titre of 1:10 000 is strongly positive, whereas a titre of 1:10 is unlikely to be of significance. Antinuclear antibodies in low titre are found in 1–5% of healthy adults, the percentage rising with age.

Testing for antinuclear antibodies as described is a useful 'screening test' for SLE and most autoimmune diseases. These antinuclear antibodies can be directed against a number of different cellular components. Using a variety of techniques, it is now possible to detect a number of different antinuclear antibodies, many of which are highly disease-specific. For example, anticentromere antibodies are highly specific for the limited cutaneous variant of systemic sclerosis (Ch. 9), although this is not a sensitive test (only about 50% of affected patients have these antibodies). Other autoantibodies, such as anti-Ro, anti-La, anti-Sm and anti-Scl-70, are also useful diagnostically and are referred to in Chapter 9.

Antibodies to double stranded DNA (anti-dsDNA)

These merit particular mention here because they are useful in monitoring disease activity in SLE. Anti-dsDNA antibodies are highly specific for SLE, being rarely found in other diseases. As a generalisation, the higher the level, the more active the clinical disease activity.

Other specific autoantibodies

A number of other autoantibodies can be detected in different rheumatic diseases, among them:

- antineutrophil cytoplasmic antibodies (ANCAs) – two patterns of staining by immunofluorescence are described:
  — cytoplasmic (cANCA), which is highly specific for Wegener's granulomatosis (Ch. 9)
  — perinuclear (pANCA), which is less specific and is found in other forms of vasculitis and other conditions
- antiphospholipid antibodies – when present in high titre, these can be associated with antiphospholipid syndrome, a disorder with a variety of clinical features, including
  — thrombosis
  — recurrent fetal loss
  — thrombocytopenia (Ch. 9).

Complement

The complement system is a group of proteins which play an important role in the immune system. Its functions include activation of inflammatory cells, killing of infected cells, and opsonisation of foreign debris prior to phagocytosis.

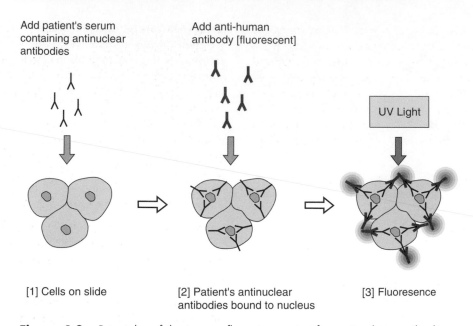

Figure 4.3   Principles of the immunofluorescence test for antinuclear antibodies.

The components most commonly measured are C3 and C4. Low complement levels are found in diseases associated with circulating immune complexes, such as SLE and vasculitis. Monitoring complement levels may be useful as a gauge of disease activity.

Hypocomplementaemia may be a result of genetic deficiency. Some patients with SLE have deficiencies particularly in the early components of the complement cascade. This is most often a result of the disease process (active disease is associated with complement consumption) but more rarely reflects a genetic deficiency.

HLA-typing

In recent years, considerable attention has focused on the immunogenetics of the different rheumatic diseases. Specific HLA polymorphisms are associated with several rheumatic diseases. In case you are not familiar with the concept of HLA molecules, this is described briefly in Chapter 8. At present, the only association which is sometimes exploited in the clinical setting is the association between HLA-B27 and the spondyloarthropathies, in particular ankylosing spondylitis. For example, if a young man presents with symptoms which are suggestive of ankylosing spondylitis, then, if he is HLA-B27-positive, this is in favour of this diagnosis (although it is important to stress that this test is not in itself diagnostic).

URINE TESTS

The urine may give the first clue to the presence of renal involvement of disease, or of an adverse drug effect. The presence of protein or blood on Dipstix testing must be explained. Possible causes would include a urinary tract infection, glomerulone-

Figure 4.4   Postive antinuclear antibody in a patient with SLE (Courtesy of S. Ferrand).

phritis (which can occur as part of many rheumatic diseases including rheumatoid arthritis and SLE), renal infarction (which can occur in vasculitis and result in haematuria), or drug toxicity (e.g. gold and penicillamine can cause nephrotic syndrome).

Therefore if blood and/or protein is found on Dipstix testing, or if there is a clinical suspicion of renal involvement of disease, the following should be requested:

- urine microscopy – looking for red blood cells and casts, which may indicate glomerular disease
- urine culture – looking for infection
- a 24 h urine collection – for quantitation of protein excretion and creatinine clearance.

Depending on results of these tests and the clinical setting, further investigations, e.g. renal ulrasound, estimation of glomerular filtration rate or renal biopsy, may be indicated.

If there is a clinical supicion of myeloma, e.g. in a patient with osteoporosis and a high ESR (see Case history), the urine should be sent for estimation of Bence–Jones' protein.

SYNOVIAL FLUID ANALYSIS

The one absolute indication for synovial fluid analysis is clinical suspicion of infection (Ch. 7). However, examination of the synovial fluid can give important information in many other clinical settings, e.g. in the diagnosis of crystal arthritis or in the differentiation of an inflammatory from a non-inflammatory effusion.

Synovial fluid should be aspirated using an aseptic or 'no-touch' technique, in order to minimise the risk of introducing iatrogenic infection into the joint. Once the fluid has been aspirated, the following need to be requested or taken into account.

Macroscopic appearance. Normal synovial fluid is viscous and clear. 'Inflammatory' synovial fluid, e.g. from a patient with active rheumatoid arthritis, is non-viscous and turbid (often straw-coloured). Frank pus may be aspirated from a septic joint. Blood staining often reflects a 'traumatic tap', but if uniform it indicates a haemarthrosis.

Gram stain and culture. These must be requested if there is any clinical suspicion of infection.

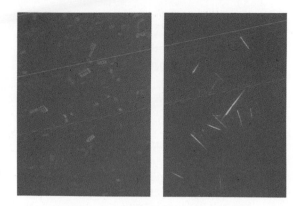

Figure 4.5 Pyrophosphate (left) and urate (right) crystals in synovial fluid viewed under polarising light. Courtesy of Professor A.J. Freemont.

Organisms on microscopy indicate infection, although the absence of organisms does not exclude this. With respect to culture, the synovial fluid should be sent immediately to the microbiology laboratory. If tuberculosis or other unusual organisms are suspected, then this should be discussed in advance with the microbiologist.

Cell count and differential cell count. The total cell count is useful in broadly differentiating between inflammatory and non-inflammatory fluid. In non-inflammatory effusions, the white cell count is less than 2000 cells/mm³ (often less than 200), whereas a cell count of greater than 2000 cells/mm³ would be expected in inflammation. The greater the degree of inflammation, the higher the white cell count. High proportions of polymorphs (>90%) are found in septic and crystal arthritis, and in active rheumatoid arthritis. Very high cell counts greater than 50 000/mm³ (with >90% polymorphs) are found in septic and crystal arthritis.

Polarised microscopy. Crystals are best identified by polarising microscopy. Urate crystals are usually needle-shaped and strongly negatively birefringent, whereas pyrophosphate crystals are more variable in shape and weakly positively birefringent (Fig. 4.5).

RADIOLOGY

A large number of imaging techniques are now available to the rheumatologist and orthopaedic surgeon for the assessment of disease and of injury.

These continue to be developed and refined. For example, in the last 5 years spinal imaging has been revolutionised by the increasing availability of computed tomography (CT) scanning and MRI.

The main imaging modalities used in musculoskeletal disorders are discussed below.

Conventional radiography

Plain X-rays are best at showing bone. Most fractures are obvious on plain X-ray. Adequate X-rays of a suspected fracture should include two views in planes at right angles, usually anteroposterior (AP) and lateral. X-rays of an injured bone should include views of the joint at each end; failure to do this may result in missing associated injuries such as dislocations. In patients with early inflammatory joint disease such as rheumatoid arthritis, plain X-rays may be normal (other than showing soft tissue swelling), but as the disease progresses, periarticular osteopenia, loss of joint space and bone erosion occur and serial plain X-rays may be used to monitor disease progression. A number of musculoskeletal conditions can be diagnosed or suspected from the X-ray appearances in conjunction with the clinical setting, e.g. bone infections, avascular necrosis and bone tumours.

Computed tomographic (CT) scanning and magnetic resonance imaging (MRI)

CT scanning is excellent for the evaluation of bony structures; it allows X-ray sections of such areas as the spine and pelvis. In the spine, spinal canal and foraminal stenosis can be readily identified. It is less good at identifying disc protrusions, as these are soft tissue structures. It is of great value in imaging fractures in complex bones such as the calcaneum, pelvis and tibial plateau, where adequate evaluation of joint disruption is often impossible on plain X-rays. In patients with rheumatic disease, high-resolution CT scanning of the thorax is being used increasingly to diagnose interstitial pulmonary fibrosis. A disadvantage of CT scanning is the dosage of radiation involved, which may be relatively high.

A major advantage of MRI is the ability to visualise soft tissue. Moreover, no radiation is

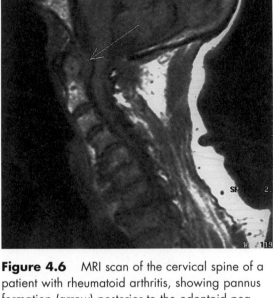

Figure 4.6   MRI scan of the cervical spine of a patient with rheumatoid arthritis, showing pannus formation (arrow) posterior to the odontoid peg causing mild cold compression. There are marked degenerative changes of the lower cervical spine. Courtesy of Dr C. Hutchinson.

involved. MRI of the spine allows visualisation of disc protrusions and intradural abnormalities such as tumours or arachnoiditis. An important role for MRI in rheumatoid arthritis is evaluation of the cervical spine pathology in patients with probable cord compression (Fig. 4.6). Other applications of MRI in patients with musculoskeletal problems include assessment of the knee (to investigate the menisci and ligaments) and shoulder. Diagnostic arthroscopy for meniscal problems has been partly superseded by non-invasive MRI, although there is concern that the sensitivity of MRI may be too high, so that menisci shown to be abnormal at scanning may in fact prove normal at arthroscopy.

Isotope bone scanning

Isotope bone scanning uses 99-technetium-labelled, phosphonate-containing compounds which are taken up by osteoblasts. One advantage of the technique is that the whole skeleton may be easily visualised. Useful applications include detection of metastatic bone disease, when multiple 'hot-spots' may be apparent (Fig. 4.7). A few types of tumour (notably multiple myeloma) are not detected by bone scans. This technique may be used to evaluate prostheses when loosening or infection is suspected. White cell scanning, which involves labelling a sample of a patient's white cells with a radiolabel and then reinjecting them into the patient, may be useful in identifying areas of infection.

Measurement of bone density

Plain X-rays are insensitive in detecting bone loss. However, there are now several different techniques by which bone density can be accurately evaluated (Ch. 11). The most commonly used is dual energy X-ray absorptiometry (DEXA), which quantifies bone mineral density using extremely low doses of ionising radiation. The sites most commonly examined are the lumbar spine and the proximal femur, where osteoporotic fractures frequently occur.

Another technique of bone density measurement is quantitative computed tomography. This has the disadvantage of a relatively high radiation dose compared with DEXA.

ARTHROSCOPY

Arthroscopy and other endoscopic procedures are now widely used, the knee being the joint most commonly arthroscoped (Fig. 4.8). Recent developments in optical and video systems have vastly improved the range of diagnostic and therapeutic

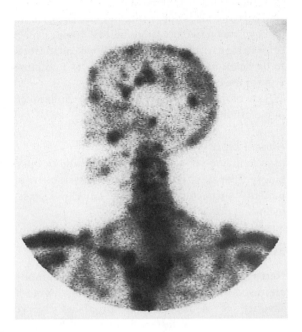

Figure 4.7　Isotope bone scan showing multiple hot spots. This patient had metastatic bone disease. Courtesy of Dr C. Hutchinson.

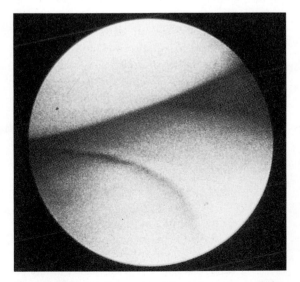
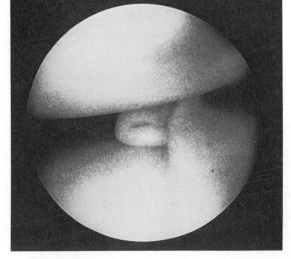

Figure 4.8　Arthroscopy. Normal meniscus (left); meniscal tear (right).

procedures that can be performed. However, the advent of MRI scanning has obviated the need for many diagnostic arthroscopies. The major indications for diagnostic arthroscopy are:

- evaluation of mechanical derangement, e.g. meniscal injury
- synovial biopsy
- septic arthritis, although often the diagnosis is made from synovial fluid obtained by aspiration.

PATHOLOGY

Histological examination of tissue may be indicated in many musculoskeletal disorders and from a variety of sites. For example, in a patient who presents with multisystem inflammatory disease, a diagnosis of vasculitis may be made/confirmed by histological examination of one of a number of tissues including kidney, nasal mucosa, bowel (if the patient has developed bowel infarction requiring resection) or sural nerve. However, tissues most frequently biopsied in the context of musculoskeletal disease are as follows.

Synovial biopsy

Synovial biopsies are usually obtained during arthroscopy. This is most commonly indicated in the patient who presents with an undiagnosed monoarthritis. One major concern is that this may be tuberculous. Synovial fluid cultures are frequently sterile in tuberculous arthritis – hence the value of biopsy.

Bone biopsy

Usually bone is obtained from the iliac crest. Bone biopsy is useful in diagnosis and assessment of severity of osteomalacia and renal osteodystropy. Occasionally it may be indicated in the investigation of osteoporosis in young patients. 'Tetracycline-labelling' of bone, by prescribing tetracycline on two occasions at least 10 days apart prior to biopsy, allows the rate of bone calcification to be determined (tetracycline binds to immature bone at the calcification front).

Bone biopsy (of lesions) may also be undertaken in metastatic disease.

Muscle biopsy

Muscle may be obtained by either needle or open biopsy. Biopsy is indicated in the assessment of patients suspected of having muscle disease, including polymyositis.

ELECTROPHYSIOLOGY

Nerve conduction studies and electromyography are used in the diagnosis and assessment of severity of neuromuscular problems. Nerve conduction studies test both motor and sensory function. In musculoskeletal disease, they are particularly useful in the localisation and assessment of severity of peripheral nerve problems including entrapment neuropathies (e.g. carpal tunnel syndrome). Electromyography is used in the assessment of myopathy. This technique records spontaneous and voluntary electrical activity of muscle. The patterns of activity are used to differentiate between primary muscle disease and neuropathic disorders.

5 | Principles of management of musculoskeletal disease

Case history — trauma

A 20-year-old plasterer was brought to the A & E department having sustained an open tibial fracture as a result of a fall from a motor bike. This was treated by external fixation, while the open tibia was covered with a local muscle flap and a skin graft by the plastic surgeons. The fracture was slow to unite, although it did so after some 8 months; there was no infection. The fracture continued to be persistently painful. It was thought that he had developed reflex sympathetic dystrophy (complex regional pain syndrome) which was treated for a period by the anaesthetists in the pain clinic. During this time he needed physiotherapy on a twice per week basis; the emphasis was on encouraging normal ankle movement. Subsequently he needed further therapy to regain a normal gait without crutches. He was able to return to work 1 year after his accident.

Case history — non-trauma

A 40-year-old woman initially presented with a 1-year history of joint swelling in the hands. She was referred to a rheumatologist who diagnosed rheumatoid arthritis. For 5 years she was treated with NSAIDs, initially alone and then in combination with gold injections. Prior to each gold injection her full blood count and urinalysis were checked. Excellent control of her joint swelling and pain was achieved, although she always had some pain in her right knee. Eventually the knee pain became severe and she was referred to an orthopaedic surgeon, who explained that the knee joint was badly damaged and proposed a total knee replacement. Unfortunately, shortly before this she had been diagnosed as having angina, which proved difficult for her GP to treat. Following the consultation in the pre-operative clinic, the operation had to be delayed while a cardiology outpatient appointment was arranged, after which she underwent coronary angiography and angioplasty. After this her angina improved. Eventually the knee replacement was carried out uneventfully under regional anaesthetic, which was employed because of atlanto-axial instability identified on pre-operative X-rays (flexion and extension views) of the cervical spine.

The most burning needs of most patients with musculoskeletal disease are the relief of pain and the restoration of function. The doctor should ideally understand the nature of the patient's disease and put it right, in the expectation that satisfaction will follow. However, this is often not possible. In most cases, the best quality care consists of a combination of specific medical or surgical treatment aimed at the underlying disease process plus treatment of the pain and a programme of functional rehabilitation (Box 5.1). Treatment of pain is discussed in Chapter 6. This chapter gives an overview of the principles of medical and surgical treatment and of rehabilitation. Specific treatments for particular conditions will be described in later chapters.

THE MULTIDISCIPLINARY TEAM

Rehabilitation, in the full sense, can only be achieved by a team (Box 5.2). The skilled musculoskeletal doctor, in addition to making correct diagnoses and delivering skilful medical or

Key points

- The primary aims of management of patients with musculoskeletetal disease are to relieve pain, reduce inflammation (where appropriate), reduce deformity and restore function.

- A wide variety of drugs is available to treat rheumatic disease. Some of these are used primarily to relieve symptoms, others to control the underlying disease process.

- Surgery can result in dramatic benefits to patients with arthritis and other musculoskeletal diseases. However, there are risks inherent in all types of surgery and it is important that all patients are as fit as practicable before operations, and that the risks, benefits and alternatives to surgery are discussed pre-operatively.

- Trauma is an important cause of morbidity at all age groups. It is vital to consider the overall state of the patient in trauma management, and not to become solely fixated on the musculoskeletal injuries.

- Musculoskeletal patients require multidisciplinary care. It is important to understand the contributions of doctors, physiotherapists, occupational therapists, nurses, podiatrists and others to the overall care of the patient which allow clinicians to achieve the best possible outcome.

Box 5.1   Elements of musculoskeletal management

- Specific medical or surgical treatment of the underlying disease process

- Relief of pain

- Rehabilitation

- The multidisciplinary approach

Box 5.2   The multidisciplinary team

- Doctors
  — rheumatologist
  — orthopaedic surgeon
  — general practitioner
  — other specialists, e.g. ophthalmologist

- Nurses

- Physiotherapist

- Occupational therapist

- Chiropodist (podiatrist)

- Social worker

- Psychologist

- School teacher

- The family

---

surgical treatments, ensures that each patient receives the relevant multidisciplinary support to encourage the fullest possible recovery. There may be major impairment of physical and psychological well-being, as a result of the effects of chronic inflammatory joint disease, severe osteoarthritis, low back pain or major injury. For these patients, 'cure' may not be possible and rehabilitation becomes an even more important aspect of management. While a full-blown multidisciplinary approach may not be necessary for patients with minor or self-limiting disease or injury, nonetheless the same holistic philosophy of care should always lie behind the approach to management.

The medically qualified members of the musculoskeletal multidisciplinary team are some combination of rheumatologist, orthopaedic surgeon and general practioner. Many cases of both traumatic and non-traumatic nature are dealt with entirely in general practice. In hospital practice most patients' care is led by either a rheumatologist or an orthopaedic surgeon, but a significant number of the most challenging cases need combined care from both. Some patients have multisystem involvement of their disease, and other hospital specialists may need to be involved. For example, most children with juvenile chronic arthritis require regular checks by an ophthalmologist.

Nursing staff, especially clinical nurse specialists, often play a key coordinating role in the delivery of care by the multidisciplinary team, in both the ward and the outpatient setting. Clinical nurse specialists also liaise with practise nurses in the community, thus optimising continuity of patient care between hospital and community.

Physiotherapists and occupational therapists now often work together in departments of rehabilitation and play a key role in the multidisciplinary team. The division of labour between them varies between hospital; as a crude generalisation, physiotherapists aim to overcome impairment; occupational therapists aim to overcome disability.

Many patients with rheumatic disease have foot problems, and therefore benefit from the skills of the chiropodist (podiatrist). For example, patients with rheumatoid arthritis often have severe metatarsalgia as a result of subluxation at the metatarsophalangeal joints. Provision of moulded insoles may significantly improve their mobility.

Clinical psychologists may be of help because patients with pain and disability often benefit from coping strategies, which allow them to feel that they have some degree of control over their disease. Social workers are key members of the team for patients with musculoskeletal disease who require social services support. The school teacher needs to be involved in the care of children with chronic musculoskeletal disease. It is important that the child is allowed to join in with activities as much as possible.

The patient's family can be considered as part of the management team. Whether or not a disabled patient has a supportive family can have a major impact on their physical and psychological well-being.

PRINCIPLES OF MANAGEMENT

There are certain basic principles of management which can be applied to most patients with musculoskeletal problems (Box 5.3). Of course, the appropriateness of these principles in individual cases will depend upon the nature of the patient's disease or injury. For example, management of a patient who has fractured a metacarpal as a result of a boxing injury will not require the intensive multidisciplinary approach necessary in a patient with severe rheumatoid arthritis. Remember also always to evaluate the likely impact of a patient's disease or injury on their life.

Box 5.3   The main steps in musculoskeletal management

- establish the diagnosis
- assess disease activity/severity
- explain the nature of the problem to the patient
- identify, and if possible remove, precipitating/aggravating factors
- prescribe specific therapy
  — drug therapy
  — orthopaedic surgery
- rehabilitate

Management of many patients with inflammatory musculoskeletal diseases, e.g. rheumatoid arthritis, is complicated by the fact that treatment is not curative. However, this does not mean that there is nothing that can be done for the patient. There is often a great deal that can be done to delay disease progression and minimise the effects of disability.

Establish the diagnosis

For most patients, effective therapy will depend upon a correct diagnosis having been made. This is done on the basis of the history and examination, along with investigations as necessary, as described in the preceding chapters. For some patients with musculoskeletal symptoms, it is not possible to make a diagnosis at first presentation. It is best not to 'label' such patient as having a specific disease, but rather to observe them until their symptoms settle or until the diagnosis later becomes apparent, in the meantime treating the clinical symptoms as appropriate. It is not always possible to reach a conclusive diagnosis before treatment starts, and the response to particular treatments may point to a particular diagnosis.

Assess disease activity/severity

Treatment may depend not only upon diagnosis but also upon how active or how severe the disease is. This applies both to patients with inflammatory disease and to those who have sustained injury. For example, in rheumatoid arthritis or SLE, patients with very active inflammation may require potentially toxic steroid and/or immunosuppressant therapy in order to prevent disease progression. Such therapy would be quite inappropriate for a patient with only very mild disease, in whom the risks of this therapy would outweigh any advantages. Also, a patient may have inflammatory disease which has caused severe joint damage but which has now become inactive. For example, a patient may have had rheumatoid arthritis for years and, although the disease is no longer active (no swollen and/or tender joints, normal ESR), may be left with major joint deformity and be severely disabled as a result of this. Potentially toxic drug therapy to control inflammation would be inappropriate for this patient. What is required is a rehabilitative approach to care, including surgical reconstruction of severely damaged joints.

Similarly, the safest way to treat a tibial shaft fracture depends on the severity of the injury. Internal fixation of the bone has many advantages and is safe in low-energy injuries, but there is a much higher risk of causing iatrogenic complications in high-energy injuries where the degree of soft tissue damage is greater.

Methods of measuring disease activity depend on the disease in question. In a patient with rheumatoid arthritis the duration of morning stiffness, the number of swollen, tender joints and the erythrocyte sedimentation rate (ESR) can all be used to monitor disease activity. Many injuries have grading systems, e.g. the Gustilo grading of compound fractures or the Garden classification of femoral neck fractures. These are presented in the appropriate chapters later in the book.

Assessment of severity of joint damage is based on a combination of X-ray appearances and functional assessment. In most osteoarthritic conditions, the patient's symptoms are more important than the severity of X-ray changes or other investigations. Thus the principal indication for total hip replacement is unremitting hip pain which is not relieved by other measures, in the presence of radiologically proven arthritis.

Patient education

Explaining the problem to the patient is always an important part of management. This is especially true for the patient with chronic rheumatic disease. The implications of the disease and its treatment need to be discussed. Usually it is best to adopt a cautiously optimistic approach, but the goals of therapy must be realistic. It is essential that patients receive a balanced view of the pros and cons of surgery in particular; most surgical procedures are irreversible and patients may have unrealistically positive or negative views of what surgery can offer them. Patient education for those with chronic disease is a continuing process. Similarly many patients about to undergo surgery may need the procedure explained on more than one occasion, and much evidence indicates that even then their long-term recall of what they have been told is relatively poor.

For some patients, education may be the single most important aspect of management. For example, a patient with mechanical back pain may find that the problem resolves after being taught back protection measures. Information leaflets describing musculoskeletal diseases and their treatments are found to be helpful by many patients.

Identification of precipitating or aggravating factors

Once a musculoskeletal condition has been diagnosed, any precipitating or aggravating factors should be identified and, if possible, removed. Sometimes this is the single most important part of management. For example, a heavy drinker who develops gout should be told to curtail their alcohol consumption. Manual workers with back problems should, if possible, switch to lighter duties.

Few musculoskeletal diseases are amenable to primary prevention. However, in recent years, increasing attention has been paid to the early detection of osteoporosis (Ch. 11). Effective treatment of osteoporosis will reduce the incidence of fractures. Prevention of accidents in the home, in the workplace or outside can reduce the incidence of injuries.

Specific treatment for the disease/injury

This includes not only drug treatment and surgery but also other modalities of treatment, e.g. physiotherapy and chiropody, which may be indicated for a specific condition. For example, treatment of an adhesive capsulitis of the shoulder ('frozen shoulder') may include intra-articular injection of steroid and local anaesthetic, physiotherapy and (in refractory cases) manipulation under anaesthesia by an orthopaedic surgeon. The broad principles of drug treatment and surgery are outlined in this section, while other modalities of treatment are described in the section rehabilitation on (p. 84).

Drug therapy (Box 5.4)

Patients with musculoskeletal disease are often prescribed analgesics to control pain and/or NSAIDs, which control pain and inflammation. These groups of drugs control symptoms, but do not affect the underlying disease process. They are described in more detail in Chapter 8. Drug treatment of pain is described in Chapter 6.

More specific drug therapy is required to cure or modify the underlying disease process. This is described for individual rheumatic diseases in the relevant sections of this book. The main groups of drugs used by rheumatologists are:

- 'Disease-modifying agents' for patients with inflammatory arthritis and connective tissue disease. These include immunosuppressant drugs (Ch. 8).
- Corticosteroids. These are powerful anti-inflammatory agents. They can be administered by a variety of routes: oral, intravenous, intra-articular and periarticular. In patients with life-threatening connective tissue disease, they are often given in combination with immunosuppressant drugs. An intra-articular steroid injection can very successfully reduce inflammation in a single joint, but is contraindicated if there is any suspicion of infection. Periarticular steroid injections may be useful for localised soft tissue inflammation (e.g. in lateral epicondylitis: 'tennis elbow').
- Antibiotics in the treatment of septic arthritis, osteomyelitis and soft tissue infections.
- Drugs used in the treatment of gout (in the acute attack and as prophylaxis against further attacks).
- Drugs used in the prevention and treatment of osteoporosis.

Because many rheumatic diseases are multisystem, other drugs are required to treat specific aspects of disease. For example, although currently there is no effective 'disease-modifying therapy' for systemic sclerosis, drugs play an important role in its management, e.g. vasodilators for Raynaud's phenomenon and proton-pump inhibition for gastro-oesophageal reflux (see Ch. 9).

Many drugs used in the treatment of rheumatic diseases are potentially toxic. This applies especially to immunosuppressant and cortico-steroid drugs. Therefore, the decision as to whether to prescribe a drug depends upon careful assessment of the probable risk–benefit ratio for that particular patient. This includes consideration of:

Box 5.4   Drug treatment in musculoskeletal disease

1. Drugs may be prescribed:
- to relieve symptoms
- as specific treatment of the underlying disease process

2. Major groups of drugs used in patients with musculoskeletal disease are:
- analgesics
- non-steroidal anti-inflammatory drugs (NSAIDs)
- 'disease-modifying drugs' including immunosuppressants
- corticosteroids (including intra-articular and periarticular steroids)
- antibiotics
- drugs used to treat gout
- drugs used to prevent and treat osteoporosis

3. All drugs are potentially toxic: before prescribing weigh up benefits and risks

4. Drug treatment is only one aspect of management in musculoskeletal disease

Principles of management of musculoskeletal disease

- other drugs the patient is currently taking – drug interactions must be avoided
- any other medical conditions the patient may have – certain antirheumatic drugs may be contraindicated or require particular caution if the patient has, for example, renal or hepatic impairment or recent peptic ulceration.

Surgical treatment

For many musculoskeletal disorders, initial treatment is purely surgical, e.g. in many cases of trauma. The principles of trauma management are somewhat different from those of management of chronic orthopaedic conditions. The aim in acute (especially traumatic) musculoskeletal conditions is to restore the patient to the degree of function obtained before the injury. This is not always possible, but should always be considered the ultimate goal. To this end, management of trauma now routinely includes bony fixation to permit early movement. This minimises the risk of soft tissue and joint problems (e.g. stiffness) arising secondary to prolonged immobilisation. Such treatment is nearly always followed by active rehabilitation regimes to ensure rapid resumption of function in the injured part.

Treatment of chronic conditions, on the other hand, often has more modest goals of attaining a better, but still not normal, level of function. It is vital to dicuss with the patient before surgery the realistic prospects for improvement in symptoms. An almost guaranteed cause for patient dissatisfaction is a surgeon who has relatively modest (but still possibly worthwhile) goals and a patient who thinks that the surgery will result in a complete resolution of all symptoms.

Operations may be intended to relieve pain, to correct deformity, to prevent arthritis, or to permit restoration and mobilisation after injury. Surgical treatments can be classified as follows:

- Arthroplasty – literally a new joint; can be excision arthroplasty (e.g. excision of first metatarsophalangeal joint, Keller's procedure) or joint replacement arthroplasty (e.g. total hip replacement)
- Arthrodesis – permanent stiffening of a joint (also known as 'fusion')

- Arthrotomy – opening a joint; usually performed to permit access for some other procedure
- Arthroscopy – inspection of a joint using an arthroscope (telescope); may be combined with performance of an intra-articular procedure under arthroscopic control
- Osteotomy – cutting of a bone, usually combined with repositioning or realignment
- Fixation – of fractures, of an osteotomy or of cartilage or ligament structures
- Soft tissue release – of tight tendons or a soft tissue contracture (e.g. Dupuytren's disease)
- Decompression of soft tissue structure – usually either a nerve (e.g. median nerve in the carpal tunnel) or a muscle (e.g. supraspinatus at the shoulder)
- Excision of lesion, e.g. tumours such as sarcoma
- Amputation.

Some specific examples of these procedures will be described in later chapters.

Preparation of patients for theatre. One of the most important tasks which you will undertake as a house officer is preparation of patients for surgical operations. The responsibility for a successful outcome from these procedures is shared by members of the surgical team, of which you will be one. There are several questions which need to be asked about any patient going to theatre.

Is the patient fit for the procedure? This needs to include an assessment of the severity of the undertaking; an operation for a carpal tunnel release performed under local anaesthetic is much less risky than a revision hip replacement. Likely areas of problems in orthopaedics include:

- blood pressure
- cardiovascular problems, including angina, cardiac failure and the risk of stroke
- chest problems (chronic bronchitis, asthma etc.)
- intercurrent sepsis, even if minor – in joint replacement surgery the results of sepsis are so devastating that even very minor sepsis may be a cause for postponement of a procedure; thus joint replacements may be postponed while severe dental caries or periodontal disease is sorted out
- bleeding problems or taking anticoagulants.

It is important that the more obvious causes of problems at the time of surgery are screened for at the time of listing. These include hypertension and dental disease. Medical management of patients, whether pre- or postoperative, is often carried out in consultation with physician colleagues. The ultimate decision about whether a patient is fit for an anaesthetic lies with the anaesthetist, who may have an opinion about the best line of medical management. It is therefore appropriate to consult an anaesthetist at an early stage if a particular patient is thought likely to pose problems. The problems of the elderly patient with a fracture are considered in more detail in Chapter 21.

Many hospitals now use a system of 'pre-operative clinics'. These allow patients to be assessed with more care than may be possible if patients are clerked on admission the day before surgery. This approach also allows a more efficient use of operating time with less risk of operating lists being wasted due to last minute cancellation of patients for medical reasons. A further advantage is that the decision to defer or cancel an operation on medical grounds is associated with less pressure and stress on both staff and patient if it is taken before admission in the pre-operative clinic.

Is the patient adequately informed about the procedure and has consent been given? Orthopaedic surgery is usually for pain rather than being life-saving. Thus patients frequently have a difficult choice to make about whether, in their eyes, the likely benefits of surgery outweigh the risks involved. This will include being informed of the other choices available and of the risks and likely benefits of the procedure on offer. Evidence shows that patients frequently do not retain much of the information proffered to them during sessions to explain operations. It is therefore important to:

- make sure that *you* understand the procedure and its risks etc; if not, seek more senior help
- keep your explanations within the abilities of the patient to comprehend; it is difficult to strike a balance between this and being unintentionally patronising on occasion
- ask the patients if they have any questions after your explanation

- check that written information to reinforce your message is available for the common procedures
- make sure that a consent form is signed.

Are the appropriate investigations available? It is very difficult to give hard and fast rules about what will be required. In general the following hold true:

- Full blood count – nearly all patients undergoing general anaesthetic.
- Urea and electrolytes, blood sugar – patients over the age of 60; patients with renal disease, diabetes, cardiac disease (especially if on diuretics) and any other condition likely to cause biochemical abnormality.
- Blood cross match – it is worth grouping and saving serum on most patients undergoing more than minor surgery. Modern methods of blood grouping allow early identification of most likely problems with antibodies against blood components before cross-matching is carried out. This allows a decision to be made to order blood early if such problems are likely.
- ECG – patients over the age of 40; anyone with known cardiac disease.
- Pulmonary function tests – anyone with known or suspected lung disease.
- Chest X-ray – indicated only in patients with cardiopulmonary disease likely to be a problem at anaesthetic.
- X-ray of affected part (recent) – all patients undergoing bone (or fracture) or joint surgery.
- Recent cervical spine X-ray (including flexion and extension views) – patients with rheumatoid arthritis undergoing general anaesthetic.
- Scans (bone, CT, MRI) – usually obtained before admission.

Have the following risks, general to all procedures, been considered on all patients admitted (elective or emergency)?

- Risk of deep venous thromboses (DVTs) and thromboembolism (Box 5.5). You need a preventative strategy, and you need to assess all patients. Not all patients will then need prophylaxis (Box 5.6), but most do. All of these

---

Box 5.5   Venous thromboembolism

Incidence

- Very common postoperatively; also occurs spontaneously
- 10% of all hospital deaths are due to pulmonary embolism (PE)
- Risks vary substantially between patients
  - low risk patients: <10% incidence of DVTs
  - moderate risk: >10% incidence of DVTs
  - high risk: >40% incidence of DVTs

Risk groups

- **Low risk**
  - minor surgery; no risk factors other than age
  - major surgery; <40 years; no other risk factors
- **Moderate risk**
  - major non-lower limb surgery, age >40, or any other risk factor
  - major medical illness (heart or lung disease, cancer, inflammatory bowel disease)
  - major trauma
  - minor surgery in any patient with thrombophilia, history of DVT or PE, oral contraception
- **High risk**
  - fracture or orthopaedics of lower limb
  - pelvic or abdominal cancer surgery
  - major surgery in any patient with a history of DVT or PE
  - lower limb paralysis

Risk factors

- **Thrombophilia (anti-thrombin III, protein C or S defiency)**
- **Lupus anticoagulant**
- **Age**
- **Obesity**
- **Varicose veins**
- **Immobility**
- **Pregnancy/puerperium**
- **History of DVT or PE**
- **Polycythaemia**
- **Nephrotic syndrome**
- **Paraproteinaemia**
- **Infection**
- **Malignancy (pelvic, abdominal or metastases)**
- **Heart failure**
- **Oral contraceptive and hormone replacement therapy**

Box 5.6   Methods of prevention of venous thromboembolism

- Mechanical methods
- Graduated compression stockings
- Foot pump or calf compression
- Dextran
- Warfarin
- Ca heparin
  - low dose
  - adjusted dose
- Low molecular weight heparin

---

methods have pros and cons – it is most unlikely as a house officer that you will be asked to choose between the different strategies, although you should know the contraindications for the different methods. The most important thing is to understand the strategy of your unit *and apply it rigorously.* Note that most anaesthetists will not use spinal or epidural anaesthesia in any patient who has recently had ANY form of anticoagulant, so starting patients on some forms of prophylaxis pre-operatively needs careful consideration.

- Need for antibiotics – are prophylactic antibiotics needed? Most surgeons use two or three doses of a broad-spectrum antibiotic active against staphylococci as prophylaxis. This is needed for any operations where metal or other devices are being implanted or where there is an above average risk of infection.
- Risk of chest infections – does the patient need early physiotherapy?
- Risk of pressure sores – is the patient thin, malnourished, bony?

Rehabilitation

A rehabilitation programme is a major part of therapy for patients who are disabled as a result of injury or after surgical treatment, or as a result of disabling rheumatic disease such as rheumatoid arthritis. For some patients, what is required is a relatively short period of rehabilitation, e.g. after a hip replacement for osteoarthritis, to enable a return to a relatively normal lifestyle. Other patients will be left disabled by their injury or disease and will, as old problems persist or new problems present themselves, require continuing support from the multidisciplinary team which is the backbone of the rehabilitation approach to treatment.

The philosophy behind the rehabilitation approach to treatment is that disability should be prevented as far as possible, and that when disability is present, its impact on the individual should be minimised. Goals include:

- to achieve the highest possible level of function
- to minimise pain
- to involve the patient in decision-making.

The aims of the rehabilitiative approach for each patient will depend upon their aspirations, age and life situation. For example, the aims for a young mother will be different from those for an elderly patient with other medical problems. Similarly children have their own specific needs. Schooling, occupation and family responsibilities all need to be taken into account.

Physiotherapy

This includes teaching the patient joint protection measures and/or exercises to regain muscle power and to maintain and increase the range of movement (Fig. 5.1). After a period of immobility, e.g. as a result of an injury or an exacerbation of inflammatory arthritis, the physiotherapist will work with the patient to help regain mobility. Physiotherapy may be the single most important aspect of management, e.g. in the patient with ankylosing spondylitis when long-term prognosis is dependent upon spinal mobility and therefore upon strict adherence to an exercise programme.

A variety of modalities of treatment are used by physiotherapists. For the patient with joint inflammation, heat treatment may provide symptomatic relief but is unlikely to have any long-term benefit. Hydrotherapy is used as an adjunct to muscle strengthening and range of motion exercises: in a warm pool patients relax and the effects of gravity are reduced (Fig. 5.2).

Physiotherapists or other members of the rehabilitation team may try transcutaneous nerve stimulation (TNS) for patients with refractory pain. In a proportion of patients, TNS will relieve pain. The theory is that by stimulating large diameter nerve fibres, TNS reduces the effects of nociceptive fibre stimulation.

Splinting is an important aspect of the management of musculoskeletal disease, which may be supervised by the physiotherapist or the occupational therapist. In a patient with an exacerbation of inflammatory arthritis, acutely swollen joints are splinted (Fig. 5.3). As the inflammation settles, the physiotherapist will gradually begin to exercise the joint.

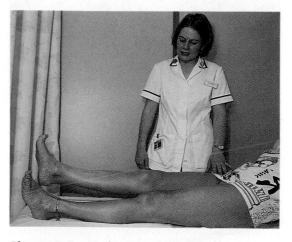

Figure 5.1 A physiotherapist showing a patient quadriceps exercises.

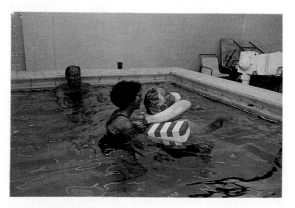

Figure 5.2 The hydrotherapy pool.

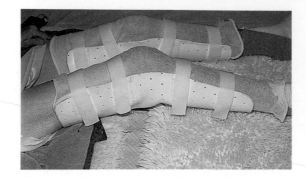

Figure 5.3 Resting knee splints.

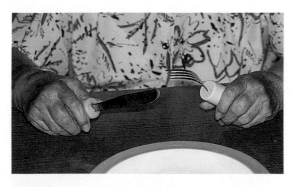

Figure 5.4 Occupational therapy aid: many patients with hand problems find using normal cutlery difficult.

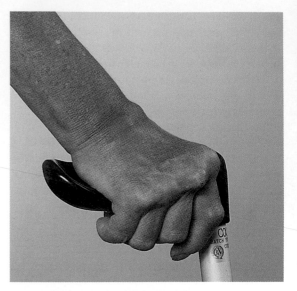

Figure 5.5 A walking aid with a specially moulded handle for a patient with rheumatoid arthritis.

One particular type of splint is the Plaster of Paris cast. Because of its ready availability, low cost and ease of moulding, it is widely used in acute splinting of fractures. The effective use of this and other casting materials depends on adequate experience and training; you should try to have the rudiments of plaster cast application demonstrated to you during your orthopaedic attachment, possibly by a plaster room technician.

Occupational therapy

Provision of simple or more complicated aids allows patients to perform tasks they would otherwise be unable to do, and to retain mobility. This aspect of management should not be forgotten: a visit from the occupational therapist may allow a disabled patient to retain an independence which would otherwise be lost (Fig. 5.4).

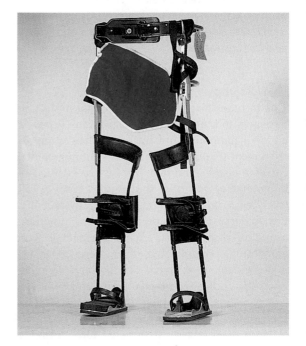

Figure 5.6 Hip guidance orthosis.

There are a wide variety of aids and appliances available, including walking aids. Remember that the patient with inflammatory joint disease often has problems with many joints; a walking aid may therefore need to have a specially adapted handle to accommodate hand deformity (Fig. 5.5).

Some patients may require aids or splints which require greater facilities to produce than are customarily available within hospital departments. These range from surgical shoes (e.g. with especially wide toe boxes for broad feet) to splints, to more complex devices such as walking frames for patients with cerebral palsy or Duchenne muscular dystrophy (Fig. 5.6). Arrangements for provision of these aids vary between hospitals, but one common system in the UK is for *fitters/orthotists* from external commercial companies to visit hospitals on a regular basis. This means that the fitter is not based within the hospital, and adequate liaison concerning patients with unusual problems may be difficult and require special arrangements.

Principles of management of musculoskeletal disease

6 | Musculoskeletal pain

Case history — trauma

A middle-aged woman stood on a stool to hang some heavy curtains and suffered a fall, which resulted in pain in her left lower limb. At the casualty department she told the doctor the pain was mainly in her knee, but when the doctor examined this joint, nothing abnormal was found. But the pain was severe and the lady was sure she would not be able to walk. The orthopaedic registrar was called and took a more detailed history of the accident. It seemed the lady fell mainly onto the side of her hip. The registrar knew that pain felt in the knee is commonly referred from the hip, so she asked for an X-ray of the pelvis, with a lateral view of the left hip. Sure enough, a minimally displaced fracture of the neck of the femur was revealed.

While the woman was waiting to go to theatre to have the fracture fixed, her pain was treated with a combination of morphine and an NSAID. With this pain relief, together with the knowledge that a definite cause of her pain had been established, she was much relieved and only slightly apprehensive about the prospect of surgery. After a straightforward operation to stabilise the fracture with screws, she was treated by patient-controlled analgesia (PCA), again using morphine. Gentle movement of the hip under the supervision of the physio-therapist was possible from an early stage using this regime. As the wound pain settled down, the PCA was discontinued and she was given tablets of codeine and paracetamol, while still continuing the NSAID. Her rehabilitation progressed satisfactorily and she went home on crutches after a few days, taking a supply of tablets to use as she needed them.

Case history — non-trauma

A 32-year-old driving instructor developed pain at the back of his right lower leg and at the outer (lateral) border of his right foot. This seemed to come out of the blue one day, for although he had been doing some heavy lifting while helping his sister to move house he was not conscious of having injured his ankle or foot in any way. He noticed that coughing made the pain worse and he began experiencing some tingling of the leg and foot as well. He attended his GP who to his surprise asked him several questions about his back, where he had no pain.

On examination, movements of the foot and ankle were full and pain-free. The straight leg raising test (Ch. 3) provoked pain at 40° on the right. The right ankle jerk was absent, ankle plantarflexion was weak and there was diminution of light touch and pinprick sensation of the lateral border of the foot and ankle. His doctor explained that the pain was probably due to a 'trapped nerve' in his lower back. He was referred to the hospital. An MRI scan showed a prolapsed disc at the L5/S1 level with compression of the right S1 nerve root.

Pain is one of the commonest presenting symptoms in musculoskeletal medicine. It is also the most informative: much can be learned about the nature of the underlying problem if enough time and care is given to eliciting exactly what the patient is feeling. Do not be in too much of a hurry to proceed to examination of the affected part, or inspection of X-rays: in many cases these stages of the assessment should be aimed at confirming or

---

Key points

- Pain is both a clue to diagnosis of an underlying condition and a problem to be solved in its own right

- Effective treatment of pain, in parallel with treatment of the underlying musculoskeletal problem, is essential for maximum recovery and rehabilitation

- The sensation of pain can arise both as a consequence of tissue damage (nociceptive pain) and through damage to or malfunction of the nerves themselves (neurogenic pain). Treatments for these two types of pain are completely different

- There is always an emotional component to pain. Understanding and reassurance are as important as operations and drugs

---

refuting the diagnostic hypotheses you have formulated in listening to the patient's description. Furthermore, pain is designed to worry the person experiencing it and most patients will feel, quite rightly, that their problem is not being taken seriously until they have had the chance to describe their pain fully.

Even if your analysis of a patient's pain leads you immediately to prescribe effective treatment for the underlying problem, it is necessary also to direct prompt and decisive treatment at the symptom of pain itself. Not to do so is not only inhumane but also inefficient, because an essential component of all musculoskeletal therapy is rehabilitation of the affected part through movement. Pain is a great inhibitor of movement.

This chapter therefore deals both with the analysis of pain (including assessment of its severity) and an approach to its treatment. Its structure is of necessity different to that of most other chapters. While most of the conditions described in this textbook can be associated with pain, in this chapter we specifically discuss fibromyalgia, a condition in which the major characteristic is widespread pain, and briefly mention back pain. Back pain deserves highlighting here as it is an extremely common problem both in hospital and community based practice.

THE ANALYSIS OF PAIN

Patients may have more than one pain, and frequently do, even when there is only one underlying lesion. Find out straight away how many distinct pains are present and take the history of each one separately, otherwise confusion and apparent inconsistency will arise. For each pain you have to make (1) a qualitative assessment (Box 6.1), which will give clues as to the underlying diagnosis, and (2) an assessment of severity, which will guide decisions about treatment. Questions to help you in the assessment of the patient with pain are outlined later in this section.

Pain is almost always a complex phenomenon, especially when it has been present for some time. All levels of the CNS respond to a continued barrage of painful afferent signals. The presenting picture is therefore infinitely variable and may be difficult to analyse. A useful model (which will probably be laughed at in 100 years' time) is to think in terms of nociceptive and neurogenic mechanisms.

Nociceptive pain

Nociceptive pain is what people usually think of when they talk about pain. Damaged tissue releases irritant chemical mediators which

---

Box 6.1   Qualitative analysis of pain

Nociceptive vs neurogenic

- **Nociceptive pain is due to local tissue damage**
  - **it is often made worse by movement**
  - **it responds to analgesics and anti-inflammatory drugs**

- **Neurogenic pain is due to peripheral nerve or nerve root dysfunction**
  - **its severity is out of proportion to apparent local tissue damage**
  - **it is unresponsive to analgesics**

Localised vs referred

- **Both nociceptive and neurogenic pain may be felt at a site remote from the causative lesion** stimulate high-threshold receptors (nociceptors) whose job it is to serve the sense of pain. The resulting afferent signals pass to the CNS along dedicated 'pain pathways' and elicit appropriate behavioural responses. On its own, this concept provides an adequate explanation of symptoms in many acute conditions and is relatively easy to analyse. In most cases, there will be other evidence of the tissue damage causing the pain, such as swelling, redness and tenderness. Furthermore, the patient will usually report that attempts to move the damaged part worsen the pain and that rest tends to relieve it. Tissue damage can arise in many ways, e.g. as a result of trauma or inflammation.

The sensation of this kind of pain is usually localised to the area where the tissue damage has occurred but, as with the 'visceral' pain which occurs in other body systems, there are recognised patterns of *referral* (or *radiation*) of pain. The reason that pain may be referred is that it can be felt in areas which share the same innervation as the injured part. For example, pain arising from the hip may be referred to the knee, and lumbar disc pain may be referred to the buttock. This is because the sensory cortex perceives the noxious stimuli arising, for example, from the hip, but cannot localise it so precisely. However, such referred pain is still fairly described as nociceptive because it is mediated by nociceptors responding to tissue damage. Remember that referred pain may arise from non-musculoskeletal pathology. For example, a patient presenting with shoulder pain may have a subdiaphragmatic abscess, referred to the shoulder because of the shared root origin of the phrenic and supraclavicular nerves. Sometimes pain is not felt at the injured site, but only at the site of referral.

Further clues to the aetiology of nociceptive pain can be gained from knowing when the pain tends to be worse. Pain that is worse during daytime activity is likely to have an underlying mechanical cause, while pain that is worse at night suggests an inflammatory or neoplastic aetiology. Arthritis, however, can display features of both, limiting mobility and also disturbing sleep. Another characteristic of pain due to inflammation is that it is often at its worst after a period of rest or sleep, when the patient gets up.

Neurogenic pain

Neurogenic pain (or 'neuropathic pain') is due to a pathological process affecting the peripheral nerves supplying the part where the pain is felt. Such pains are often more severe than nociceptive pains and are particularly alarming because there is no visible sign of tissue damage to explain them. They tend to have a peculiar and unfamiliar quality so that patients use unusual words to describe them – 'drawing', 'shooting', 'a numb pain' and so on. One classic descriptor is 'burning' pain, which has long been recognised to occur after injuries of peripheral nerves and is known as *causalgia*. Unlike nociceptive pain, neurogenic pain may be felt as a result of impulses in any afferent nerve fibre, myelinated or unmyelinated, due to the establishment of abnormal connections between nerve cells in the spinal cord. Patients often experience odd sensations and the affected area can become hypersensitive, such that a light stroking touch or other stimulus which would normally be painless is extremely painful. This last symptom is known as *allodynia*; patients find it extremely distressing.

Limbs affected by neurogenic pain often display features of autonomic disturbance. Dramatic colour changes occur – the limb may go purple or livid pink. In some cases it will go white, especially when exposed to even minor degrees of cold and this may be associated with worsening of the pain. This is known as *cold intolerance*. There may be a change in the pattern of sweating or *trophic* changes in the quality of the skin or growth of nails. Such combinations of severe pain, vasomotor instability (colour changes), swelling and stiffness are known as *algodystrophy, reflex sympathetic dystrophy (RSD)* or *complex regional pain syndrome* (Fig. 6.1).

In most cases of neurogenic pain, the lesion is in a different location from where the pain is felt. A good example of this is nerve root compression. Pressure on a lower lumbar nerve root from a prolapsed disc causes severe pain felt in the leg (below the knee) in the territory supplied by the nerve root – this classic symptom is known as *sciatica*. This could be described as a referred pain but it is more meaningful to call it a *radicular* pain since this conveys the specific information that a nerve root is the seat of the problem. In the same

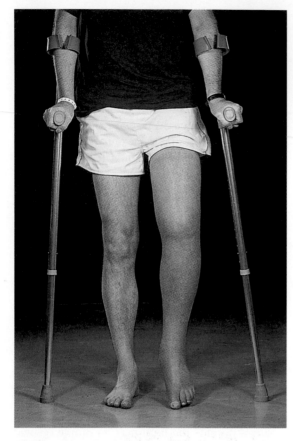

Figure 6.1 Patient with reflex sympathetic dystrophy affecting lower limb.

way, upper limb pain can be caused by cervical root entrapment. In other cases the distribution of the pain corresponds to that of a more peripheral nerve; the painful paraesthesiae caused by median nerve compression in carpal tunnel syndrome are the commonest example. However, many neurogenic pains have a distribution which does not correspond to any peripheral nerve or root, arising as a poorly understood, but potentially disastrous, addition to the nociceptive pain following an injury, which may be quite minor.

Implications for treatment

The reason why it is so important to distinguish nociceptive from neurogenic pain is that the available options for treatment of the two are quite different. In many cases of nociceptive pain, the

underlying tissue damage may be amenable to surgical treatment. Surgery may also help a root or nerve compression but in other cases of neurogenic pain it can only make matters worse. Anti-inflammatory drugs are often effective in nociceptive pains, because they damp down the chemical mechanisms by which tissue damage stimulates nociceptors. They are totally ineffective in neurogenic pain which is far more likely to respond to drugs that act on neurones directly, such as tricyclic antidepressants or anti-epileptic agents. Centrally acting analgesics are also far more likely to be effective in nociceptive pain. Generally it is advisable to consult a pain specialist in treating neurogenic pain not attributable to an operable lesion.

Questions to determine the qualitative characteristics of a pain

Where is the pain; does it spread anywhere?
Ask the patient to point to where the pain is felt. If the pain is well-localised, patients tend to indicate the site with one finger, whereas if it is more diffuse they will use the whole hand to indicate an area. Consider what structures lie deep to a well-localised pain: are they tender, does stressing them mechanically worsen the pain? Does the painful area show signs of inflammation?

When did the pain start: did anything start it off?
In particular, find out whether the onset of pain was related to a traumatic incident, or whether it was 'spontaneous'.

What is the pain like; are there colour changes in the skin?
Ask the patient to describe the quality of the pain. Nociceptive pains produce 'ordinary' words such as 'aching' or 'sharp'. Neurogenic pains produce more unusual and emotionally loaded words such as 'burning' or 'shooting'. Colour changes indicate associated vasomotor disturbance, and are also an indication of a neurogenic mechanism for the pain. Is the limb sensitive to cold? Has there been an increase in sweating or nail growth?

When is the pain worst; what exacerbates it?

Find out if the pain is related to activity. If so, is there a specific movement that triggers it or is it movement in general? Is it movement of joints or weight-bearing (gripping in the upper limb) that hurts? Many inflammatory conditions, although essentially non-mechanical, will be somewhat easier when resting. Truly unrelenting pain by day and night is characteristic of bone malignancy.

What are you taking for the pain; is it effective?

Knowledge of whether simple analgesics or NSAIDs have a significant effect on the level of pain helps to define the mechanism of pain production. Knowledge of the doses being used gives an indication of severity.

ASSESSING THE SEVERITY OF PAIN

In making treatment decisions, it is often necessary to have an estimate of the severity of a patient's pain. Since people use language differently, it is best to do this by asking behavioural questions such as how much disturbance of sleep is occurring, how many analgesic tablets (and of what strength) are being used, and how much function is being limited. This approach does not get round the essentially subjective nature of pain completely (which is neither possible nor desirable) but is better than nothing.

It is also important to assess the severity of the pain in relation to any other medical problems which the patient may have. Take for example, two patients with osteoarthritis. They both have severe knee pain, in one the pain in the knee limits walking to a few yards and prevents restful sleep; in the other, although the knee does hurt, it is actually angina pain which limits the walking distance and sleep is not a problem. For which patient would you advise total knee replacement?

Questions to assess the severity of a pain

Does the pain disturb your sleep?

No pain is pleasant, but pain which regularly prevents sleeping is really miserable. Lack of sleep undermines patients' ability to cope. For this reason, sleep disturbance may have a big influence on treatment decisions, e.g. in tipping the balance towards surgery which may be risky in an elderly patient. However, insomnia may also reflect depression – which is common in patients with musculoskeletal disease – and may indicate a quite different line of treatment. Therefore, you need to establish quite clearly exactly why sleep is being disturbed.

How does the pain limit your activities?

Find out what activities the pain is preventing. Is it pain that limits walking and, if so, after what distance? Find out, for the upper limb, what sort of movements are now impossible – this is often most easily deduced from what jobs can no longer be done.

How has the pain affected your quality of life?

Ask the patient if the pain has prevented them from working and whether their job is therefore at risk. Have recreational activities been given up? Is the pain having a bad effect on relationships?

AN APPROACH TO THE TREATMENT OF PAIN

Nociceptive pain

Patients with nociceptive pain resulting from an injury or some curable condition rehabilitate much faster if the pain is controlled. This can be done much more completely and with lower doses of analgesics if enough analgesia is given early, so as to prevent the pain from building up.

Most nociceptive pain can be controlled by opioids. However, opioids are used mainly in the treatment of post-injury, postoperative or malignant pain, and are seldom used in chronic inflammatory disease:

- Morphine is the drug of choice for moderate or severe pain. It can be given orally, intramuscularly or intravenously. In hospitals, particularly peri-operatively, it is usually given parenterally (i.m. or i.v.). Conversely, during outpatient treatment oral administration is commoner.

- Morphine is extremely safe provided it is titrated to effect. Its effects are easily reversed by small doses of naloxone.
- There is a minimal risk of addiction in giving appropriate doses of opioid to control nociceptive pain. Withholding adequate analgesia is more likely to result in drug-seeking behaviour.
- During treatment of chronic conditions or as an outpatient, immediate-release tablets or solutions of morphine are best for starting treatment, as they allow easy titration. The oral dose must be twice the parenteral dose to allow for first-pass liver metabolism.
- When the situation is stable after initial treatment, modified-release preparations such as MST are appropriate, supplemented by additional doses of immediate-release preparations for breakthrough pain. These latter preparations should amount to approximately 10% of the total daily dose. Opioids can lead to a variety of side-effects (e.g. dizziness, drowsiness, hallucinations) by all routes. In addition, oral treatment may cause constipation.
- There is a useful synergism between morphine and NSAIDs, especially in musculoskeletal nociceptive pain. However, bear in mind the side-effect profile of NSAIDs – bleeding in postoperative patients, gastrointestinal problems (which may be more likely due to the risk of stress ulceration around the time of operation) and the risk of asthma (which in a small number of patients may be precipitated or worsened by these drugs).

Patients' sensitivity to analgesics varies widely, and it is dangerous to think too rigidly about the 'correct dose' as one would with, say, antibiotics. The correct dose for a given patient is the dose that controls the pain. This is particularly true of opiates, where children, frail or elderly patients may need less, but opioid-tolerant patients will need much more.

When discussing analgesic management, it is useful to consider two typical scenarios.

Postoperative pain relief. As a house officer you will frequently be asked to adjust a patient's postoperative pain control. Several suitable regimes are available, and the best one will depend on the nature of the operation (how painful, how long will the pain last?), the nature of the patient (old, young, confused etc.) and the available technology.

Likely methods include:

- patient-controlled analgesia (PCA) – the patient controls a pump giving parenteral opioid; as well as ensuring relatively regular doses, this gives control of the medication to the patient, relieving some of the fear of pain
- infusion analgesia – in this case the rate of delivery of the drug is fixed by the doctor
- epidural analgesia with bupivicaine (local anaesthetic) or opioid (e.g. fentanyl) p.r.n.
- Oral opioid plus regular NSAID – this works well for many acute musculoskeletal conditions and minimises the risks of drowsiness or dizziness.

Pain relief for patients in the community. This problem will frequently be encountered both when arranging discharge medication for patients as a house officer and when working in general practice. Satisfactory methods include:

- regular simple analgesia (e.g. paracetamol or compound analgesics such as paracetamol/codeine mixtures).
- regular or p.r.n. simple analgesia (paracetamol or compound analgesic) plus regular NSAID; this is frequently used in rheumatoid arthritis and other forms of inflammatory arthritis, and in patients with osteoarthritis in whom simple analgesia alone does not suffice
- oral opioids (e.g. sustained-release morphine + breakthrough preparation) — appropriate warnings should be given about the risks of drowsiness etc., particularly when patients are likely to drive or use machinery; doses initially will require titrating upwards to obtain optimal effect.

All types of pain (nociceptive and neurogenic, acute and chronic) have psychic effects. Some patients may be psychologically disturbed by the experience of pain and may benefit from psychological assessment and support. This may

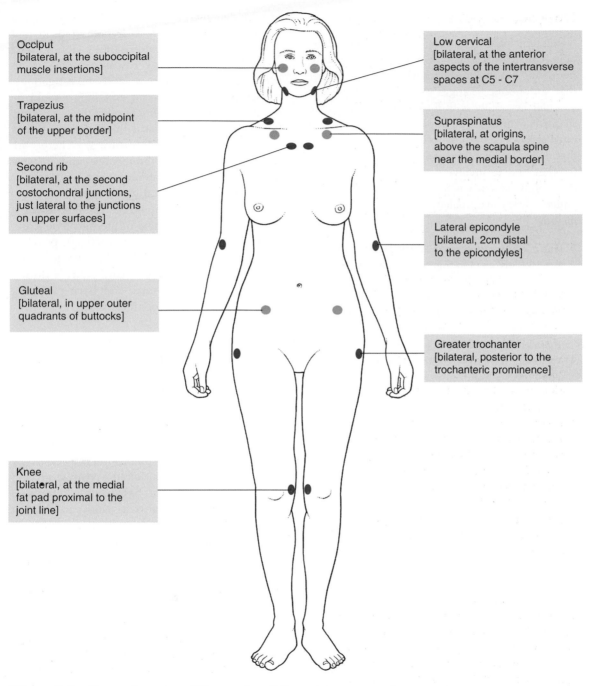

Occlput
[bilateral, at the suboccipital muscle insertions]

Trapezius
[bilateral, at the midpoint of the upper border]

Second rib
[bilateral, at the second costochondral junctions, just lateral to the junctions on upper surfaces]

Gluteal
[bilateral, in upper outer quadrants of buttocks]

Knee
[bilateral, at the medial fat pad proximal to the joint line]

Low cervical
[bilateral, at the anterior aspects of the intertransverse spaces at C5 - C7]

Supraspinatus
[bilateral, at origins, above the scapula spine near the medial border]

Lateral epicondyle
[bilateral, 2cm distal to the epicondyles]

Greater trochanter
[bilateral, posterior to the trochanteric prominence]

Figure 6.2   The tender points of fibromyalgia (18 points in nine pairs).

substantially help in pain management, as psychological effects may both arise from pain and exacerbate the experience of pain. Many patients with chronic pain prove to have inadequate methods to deal with it, and some have an inappropriate reaction to the pain. Such patients may be helped by counselling in pain control strategies.

Neurogenic pain

Neurogenic pain is characteristically unaffected by opioid analgesics. This type of pain is, regrettably, frequently not recognised for what it is. Remember that autonomic changes (sweaty or dry skin, vascular instability with flushes or blanching) are frequent with this type of pain, and that there are often sensory changes as well. It is worth knowing that there are several possible lines of treatment. It is often best to involve a pain control specialist (frequently an anaesthetist) in the management of patients with this problem. Methods of treatment include:

- Tricyclic antidepressants. Amitriptyline is the most widely used in this context. It may be important to emphasise to the patient that use of this drug does not mean that you think that the pain is 'all in the mind'. Doses prescribed to suppress pain are lower than those used in the treatment of depression.
- Anticonvulsants. A typical example of this would be the use of carbamazepine for trigeminal neuralgia.
- Transcutaneous nerve stimulation (TNS).
- Nerve blocks.
- Physiotherapy.

FIBROMYALGIA

This is a common condition characterised by widespread pain, which has gained increasing attention in recent years. Patients with fibromyalgia complain of generalised pain (hence its inclusion in this chapter), the other cardinal feature being the presence of multiple tender points on examination. For the diagnosis to be made, a patient must have widespread pain, *in addition to* tenderness at 11 of the 18 specific points (at least) highlighted in Figure 6.2.

Other characteristic features of fibromyalgia are tiredness and 'non-restorative' sleep – patients wake feeling unrefreshed – stiffness, headaches, anxiety and depression. Fibromyalgia can be extremely debilitating.

Fibromyalgia is commonest in women. Because the clinical features are non-specific, it is important to exclude other diagnoses which may require specific treatment, such as hypothyroidism and systemic lupus erythematosus (SLE). Fibromyalgia is not an inflammatory disease – there is no synovitis or myositis – and investigations, including full blood count and ESR, should be normal. However, to complicate the issue, fibromyalgia may coexist with conditions such as SLE and rheumatoid arthritis. There are associations between fibromyalgia and irritable bowel syndrome and chronic fatigue syndrome.

Management is often difficult in those severely affected. The patient should be reassured that the condition is not deforming or life-threatening and should be encouraged to keep as active as possible. A proportion of patients benefit from low-dose antidepressants. However, many patients do not respond to these measures and have persisting severe disability and work incapacity.

BACK PAIN

While pain, either localised or generalised, is a major feature of most of the musculoskeletal conditions described in this textbook, it is worthwhile making a special mention here of back pain. Low back pain, especially when it becomes chronic, is an enormous problem. It can be a major problem to the individual, because when severe and chronic it is disabling and has significant effects on quality of life. It is also a major problem in socioeconomic terms because of the number of days lost from work and because of the burden of so much disability on society (Fig. 17.2). While we do not understand why the number of patients affected by low back pain has risen exponentially in recent years, it is a problem which general practitioners, rheumatologists, orthopaedic surgeons, specialists in pain, occupational health physicians and doctors from many other specialities have to face.

The approach to adopt for patients with back pain is described in Chapter 17. As with other conditions characterised by pain, the aim is to diagnose the underlying condition and to treat the pain. While in most patients back pain settles spontaneously, it is so common that the minority with persistent pain represents a very large number of patients. If at all possible, back pain should not be 'allowed' to become chronic, and so patients should be assessed early, before the vicious cycle of pain, immobility, disability and further pain becomes established. Many centres now offer specific back pain services which are staffed by a multidisciplinary team.

In conclusion, adequate pain management is one of the most important and rewarding tasks for any doctor. Treatment of pain requires an assessment of the nature and cause of the pain, a graded approach to therapy and a willingness to review and adjust treatment until it is optimised. Do not be afraid to ask for help and advice about pain management from more senior colleagues.

Musculoskeletal pain

7 | Acute monoarthritis

Case history

A 35-year-old man presented with a short history of a hot, red and painful knee. There was no history of trauma or previous joint disease and he was generally fit, although he drank 30–40 pints of beer per week. He had a temperature of 37.5°C and movements of the knee joint were reduced and acutely painful. He was immediately admitted to hospital with a differential diagnosis of septic arthritis or gout. Blood tests showed a normal white cell count and a raised level of uric acid. Needle aspirate of the joint produced a pale yellow, cloudy fluid. Microscopy of this fluid showed crystals and white cells, but no bacteria on Gram staining. He was treated for gout, with bed rest and indomethacin, and made a good recovery within a few days. He was advised to reduce his alcohol intake, but despite this he had three further attacks over the next year. He was therefore treated with allopurinol, initially combined with an NSAID.

This chapter outlines the approach to take with a patient who presents with monoarthritis (inflammation of a single joint). While there are several possible causes (the main ones are listed in Box 7.1), the one to worry about most is septic arthritis (bacterial infection of a joint). Here we place special emphasis on septic arthritis and crystal arthritis, as both of these most commonly present with monoarthritis (although both can be polyarticular). Most of the other conditions which can present with monarthritis are discussed more fully in other chapters. Figure 7.1 shows the hand of a patient who presented with a monoarthritis of the right middle proximal interphalangeal joint – this proved to be septic.

Key points

- Acute monoarthritis is a medical emergency because the joint may be infected

- The main causes of monoarthritis are infection and crystals

- Joint aspiration is a vital step in diagnosis

- Infection is treated with antibiotics and joint lavage – delay in treatment may result in irreversible joint damage

- Crystal arthritis is treated acutely with NSAIDs or colchicine; drugs which reduce serum uric acid levels may be needed later for prevention of further attacks

- Do not inject steroids unless you are certain there is no infection

PATHOLOGY

Monoarthritis can be infective or non-infective; the pathological effects are partly due to the host response. Monoarthritis can occur against a background of previous joint problems, but often presents acutely and without any apparent predisposing or precipitating cause.

Septic arthritis

Septic arthritis is most frequently caused by Gram-positive organisms, especially staphylococci. The classical causative agent is *Staphylococcus aureus*, but increasingly infections by *Staphylococcus epidermidis* are being recognised. Infection may be caused by a wide variety of organisms, including streptococci, Gram-negative organisms and

---

Box 7.1   Causes of monoarthritis

- Septic arthritis
- Crystal arthritis
  — gout (urate crystals)
  — pseudogout (pyrophosphate crystals)
- Trauma (especially if associated with haemarthrosis)
- Monoarticular presentation of:
  — spondyloarthropathy, e.g. psoriatic arthritis
  — rheumatoid arthritis
- Exacerbation of osteoarthritis
- Haemarthrosis associated with clotting abnormalities, e.g. haemophilia
- Juvenile chronic arthritis

Note: (1) Remember the possibility of tuberculosis, especially in chronic monoarthritis. Fungal and viral infections can also cause a monoarthritis. (2) Inflammation at or near a joint may be due to a bursitis, cellulitis, tendinitis or (rarely) osteomyelitis, rather than arthritis.

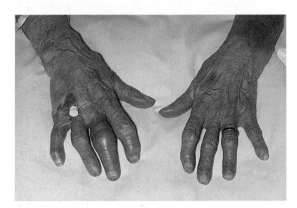

Figure 7.1   Acute monoarthritis of the right middle proximal interphalangeal joint. This proved to be a septic arthritis.

gonococci. *Haemophilus influenzae* is the commonest cause in children. Organisms may gain entry to the joint by direct introduction, which may occur due to penetrating injuries or after surgery. More commonly, infection appears spontaneously, probably due to haematogenous spread. This is particularly the case in previously damaged joints

and in immunocompromised patients, e.g. those with rheumatoid arthritis receiving treatment with immunosuppressive drugs.

Septic arthritis may cause gross joint damage; it is controversial whether the cartilage damage is caused directly by toxins and enzymes produced by the organisms, or by the inflammatory response to the infection. This response is characterised by large numbers of polymorphonuclear leucocytes in the synovial fluid, and the enzymes which they release are a probable cause of the chondral damage which occurs in this condition. This damage may result in severe residual fibrosis in the joint, which may cause permanent stiffness even when the infection has been adequately treated.

Crystal arthritis

Acute arthritis can result from the inflammatory response to crystals within a joint. When the crystals are of monosodium urate monohydrate, this is termed gout, and when they are of calcium pyrophosphate dihydrate (CPPD), it is termed 'pseudogout' (the acute form of CPPD deposition disease).

Gout

Gout is one of the results of hyperuricaemia (raised serum uric acid). Uric acid is produced from nucleic acids via hypoxanthine and xanthine, and hyperuricaemia occurs when uric acid is either overproduced or underexcreted by the kidney. The breakdown of hypoxanthine to xanthine and of xanthine to uric acid is catalysed by the enzyme xanthine oxidase. These concepts are important with respect to the management of gout. While there may be no identifiable underlying cause for hyperuricaemia, one should always be sought. Causes of overproduction of uric acid include myeloproliferative diseases and psoriasis, both of which are associated with increased cell turnover and rarely an inherited enzyme deficiency. Causes of underexcretion of uric acid include certain drugs (most importantly diuretics, which are commonly prescribed in the elderly, and low doses of aspirin) and renal impairment. Excessive alcohol consumption can also result in hyperuricaemia. Urate crystals are formed and phagocytosed within the joint and an inflammatory response initiated. However, many patients with hyperuricaemia do not develop gout, or do so only after several years of asymptomatic hyperuricaemia.

If gout is untreated the patient may develop *chronic tophaceous gout*, when urate crystals are deposited in connective tissue forming nodular lesions called tophi, or in bone causing 'punched out' erosions visible on X-ray (Fig. 7.2). Typical sites for tophi are the hands and feet (Fig. 7.3); the helix of the ear may also be affected. Deposition of urate in renal interstitial tissue can lead to a urate nephropathy. Hypertension may be associated with hyperuricaemia and gout.

Pseudogout

CPPD crystal deposition can be associated with an acute synovitis, when CPPD crystals released into the joint initiate an acute inflammatory response; a chronic arthropathy; and asymptomatic chondro-calcinosis on X-ray (Fig. 7.4). Pseudogout is a common cause of monoarthritis in the elderly and there is an association with osteoarthritis. In a proportion of patients a predisposing factor can be identified, such as hyperparathyroidism or haemochromatosis. This is especially true when pseudogout presents in a young or middle-aged adult.

Related pathologies

While the main causes of monoarthritis are sepsis and crystals, there are a number of other possible causes (Box 7.1). An acute flare-up in one joint can occur in patients with polyarthritis, e.g. rheumatoid arthritis, seronegative spondylo-

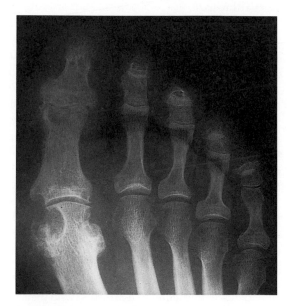

Figure 7.2   'Punched out' juxta-articular erosions of gout.

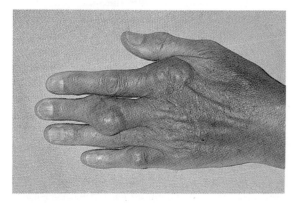

Figure 7.3   Tophaceous gout.

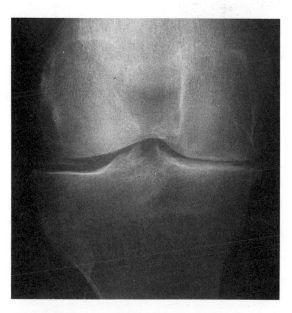

Figure 7.4   Chondrocalcinosis of lateral meniscus.

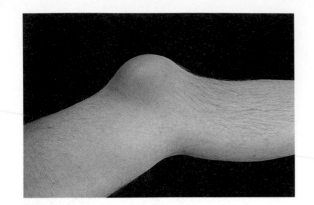

Figure 7.5   Prepatellar bursitis.

arthropathy (Ch. 8) and osteoarthritis (Ch. 10). However, patients with these conditions may also develop joint infection, so caution is needed.

Trauma to a joint can produce a picture of acute swelling and inflammation, especially if a haemarthrosis is present (Ch. 22). Osteomyelitis in bone adjacent to a joint can produce a sympathetic effusion (Ch. 11).

Inflammation and swelling of a bursa, which may or may not be caused by infection, may occur very close to a joint; it should be distinguished by clinical examination (Ch. 3). The commonest examples are prepatellar bursitis in front of the knee (Fig. 7.5) and olecranon bursitis over the point of the elbow.

CLINICAL FEATURES

History

The patient with an acute monoarthritis will complain of pain and swelling of the affected joint. The pain is exacerbated by any movement. An acute monoarthritis typically develops rapidly over 24–48 hours. This is especially true of septic or crystal arthritis. If the patient is systemically unwell with a high fever then sepsis is likely, although fever can occur in crystal arthritis. A long duration of monoarthritis (several weeks or months) may indicate tuberculosis.

Age

Septic arthritis may occur at any age. In young adults gonococcal arthritis may present with a monoarthritis, although often the arthritis is migratory. Gout is typically seen in middle-aged males (males are much more commonly affected than females), and pseudogout is primarily a condition of the elderly.

Associated symptoms

A recent genitourinary or diarrhoeal illness may indicate a reactive arthritis (Reiter's disease). Acute attacks of crystal arthritis (either gout or pseudogout) may be precipitated by illness or surgery. Trauma to the joint may indicate a haemarthrosis.

Predisposing factors

Ask about predisposing factors for septic and crystal arthritis, and for other conditions which may present as a monoarthritis. Patients who are predisposed to infection as a result of either underlying disease (e.g. diabetes or leukaemia) or drug treatment (e.g. corticosteroids or immunosuppressives) are at increased risk of septic arthritis, as are intravenous drug abusers. A penetrating injury may result in joint sepsis, and occasionally joint aspiration or injection can be complicated by bacterial sepsis. Treatment with diuretics and excess alcohol are common associations with gout.

Joint problems

In patients with rheumatoid arthritis (who may be immunocompromised) sepsis may occur in more than one joint and these patients may not mount the classical response to joint sepsis, especially if they are on treatment with steroids, when fever may be masked. It is therefore always important to have a high index of suspicion of joint sepsis in a patient with inflammatory joint disease who becomes non-specifically unwell, especially if on steroids or immunosuppressant drugs. Joint replacement infections are usually chronic and rather indolent; however, acute septic arthritis does occasionally occur in artificial joints.

When acute monoarthritis is due to gout, there may be a history of previous acute attacks. The classical scenario of a patient with untreated gout is that after a first acute attack (which classically affects the great toe metatarsophalangeal joint, although other peripheral joints may be affected), which lasts approximately 2 weeks, there is a symptom-free interval followed by another attack affecting either the same or another joint. If the patient remains hyperuricaemic then as time passes further attacks may occur, becoming more and more frequent, and the patient may go on to develop chronic tophaceous gout.

Family history

This may be relevant in certain patients with gout and seronegative spondyloarthropathy.

Examination

The affected joint is swollen and possibly red, and on palpation it is warm and tender. Movements will be painful and restricted. Look carefully at the skin, where there may be a focus of infection. Scars or rashes associated with seronegative spondyloarthropathies may be important, e.g. a plaque of psoriasis (Fig. 7.6). Perform a general examination, looking specifically for signs of infection and conditions which can be associated with monoarthritis, and of intercurrent disease. Remember to examine the other joints, looking for evidence of a generalised joint disorder.

The site of joint involvement may give a clue to the diagnosis. Large joints such as the knee are the commonest sites of septic arthritis, but no joint is exempt. Classically the great toe metatarsophalangeal joint is involved in gout, but other peripheral joints may be affected, e.g. the knee, ankle and elbow. Pseudogout affects predominantly the knee, wrist, shoulder or ankle.

Investigations

The single most important investigation in acute monoarthritis is microscopy (urgent Gram stain) (Fig. 7.7) and culture of the synovial fluid (Box 7.2). The joint must therefore be aspirated and the fluid sent to the microbiology laboratory. If facilities are available for cytological analysis of the synovial fluid, with polarising microscopy for crystal

---

Box 7.2   Microscopy of synovial fluid in acute monoarthritis (key points)

Non-inflammatory
- Clear/straw-coloured
- Cell count < 2000/mm³

Crystal-arthritis
- Cloudy/purulent
- Crystals (best seen under polarising light)
  — urate: needle-shaped, often within polymorphonuclear leucocytes, strongly negatively birefringent
  — pyrophosphate: less regular in shape, often rhomboid, weakly positively birefringent
- High white cell count, mainly polymorphs – can be > 60 000–80 000/mm³

Septic arthritis
- Cloudy/purulent
- Organisms on Gram stain (not always)
- High white cell count, mainly polymorphs – can be > 60 000–80 000/mm³

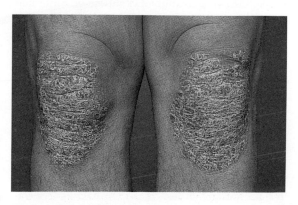

Figure 7.6   Plaque psoriasis.

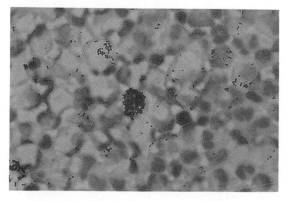

Figure 7.7   Gram stain of synovial fluid showing Gram-positive organisms. Courtesy of Professor A J Freemont.

definition, then further diagnostic information can be obtained (Fig. 4.5).

Other investigations which must be performed when the patient presents are:

- full blood count – looking mainly for a leucocytosis which suggests sepsis, although some elevation of the white count can also occur in gout
- blood cultures – sometimes the organism is isolated from the blood but not from the synovial fluid
- an X-ray of the affected joint – while, in the early stages of septic arthritis, this will be normal, or simply show soft tissue swelling, it serves as baseline. An X-ray may also be helpful diagnostically in the acute situation (e.g. showing chondrocalcinosis in an elderly patient with acute knee swelling (Fig. 7.4).

Other investigations which should be performed, but which may wait until the following day if the patient presents in the evening, are an ESR (raised in inflammatory arthritis), serum urate (which is usually high in untreated gout, but which can occasionally be normal even at the time of an acute attack), and blood biochemistry (especially renal function tests, which may show renal impairment in patients with gout). If there is renal impairment then this may influence management. If no immediate cause for the monoarthritis can be identified, check the rheumatoid factor, as rheumatoid arthritis can present as a monoarthritis (although, as discussed in Ch. 4, a positive rheumatoid factor does not equate to a diagnosis). In chronic monoarthritis, synovial biopsy and culture should be considered, looking in particular for tuberculosis.

Note that the gold standard in the diagnosis of gout is the finding of crystals in the synovial fluid. Even if only a tiny drop of synovial fluid can be obtained, this is sufficient for microscopy. However, many cases are diagnosed on the basis of a typical history and hyperuricaemia.

Certain medical conditions are associated with gout, including hypertension, hyperlipidaemia and vascular disease. These should therefore be sought, especially in a young person presenting with gout.

> **Box 7.3   Features of septic arthritis**
>
> - **Fever**
> - **An acutely inflamed joint**
> - **High white blood count in peripheral blood**
> - **Cloudy, purulent synovial fluid**
>
> **Remember: high index of suspicion of joint sepsis in patients with rheumatoid arthritis who become non-specifically unwell.**
>
> **Urgent synovial fluid analysis is mandatory when septic arthritis is suspected**

MANAGEMENT

General measures

An acutely inflamed joint should be rested and, depending upon which joint is involved, it may be necessary to splint the joint to avoid contracture. Analgesics should be prescribed and NSAIDs are often very effective in controlling inflammation.

Specific drug treatment (Box 7.4)

Septic arthritis

High-dose intravenous antibiotics should be commenced as soon as cultures have been sent whenever there is a strong index of suspicion of septic arthritis, even if the Gram stain is negative. Once culture results are available, the situation can then be reviewed. If organisms are identified on the Gram stain then these will influence the choice of antibiotic; otherwise a broad-spectrum regime, e.g. flucloxacillin and a cephalosporin, should be given. Intravenous antibiotics should be continued for 2 weeks and then changed to oral antibiotics for a further 6 weeks. The situation should be discussed with an orthopaedic surgeon: surgical drainage or lavage (wash out) may be indicated.

Gout

There are two main aspects to the treatment of acute gout.

Treatment of the acute attack.   This is usually with a NSAID such as indomethacin or ibuprofen, initially in high dose, reducing as the acute inflammation settles. If an NSAID is contra-

Box 7.4   Drugs used in the treatment of monoarthritis

General
- **Analgesics**
- **NSAIDs**

Septic arthritis
- **High-dose i.v. antibiotics, followed by oral**

Gout
- **Acute attack**
  - **NSAID**
  - **colchicine**
- **Prophylaxis (drugs are not always necessary)**
  - **allopurinol (inhibits xanthine oxidase)**
  - **uricosuric (probenecid or sulphinpyrazone)**
  - **(Both initiated under cover of NSAID or colchicine)**

indicated, e.g. in a patient with peptic ulceration, then an alternative is colchicine. Colchicine is anti-inflammatory in acute gout and has effects on leucocyte migration; not uncommonly it causes dose-dependent gastrointestinal side-effects.

Once sepsis has been excluded, an intra-articular steroid injection may be useful in the small number of cases which do not settle quickly with an anti-inflammatory. NSAIDs, colchicine or intra-articular steroids may also be used in pseudogout.

Prevention of further attacks. The first step in prophylaxis is to identify precipitating factors and to try to remove these. Advice should be given regarding alcohol consumption, weight reduction and dietary modification. It may be possible to reduce or discontinue a patient's diuretic.

Prophylactic drug therapy may be indicated if the above measures fail and the patient has further attacks; if the uric acid level is very high; or if the patient has chronic tophaceous gout. Prophylactic drug treatment should be continued indefinitely. The aim is to reduce hyperuricaemia and this can be done either by reducing production of uric acid or by increasing its renal excretion.

Allopurinol inhibits the enzyme xanthine oxidase and so reduces uric acid synthesis (xanthine oxidase catalyses the steps in nucleic

acid breakdown from hypoxanthine to xanthine and from xanthine to uric acid). It is generally well tolerated, but can cause hypersensitivity reactions. Beware of the important drug interaction between allopurinol and either azathioprine or mercaptopurine (both of which are inactivated by xanthine oxidase). If allopurinol is co-prescribed, the dosage of azathioprine or mercaptopurine must be reduced, otherwise toxicity (e.g. bone marrow suppression) may result.

Probenecid and sulphinpyrazone are both uricosuric drugs: they increase uric acid excretion. They should not be used in patients with pre-existing renal impairment.

When treatment with either allopurinol or a uricosuric drug is commenced, serum uric acid levels change and paradoxically an acute attack can be precipitated. Therefore when treatment with these drugs is initiated, either an NSAID or colchicine should be prescribed concomitantly for 2–3 months. Also, wait for an acute attack to settle before commencing allopurinol or a uricosuric, otherwise the acute attack may be prolonged.

Uric acid levels are monitored on prophylactic treatment. It is important not to commence allopurinol or a uricosuric drug until the diagnosis of gout is established, otherwise uric acid levels fall on treatment and it is then difficult to confirm a diagnosis.

While gout is a condition that can be treated very effectively, there are a number of common pitfalls in the management (Box 7.5). Ineffective treatment can lead to irreversible joint damage, which should have been preventable.

Surgical management (Box 7.6)

Acute septic arthritis is a medical emergency due to the high risk of permanent joint damage. In effect, the situation is similar to treatment of an abscess, where a collection of pus has developed; however, leaving the joint open to drain pus (as might be carried out with an abscess) is a poor option due to the risk of superinfection of the joint and the risk of cartilage necrosis due to desiccation. The blood supply and antibiotic penetration to large areas of the collection are poor. Accordingly, in addition to appropriate antibiotic

---

Box 7.5   Pitfalls in the management of gout

- The diagnosis may be incorrect
- Prophylactic treatment may be given inappropriately
- Prophylactic treatment may precipitate an acute attack (especially if given without the cover of an NSAID or colchicine)
- The patient is not told that prophylactic treatment is for life
- The patient takes prophylactic treatment intermittently, thereby causing fluctuations in the serum urate which may trigger acute attacks

---

Box 7.6   Surgical management of septic arthritis

- All patients with septic arthritis of major joints should be assessed by an orthopaedic surgeon
- Copious irrigation is a keystone of treatment of large joint septic arthritis and should be considered in all cases. It can be achieved by arthrotomy or by arthroscopic lavage
- Acute septic arthritis is common in children, where it poses additional difficulties due to the potential for long-term damage to the physis

---

treatment the pus should be physically removed as far as possible without leaving the joint open. This may be carried out by open exploration of the joint (arthrotomy), or the pus may be washed out using copious irrigation with an arthroscope. Both methods have merits: arthrotomy permits the most thorough cleaning, but arthroscopy is a less invasive procedure. Occasionally, repeat cleaning procedures are required.

There is a risk of bursitis close to the joint (prepatellar, olecranon) being confused with septic arthritis, as mentioned above. Most bursitis of this type can be managed conservatively with antibiotics, although it may take several days to settle. Some patients with bursitis fail to improve or have large collections of pus, so surgical drainage is carried out; this generally results in resolution of the infection, but may also result in sensitive scars in areas of high pressure on kneeling or leaning on the elbow.

Septic arthritis in children poses particular difficulties because of the risk of permanent damage to the physis as well as to the joint. This is exemplified by the hip, where septic arthritis may result in high intra-articular pressure, partial necrosis of the proximal femoral physis (femoral head) resulting in both osteoarthritis and growth deficiency in the lower limb with consequent limb length inequality. Because of these severe permanent effects, most surgeons tend to explore and decompress septic arthritis in children's hips, and make strenuous efforts to establish the diagnosis accurately (which may include aspiration or arthrotomy).

8 | Polyarthritis

Case history

A 40-year-old woman began experiencing joint pains shortly after returning from a holiday in France. Initially her hands felt stiff and she noticed that her rings were tighter than usual. Then she noticed that her hands were swollen, and at the same time her feet, ankles and left knee became painful. She had no back pain, but her neck felt a little stiff. Her symptoms were worst first thing in the morning and she felt tired. Otherwise she was in good health and, other than tuberculosis in childhood, she had suffered no previous illnesses. There was no family history of joint disease. Her mother had psoriasis.

She attended her GP, who noted that she had tender swelling of the MCP and PIP joints of several fingers, which meant that her grip was weak and painful. She was tender over the MTP joints and she had synovitis and a small effusion of the left knee. He took a blood sample, prescribed ibuprofen, and asked her to come back to the surgery in 2 weeks' time.

On reattending the surgery, she reported that the ibuprofen had helped a little, but she was still experiencing significant pain and stiffness, and now her right knee had become swollen. She had had to stop work as a supervisor in a local store because of the joint problems. Her GP noted that she now had moderate-sized effusions of both knees. He had received the results of her blood tests. The full blood count showed that she was slightly anaemic (Hb, 109 g/L) and the ESR was high at 55 mm/h. The GP said that she had arthritis, but he was not sure which type. He telephoned the hospital to request an urgent appointment for the rheumatology clinic, where she was seen the next day.

'Polyarthritis' means arthritis of several joints. Patients presenting with polyarthritis, e.g. the patient described in the Case history, may have any one of a number of different diseases (Box 8.1), but the two most important are rheumatoid arthritis and the spondyloarthropathies (often termed the 'seronegative' spondyloarthropathies because patients are seronegative for rheumatoid factor). Polyarthritis can also occur as a result of infection (see Ch. 7) or as a manifestation of different

Key points

- The two major subtypes of polyarthritis are: rheumatoid arthritis and the seronegative spondyloarthropathies.
- Both can cause severe joint destruction with consequent major disability.
- Both can be associated with extra-articular manifestations.
- The primary joint damage is caused by synovitis, but secondary damage occurs due to disturbance of normal joint mechanics and can produce severe deformities.
- Drug treatment is indicated early, before irreversible joint damage has occurred.
- Surgical reconstruction often requires multiple operations, whose sequence and timing must be carefully planned.
- Specific drug and surgical treatment must be combined with rehabilitation delivered by a skilled mutidisciplinary team.

> **Box 8.1   Main differential diagnosis of adult-onset polyarthritis**
>
> - Rheumatoid arthritis
> - Seronegative spondyloarthropathies
> - Other connective tissue diseases, e.g. SLE
> - Viral arthritis
> - Primary generalised osteoarthritis
> - Calcium pyrophosphate deposition disease

connective tissue diseases, e.g. SLE (see Ch. 9). Patients of any age may present with polyarthritis. Juvenile chronic arthritis is described in Chapter 13.

The spondyloarthropathies are characterised by inflammation of the axial and/or peripheral joints and can be subdivided into four major types:

- ankylosing spondylitis
- psoriatic arthritis
- reactive arthritis (often termed 'Reiter's syndrome')
- enteropathic arthritis.

While rheumatoid arthritis and the different types of spondyloarthropathy have certain features in common and share general principles of management, these should all be considered separate diseases. When a patient presents with arthritis affecting several joints, it is important to make the correct diagnosis. However, this is not always possible, especially in the early stages of disease, in which case, until further information is available, the patient should simply be labelled as having a polyarthritis.

In this chapter, to 'set the scene' we give brief descriptions of rheumatoid arthritis and the spondyloarthropathies, accompanied by 'typical' case histories. The epidemiology, aetiology and pathology of rheumatoid arthritis and the spondyloarthropathies are then described separately, as these are very different. The approach to the patient presenting with a polyarthritis is then described, highlighting key points in the history, examination and investigations which are important in diagnosis and in

assessment of disease activity/severity. The final section outlines the approach to treatment of the patient with polyarthritis. We have included some additional short 'scenarios' in the chapter to demonstrate some of the important issues.

Rheumatoid arthritis

Rheumatoid arthritis is the commonest polyarthritis. Its course is variable, characterised by exacerbations and remissions. While some patients have mild self-limiting disease, a significant proportion progress to chronic destructive joint disease (see Scenario 1). Rheumatoid arthritis is sometimes termed 'rheumatoid disease'; although the disease is mainly articular, extra-articular disease is common and internal organ involvement can (rarely), be life-threatening.

Scenario 1 – rheumatoid arthritis

A 55-year-old woman, diagnosed as having seropositive rheumatoid arthritis 8 years previously, attended the rheumatology clinic. She had been unwell recently. When she had first developed joint problems, her symptoms had been well controlled with diclofenac and she had been able to continue her work as a primary school teacher without too much difficulty. Initially her hands, wrists and feet had been mainly affected, but over the years her elbows, shoulders, neck, ankles and knees had become involved. She had had a very bad flare-up 2 years after the onset of her joint problems, when she had been admitted to hospital for bedrest and intra-articular injections of her knees and shoulders, followed by physio-therapy. At that time she was commenced on gold injections. She was very well while on gold, which unfortunately had to be stopped because of a fall in her platelet count (her full blood count and urinalysis were checked prior to each gold injection). On stopping the gold her disease flared up and she was commenced on sulpha-salazine. While on sulphasalazine she had regular blood checks. She was never convinced that the sulphasalazine really helped her. However, despite her difficulties (including

morning stiffness of around 2 hours) she managed to continue working, up until this recent severe flare-up of her joint disease. On examination at the clinic this time, she had ulnar deviation at the MCP joints and marked synovitis of several of the MCP joints and of the wrists. Wrist movement was very restricted. She had synovitis and 20° fixed flexion deformities of both elbows, painful restricted shoulder movements, restriction of neck movements, synovitis and small effusions of both knees, synovitis of both ankles and tenderness of the MTP joints (with MTP subluxation and callosities). She had a full range of hip movements.

Her haemoglobin was 101 g/L and the ESR 65 mm/h. Plasma biochemical profile showed normal renal and liver function. X-rays of her hands and feet showed erosive changes, which had progressed since the time of the last X-rays 2 years previously.

The rheumatologist explained to her that because her disease was active he recommended treatment with methotrexate, to be taken in tablet form once a week. She was also prescribed folic acid. He gave her an information leaflet on methotrexate. He also suggested that if her joint disease became any worse then a further period of in-patient care would be advisable, and that if the pain from her feet remained severe then a consultation with an orthopaedic surgeon to consider forefoot surgery would be appropriate.

Spondyloarthropathies

All spondyloarthopathies have an association with the histocompatibility antigen HLA-B27 (see below) and share certain clinical manifestations. Enthesopathies (abnormalities at the site of tendon, ligament or articular capsule insertion into bone) are a characteristic feature, but synovitis also occurs. Iritis and other extra-articular features can occur.

Ankylosing spondylitis

Ankylosing spondylitis is predominantly a disease of the axial skeleton (spine and sacroiliac joints).

The typical presentation is back pain in a young adult (see Scenario 2).

Scenario 2 – ankylosing spondylitis

A 27-year-old man presented to his GP with a 6-month history of low back pain. Initially he thought he had strained his back moving furniture and he had rested for 2 weeks. However, this had made him feel even worse, especially in the mornings when he felt particularly stiff. He found that walking eased the pain. His GP referred him to the hospital when his lumbar spine movements were found to be reduced in all planes. X-ray of the sacroiliac joints showed changes of early sacroiliitis. He was HLA-B27-positive.

The NSAID naproxen prescribed by the GP did not help very much and the rheumatologist changed this to indomethacin, which was more effective. However, the most important part of his management was physiotherapy. He was taught a home exercise programme and attended the physiotherapy department regularly. He also went swimming twice a week. With continuing exercises he remained well, and was able to continue his work as a car mechanic. The rheumatologist had been interested in the fact that his father and sister had psoriasis.

Psoriatic arthritis

There are different subtypes of psoriatic arthritis (Box 8.2), which occurs in association with the skin disease psoriasis (Scenario 3). Some patients have an inflammatory polyarthritis clinically indistinguishable from rheumatoid. In a proportion of patients the articular disease precedes skin psoriasis.

Scenario 3 – psoriatic arthritis

A 25-year-old man was referred with a 1-week history of a painful, swollen right ankle. There was no history of injury and he was otherwise well. On examination, the ankle was diffusely swollen, with synovitis. The only other

---

> **Box 8.2   Different clinical patterns of psoriatic arthritis**
>
> - An asymmetrical oligoarthritis. The fingers and toes are often involved and diffuse swelling of the digit ('sausage' digit), caused by interphalangeal joint and flexor tendon sheath inflammation, can occur. This diffuse swelling is termed 'dactylitis'
>
> - A distal arthritis involving distal interphalangeal joints
>
> - A symmetrical arthritis clinically similar to rheumatoid
>
> - Arthritis mutilans, which is a deforming, destructive arthritis
>
> - A spondyloarthopathy

abnormality was that he had a scaling rash behind both ears and at the umbilicus, which the rheumatologist diagnosed as psoriasis.

The ankle was aspirated at the rheumatology clinic. Five millilitres of straw-coloured fluid were aspirated and microscopy showed inflammation (white blood count, 15 000/mm³). The fluid was sterile on culture.

Although the ankle settled after 4 days with bedrest and ibuprofen, over the following 2 years he developed other joint problems: low back ache in the mornings (when he felt stiff for around half an hour) and painful swelling of several of his toes. He was under regular review at the rheumatology clinic, where it was noted that he had developed dactylitis of his left second and fourth, and right third and fourth toes, and that his lumbar spine movements had become slightly reduced (Schober's test 4 cm; back extension reduced). He was told that his joint problems were related to his psoriasis, and because of his increasing problems he was commenced on sulphasalazine in addition to ibuprofen.

Reactive arthritis (Reiter's syndrome)
Reactive arthritis develops in response to infection at a distant site (usually urogenital, gastrointestinal or throat) (Scenario 4). This is as distinct from septic arthritis when organisms can be isolated

from the joint itself (synovial fluid in reactive arthritis is inflammatory but sterile). The term 'Reiter's syndrome' is often used when the arthritis follows a sexually transmitted or diarrhoeal illness, the classic triad of clinical features being arthritis, conjunctivitis and urethritis. Mucocutaneous lesions including balanitis are common. While most patients recover spontaneously, the disease can pursue a chronic course. Patients infected with HIV may suffer very severe forms of reactive arthritis.

Scenario 4 – reactive arthritis (Reiter's syndrome)

A 28-year-old woman attended the A & E department with a 3-day history of painful right knee swelling. It had become so painful she was unable to bear weight. One week previously, while on holiday, she had had a diarrhoeal illness, which was only just settling. Her sister had also been affected, so it had spoiled the end of their week.

On examination she was apyrexial. The only abnormal finding was a warm effusion of the right knee, which was diffusely tender, and flexion was limited by pain to 20°. Forty millilitres of fluid were aspirated. The fluid was inflammatory (white cell count, 11 100/mm3). No crystals or organisms were identified. She was admitted to hospital and commenced on ibuprofen. The rheumatologist was confident that this was a reactive arthritis and no antibiotics were prescribed. Over the next 2 days the knee settled and she began walking again. As suspected, the 48 hour synovial fluid culture was negative. She was discharged after 3 days and had no further symptoms.

Enteropathic arthritis
In most patients this is associated with inflammatory bowel disease (Crohn's disease or ulcerative colitis) (Scenario 5).

Scenario 5 – enteropathic arthritis

A 25-year-old man, diagnosed as having ulcerative colitis 2 years previously, began experiencing joint symptoms. His knees and ankles were particularly affected, with morning stiffness in addition to pain and slight swelling. He noticed that these symptoms fluctuated, and were especially troublesome during exacerbations of his ulcerative colitis. His back also felt stiff.

The physiotherapist taught him an exercise programme, explaining that it was important to maintain his range of spinal mobility. However, over the next year he had major problems with his ulcerative colitis, culminating in colectomy at the time of a very severe exacerbation. Subsequently he had very little in the way of knee or ankle symptoms.

EPIDEMIOLOGY

Rheumatoid arthritis

Rheumatoid arthritis occurs in all racial groups. Its prevalence in the UK is approximately 1%. It is two to three times more common in women than in men. In adults, onset can occur at any age but the peak age of onset is generally considered to be between 35 and 60 years. Patients with rheumatoid arthritis, especially those with severe disease, have an increased mortality compared to the general population.

Spondyloarthropathies

Ankylosing spondylitis

The prevalence of ankylosing spondylitis in different populations is related to the frequency of HLA-B27 in these populations (the HLA is discussed below). In Caucasians, the prevalence of ankylosing spondylitis is usually in the order of 0.5–1%, and that of HLA-B27 in the order of 10%. Over 90% of patients with ankylosing spondylitis are HLA-B27-positive. Earlier studies suggested that men were around 10 times more likely to be affected than women, but with increasing recognition of milder disease the male:female ratio is now taken to be in the order of 2–3:1. Onset is usually in young adults.

Psoriatic arthritis

Approximately 1% of the population develop psoriasis. Around 5% of patients with psoriasis develop psoriatic arthritis, but the onset of psoriatic arthritis may precede that of the skin disease. Taking into account the different forms of psoriatic arthritis, equal numbers of males and females are affected, with a peak age of onset from 20 to 40 years.

Reactive arthritis

This is usually a disease of young adults. Next to ankylosing spondylitis, it has the highest HLA-B27 association of the spondyloarthropathies: in the order of 70–80% of patients are HLA-B27-positive. Men and women are equally affected.

Enteropathic arthropathy

Between 2 and 20% of patients with inflammatory bowel disease (Crohn's disease or ulcerative colitis) develop arthritis.

PATHOLOGY

Neither rheumatoid arthritis nor any of the spondyloarthopathies is known to have a specific aetiology. It is likely that the aetiology of each is multifactorial, involving both genetic and non-genetic factors, and that an antigenic 'trigger' (possibly an infectious agent) initiates an abnormal immune response in a genetically susceptible individual. That genetic factors are important is illustrated by the association between rheumatoid arthritis and the major histocompatibility complex (MHC) class II tissue type HLA-DR4 in Caucasians. HLA-B27, a class I molecule, is thought to be a disease susceptibility factor for the spondyloarthropathies.

MHC. In case you have not come across the concept of the MHC before, here is a brief background. Genetic susceptibility to many different diseases, including several rheumatic diseases, involves the MHC, which is located on the short arm of chromosome six, and includes the HLA genes. MHC genes encode many different types of molecule which are important in immune responses. These include two classes of cell surface molecules: I and II. Class I molecules include the HLA-A, -B and -C molecules which are important in transplantation and which are expressed in all nucleated cells. Class II molecules include HLA-DP, HLA-DQ and HLA-DR molecules and are found on macrophages, B-cells and activated T-

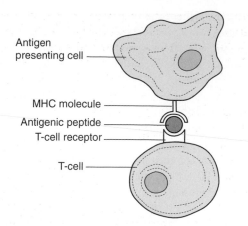

Figure 8.1 The trimolecular complex of the MHC molecule, antigenic peptide and T-cell receptor which is believed to be central in T-cell activation in the rheumatic diseases.

cells. The MHC genes which encode the class I and class II molecules are highly polymorphic. This means that multiple alleles exist and that there is a wide variety of possible gene products. This has important implications with respect to cellular interactions which initiate the immune response, because class I and class II molecules both play an important role in antigen presentation.

How environmental and genetic factors interact at the molecular level to set in motion the inflammatory cascade of rheumatoid arthritis is currently the subject of much research. Antigen binds to specific amino acids of the MHC molecule. Specific T-cell receptor sequences in turn bind to this MHC molecule-bound antigen (Fig. 8.1). As a result of this trimolecular interaction, the T-cell is activated and the inflammatory response initiated.

Rheumatoid arthritis

Rheumatoid arthritis is an inflammatory disease which can affect most body systems. The initial inflammatory response is non-specific, but is succeeded by a granulomatous response where macrophages and plasma cells produce a vigorous inflammatory process. As already stated, the precipitating cause of this immune response is not clear, with theories including a response to bacterial or viral infection and autoimmunity to various

cartilage and joint components including collagens (especially collagen II). Many of these changes are exemplified by the rheumatoid nodule. This frequently occurs at the olecranon, but also over other bony prominences, and consists of palisaded macrophages with lymphocytes. The synovium is the principal tissue involved in the inflammatory rheumatoid process, with synovitis occurring in the synovium of both joints and tendon sheaths. Synovium throughout the body is affected, so all synovial joints and many tendons may be damaged. Subsequently, articular cartilage, bone and other connective tissues are damaged. The proliferating synovium, containing many inflammatory cells, grows across the surface of articular cartilage, where it is known as pannus. Macrophages in this tissue cause connective tissue damage in several ways. First, they release enzymes such as elastase which can cause damage directly; secondly, they release signalling molecules (e.g. cytokines, growth factors and prostaglandins) which activate other cells to cause tissue damage. Tissue degradation in connective tissues is mediated by a variety of enzymes, notably metalloproteinases of various kinds (e.g. collagenase, cathepsins), which are often produced by the same cells that produce the matrix of the tissue. The enzymes are deposited in the matrix in an inactive form and subsequently activated in the matrix. Cells producing such enzymes include synovial cells, chondrocytes and fibroblasts.

These complex mechanisms result in early damage to proteoglycans and collagen in cartilage. Rheumatoid disease characteristically progresses with intermittent exacerbations (flares) of disease; eventually these may cease, leaving damaged joints (secondary osteoarthritis). Joint deformity may be severe in rheumatoid arthritis; this is usually due to damage to the joint geometry rather than damage to ligaments, which may, surprisingly, remain intact. Associated with the severe joint damage is early osteoporosis, which is generally juxta-articular. This is caused by osteoclast activation, which occurs both as a diffuse osteoporosis at the end of long bones and as erosions at the osseosynovial junction where the capsule arises from the bone.

Vasculitis may occur in patients with rheumatoid arthritis, presenting as a mild endarteritis affecting the digital vessels and causing infarcts of the finger tips or nailfolds. More seriously, an inflammatory vasculitis may affect larger vessels, causing necrosis and gangrene which may (rarely) prove fatal, e.g. if there is mesenteric artery involvement.

Spondyloarthropathies

The pathological hallmark of ankylosing spondylitis and of the other spondyloarthropathies is an enthesopathy. It is the enthesis (the site of insertion of tendon, ligament or articular capsule into bone) which is primarily affected, as opposed to the synovium in rheumatoid arthritis. Cartilaginous joints (including the intervertebral discs) and various ligamentous attachments are therefore affected as well as synovial joints. While there is an initial inflammatory, erosive phase at the enthesis, this is superseded by fibrosis and ossification. The classic spinal changes in ankylosing spondylitis are due to an initial erosive lesion at the attachment of the outer annulus of the intervertebral disc to the corner of the vertebral body, with subsequent new bone formation. These changes give rise to the initial appearance on X-ray of 'squaring' of the vertebrae, followed by growth of bony spurs called syndesmophytes across the annulus fibrosis. Upper and lower syndesmophytes fuse to form bony bridges between vertebrae, resulting in spinal fusion. Destruction of the vertebral end-plates can also occur.

Synovitis occurs in peripheral joints, and involvement of the sacroiliac joints (with progression to bony fusion) is one of the hallmarks of the spondyloarthropathies.

Pathological changes may also occur in the heart (most importantly fibrous scarring affecting aortic valve function) and lung (resulting in pulmonary fibrosis and cyst formation).

CLINICAL FEATURES
History

While rheumatoid arthritis and the spondylo-arthropathies predominantly affect joints, both can be associated with extra-articular manifestations (Boxes 8.3 and 8.4). Therefore it is important to take

---

Box 8.3   Important extra-articular features of rheumatoid arthritis

- Weight loss (in active disease)
- Anaemia
- Rheumatoid nodules
- Vasculitis, including:
  - nailfold infarcts
  - cutaneous ulceration
- Secondary Sjögren's (sicca) syndrome
- Felty's syndrome
- Cardiovascular
  - pericarditis
- Respiratory
  - pleural effusions
  - interstitial fibrosis
  - pulmonary nodules
- Renal
  - glomerulonephritis
- Nervous system
  - entrapment neuropathy
  - cervical myelopathy
  - peripheral neuropathy
- Eye
  - scleritis
- Bone
  - osteoporosis
- amyloidosis as a possible complication (causing proteinuria, hepatosplenomegaly)

Box 8.4   Important extra-articular features of spondyloarthropathies

- Iritis/conjunctivitis
- Skin lesions
- Mouth ulcers
- Small and/or large bowel ulceration
- Aortic incompetence ⎫
- Pulmonary fibrosis   ⎬ in ankylosing
  (upper lobes)   ⎪ spondylitis
- Amyloidosis as a   ⎭
  complication (rare)

a full history and perform a full examination. Taking a full history may also provide diagnostic clues in a patient presenting for the first time with polyarthritis, and may identify symptoms which reflect side-effects of therapy.

Musculoskeletal

The key points to ask about are:

- *Are symptoms of joint inflammation present?* Patients with polyarthritis will complain of pain, swelling and stiffness of several joints, often resulting in loss of function (Ch. 2). Prolonged morning stiffness is a major feature of inflammatory arthritis, and patients also experience post-inactivity gelling.
- *What is the pattern of the joint involvement?* Rheumatoid arthritis commonly affects firstly the wrists and small joints of the hands and feet (proximal IP, MCP and MTP) progressing to involve other synovial joints, as in Scenario 1. No synovial joint is exempt although the distal IP joints of the hand are often spared. Involvement of the temperomandibular joints causes pain on chewing. In a small proportion of patients, rheumatoid arthritis may present as a monoarthritis.

  The spondyloarthropathies may present with a peripheral arthritis, with axial skeleton involvement (spondylitis and/or sacroiliitis), or with both (as in Scenarios 2–5). The peripheral arthritis of the spondyloarthropathies, with the exception of psoriatic arthritis, tends to be predominantly lower limb, asymmetrical, and affecting large joints (hip, knee, ankle). While this pattern does occur in psoriatic arthritis, joint involvement can be symmetrical, and the distal IP joints of the hands may be affected. There are generally considered to be five clinical patterns of psoriatic arthritis (Box 8.2).
- *Was the onset of arthritis acute or insidious, and were there any associated features?* Rheumatoid arthritis is classically of insidious onset, although a small proportion of patients experience an acute onset. The spondyloarthropathies also are usually of insidious onset, although onset of peripheral arthritis in reactive arthritis (following a recent genitourinary or diarrhoeal illness) is usually acute (as in Scenario 4).

- *What has been the pattern of the disease over time in the patient with long-standing disease?* Rheumatoid arthritis is a relapsing, remitting disease. A significant proportion of patients suffer recurrent exacerbations or 'flares', at the same time progressing towards irreversible joint destruction. Others have mild, self-limiting disease.

  Many patients with spondyloarthropathies have mild disease but a proportion will progress to joint destruction. Flares of peripheral arthritis associated with ulcerative colitis or Crohn's disease often coincide with flares of the gut disease.
- *Are there features suggestive of an enthesopathy?* These include heel pain due to Achilles tendinitis or plantar fasciitis, or chest wall pain due to costochondritis and are suggestive of a spondyloarthropathy.

Systemic enquiry

Patients with active joint disease may have non-specific systemic symptoms, e.g. lassitude and weight loss. More specific symptoms are described below.

Cardiovascular and respiratory. Ask about breathlessness, which may be a symptom of pulmonary fibrosis in the patient with rheumatoid arthritis or, rarely, ankylosing spondylitis. Breathlessness may also occur as a result of drug treatment (e.g. pneumonitis with methotrexate) or infection (including opportunistic) occurring as a complication of disease and/or drug treatment. Symptomatic cardiac involvement can occur in rheumatoid arthritis and ankylosing spondylitis but is rare.

Gastrointestinal. Lower gastrointestinal symptoms may point to a diagnosis of reactive arthritis or enteropathic arthritis. Many drugs used in the treatment of arthritis (particularly NSAIDs) can cause gastrointestinal side-effects.

Genitourinary. Recent cervicitis or urethritis may indicate reactive arthritis.

Neurological. Neurological symptoms occur in rheumatoid arthritis for a number of reasons: entrapment neuropathy (e.g. median nerve compression, see Ch. 15), cervical myelopathy and peripheral neuropathy. Symptoms can be difficult to interpret, because patients may have combinations of these problems and may be weak secondary to joint inflammation/destruction as well as to neurological disease. Rarely, a cauda equina syndrome can occur in ankylosing spondylitis.

Mucocutaneous. Always ask about rashes, which may occur as a result of the disease (e.g. psoriasis) or as a side-effect of drug treatment (e.g. gold). Mouth ulcers can occur in reactive arthritis. Stomatitis may be due to methotrexate.

Eyes. Ask about dry eyes (and a dry mouth), suggestive of secondary Sjögren's syndrome (Ch. 9) which can occur in rheumatoid arthritis. A history of a painful red eye is suggestive of iritis and therefore of a spondyloarthropathy. Conjunctivitis is a feature of reactive arthritis (Reiter's syndrome).

Drug history

In a patient with long-standing disease, ask about previous drug treatment and why this was discontinued. Was this because of lack of effect or adverse effects? In Scenario 1, gold was stopped because of a fall in the platelet count. It is important to know the current drug treatment, in order to assess efficacy and toxicity.

Family history

There is an increased incidence of rheumatoid arthritis, especially in first-degree relatives. Ask about a family history of HLA-B27-related disorders (psoriasis, inflammatory bowel disease, ankylosing spondylitis): if present this increases the likelihood of the patient having a spondyloarthropathy.

Social history

The patient with polyarthritis is often disabled, and so it is important to ask about support at home and about housing.

Examination

A full physical examination must be performed in the patient with polyarthritis.

Musculoskeletal

It is important to distinguish between the patient with active disease, when there is synovitis but possibly little or no deformity, and the patient with 'burnt-out', inactive disease, when there is deformity but no ongoing inflammation (there may, however, be elements of both, i.e. synovitis at sites of obvious joint damage). Patients with inflammatory arthritis may develop contractures, a result of resting an inflamed joint in the position of maximum comfort.

Principles of musculoskeletal examination are outlined in Chapter 3. The pattern of joint involvement is important as already noted in the section on 'history'. Some specific and characteristic features of rheumatoid arthritis and the spondyloarthropathies are discussed below.

Hands and wrists

Rheumatoid arthritis. There are a number of classical appearances and deformities of the hand in rheumatoid arthritis. In the early stages of disease 'spindling' of the fingers occurs as a result of synovitis of the proximal IP joints (Fig. 8.2). Synovitis affects not only the proximal IP, MCP and wrist joints, but also the tendon sheaths of the fingers and wrist. Rupture of the finger extensor tendons can occur, and synovitis of the wrist flexors can lead to carpal tunnel syndrome, with signs of median nerve entrapment.

As the disease progresses, the following deformities can occur:

- ulnar deviation and flexion at the MCP joints (Fig. 8.3)
- boutonnière deformity, with flexion at the proximal IP joint and extension at the distal IP joint (Fig. 8.4)

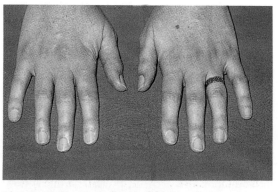

Figure 8.2 'Spindling' of fingers due to proximal IP joint swelling in early rheumatoid arthritis.

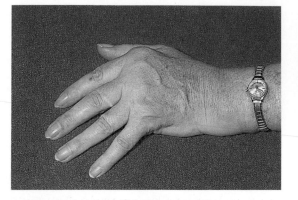

Figure 8.3 Ulnar deviation at the MCP joints in rheumatoid arthritis.

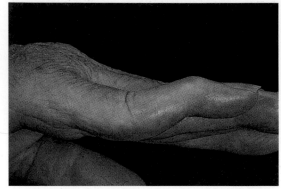

Figure 8.5 Swan neck deformity in rheumatoid arthritis.

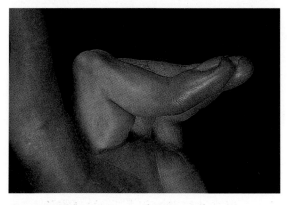

Figure 8.4 Boutonnière deformity in rheumatoid arthritis.

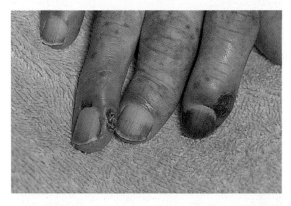

Figure 8.6 Digital vasculitis in a patient with rheumatoid arthritis.

- swan neck deformity, with hyperextension at the proximal IP joint and flexion at the distal IP joint (Fig. 8.5)
- Z-thumb, with flexion at the MCP joint and hyperextension at the IP joint
- dorsal subluxation of the ulnar head.

Other signs of rheumatoid arthritis which may be seen in the hands include nailfold infarcts (indicative of a vasculitis) (Fig. 8.6) and palmar erythema.

Spondyloarthropathies. Hand involvement is most common in psoriatic arthritis but may also occur in the other spondyloarthropathies. Distal IP joint inflammation can occur in psoriatic arthritis (Fig. 8.7), in contrast to rheumatoid when these joints are usually spared. Dactylitis is typical of the spondyloarthropathies (Fig. 8.8). Characteristic nail

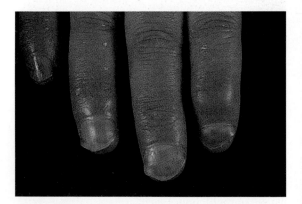

Figure 8.7 Distal IP joint involvement in psoriatic arthritis.

changes may be seen in psoriatic arthritis, e.g. nail pitting, onycholysis and hyperkeratosis (Fig. 8.9).

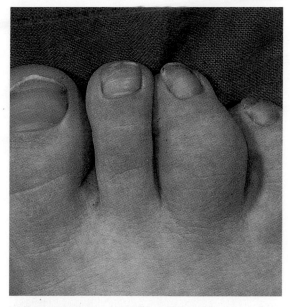

Figure 8.8   Dactylitis of third toe.

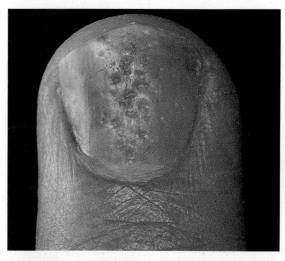

Figure 8.9   Nail changes in psoriasis.

Feet

Rheumatoid arthritis. Foot involvement is a major cause of pain and disability in patients with rheumatoid, primarily due to involvement of the MTP joints. Persisting synovitis at these joints can lead to subluxation, so that the patient walks on the metatarsal heads, leading to the symptom of 'walking on pebbles'; callosities and ulcers beneath

the metatarsal heads can result and hallux valgus is common (Fig. 8.10).

Spondyloarthropathies. Specific features include dactylitis (as in the fingers), Achilles tendinitis (tenderness over the Achilles tendon, and pain on standing on tip-toe) and plantar fasciitis (tenderness over the insertion of the plantar fascia into the calcaneus).

Knee. Knee involvement is common in both rheumatoid arthritis and the spondyloarthropathies. Examination of the knee should always include palpation posteriorly: popliteal cysts can occur and may rupture ('ruptured Baker's cyst'). When this happens, irritant synovial fluid tracks down into the calf and the patient complains of a painful, swollen calf, which may be misdiagnosed as a deep venous thrombosis.

Hip

Rheumatoid arthritis. Hip involvement is usually a late manifestation of rheumatoid arthritis but can be severe with marked restriction of movement.

Spondyloarthropathies. A proportion of patients with ankylosing spondylitis develop severe hip involvement, especially those with early onset disease (in their teens).

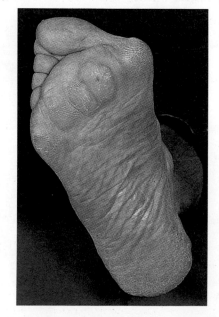

Figure 8.10   Callosities beneath subluxed MTP joints in rheumatoid arthritis, with hallux valgus.

Cervical spine

Rheumatoid arthritis. Cervical spine involvement is common in rheumatoid arthritis, especially subluxation at the atlanto-axial level (Fig. 8.11). The transverse ligament of the atlas is damaged which means that the odontoid peg is no longer in close apposition to the posterior aspect of the anterior arch of the atlas, especially in flexion. This leads to instability, which can be asymptomatic (Scenario 6) or, at worst, lead to cord compression. Instability can also occur at lower levels. On examination, neck movements may be restricted and painful. Careful assessment of the cervical spine is mandatory before anaesthesia.

Scenario 6 – Rheumatoid neck

A 49-year-old woman with rheumatoid arthritis was admitted for varicose vein surgery. As part of her pre-operative assessment, the house officer arranged flexion and extension views of the cervical spine. These showed 10 mm of atlanto-axial subluxation on flexion. This surprised the house officer, because the patient had very little neck pain and no neurological signs. The anaesthetist decided against a general anaesthetic and employed a spinal anaesthetic instead.

Spondyloarthropathies. Cervical spine involvement can occur in all forms of spondyloarthropathy. All planes of movement are restricted in the patient with advanced ankylosing spondylitis.

Axial skeleton involvement in the spondyloarthropathies. Cervical spine involvement has already been mentioned. Chest expansion is reduced when the thoracic spine is involved. All planes of lumbar spine movement may be reduced, as in Scenario 2, and if ankylosis has occurred then there is virtually no movement as demonstrated in Figure 8.12. Tenderness over the sacroiliac joints may indicate sacroiliitis. The sacroiliac joints and lumbar spine tend to be involved early, inflammation later extending up the thoracic and cervical spine.

Temperomandibular joint. This is commonly affected in rheumatoid arthritis, when tenderness can be elicited and the patient experiences pain on opening the mouth.

Extra-articular features (Boxes 8.3 and 8.4)
Clinical signs of extra-articular disease should be looked for carefully.

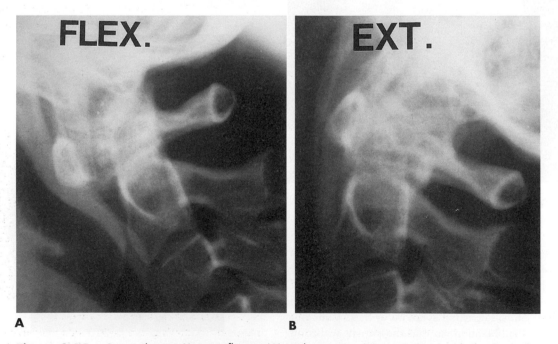

A **B**

Figure 8.11 Cervical spine X-ray in flexion (A) and extension (B) in a patient with rheumatoid arthritis, showing atlanto-axial subluxation on the flexion view.

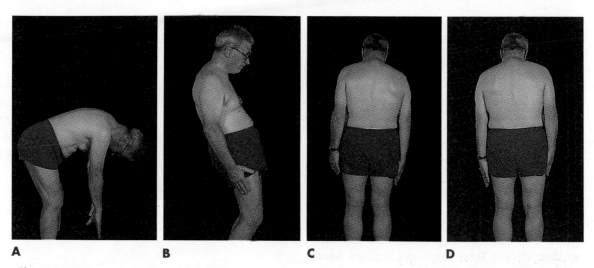

A   **B**   **C**   **D**

Figure 8.12   Severely restricted lumbar spine movements in a patient with advanced ankylosing spondylitis **A.** flexion. **B.** Extension. **C.** Lateral bending to the right. **D.** Lateral bending to the left.

Cardiac. While pericardial involvement is common in rheumatoid arthritis, this is usually asymptomatic and not associated with clinical signs. However, in a minority of patients, pericardial tamponade occurs. Around 1% of patients with ankylosing spondylitis develop aortic incompetence; this is even less common in rheumatoid arthritis.

Respiratory. Rheumatoid arthritis can be associated with pleural effusions (exudate), interstitial fibrosis (with bilateral basal crepitations on examination) and pulmonary nodules. Pulmonary fibrosis can also occur as a result of drug treatment, e.g. gold or methotrexate (Fig. 8.13). Pulmonary fibrosis can be a feature of ankylosing spondylitis but is then usually apical, as opposed to the fibrosis in rheumatoid arthritis which is initially basal.

Abdomen. Splenomegaly in a patient with rheumatoid arthritis may indicate Felty's syndrome (splenomegaly and leukopenia in a patient with rheumatoid arthritis). Patients with Felty's syndrome usually have severe rheumatoid arthritis, and may have leg ulceration and lymphadenopathy. Rarely a patient with long-standing polyarthritis (especially rheumatoid arthritis) may have hepatosplenomegaly as a result of amyloidosis. Mild hepatomegaly can occur in patients with rheumatoid arthritis (fatty change).

Neurological. Neurological examination is often difficult in the patient with polyarticular disease, because of pain on movement and muscle wasting and weakness secondary to joint disease. However, it is important to look for evidence of entrapment neuropathy, cervical myelopathy and peripheral neuropathy, which can occur particularly in the patient with rheumatoid arthritis. Carpal tunnel syndrome is the commonest entrapment neuropathy in patients with rheumatoid arthritis (Scenario 7) although those with severe elbow involvement may develop ulnar neuropathy.

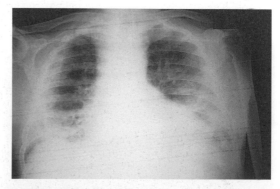

Figure 8.13   Chest X-ray showing basal interstitial shadowing in a patient with rheumatoid arthritis. This patient had a methotrexate-induced pneumonitis.

Polyarthritis

Scenario 7 – Carpal tunnel syndrome in a patient with rheumatoid arthritis

A 69-year-old woman with long-standing rheumatoid arthritis developed tingling in the fingers of her right hand. All fingers were affected, but especially the thumb, index and middle fingers. The tingling sometimes woke her in the early hours of the morning. She also found that she was having difficulty grasping her walking stick in her right hand.

On examination she had marked muscle wasting of the thenar eminence. Power was difficult to evaluate because of the rheumatoid hand deformities. There was no obvious sensory deficit. Tinel's sign was positive. Nerve conduction studies confirmed the clinical impression of median nerve compression and her symptoms improved after surgical decompression, which was performed under local anaesthetic.

Mucocutaneous

Rheumatoid arthritis. The classic lesion of rheumatoid arthritis is the rheumatoid nodule (Fig. 8.14), which typically occurs at points of mechanical stress such as over the olecranon. Nodules can ulcerate, and if this occurs over the sacrum can be very difficult to heal. Patients with nodules tend to be strongly seropositive for rheumatoid factor. In addition to nailfold infarcts, patients with vasculitis may develop cutaneous ulceration (Fig. 8.15).

Spondyloarthropathies. The rash of psoriasis may be very mild and unrecognised by the patient and so

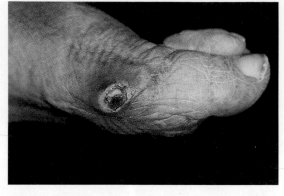

Figure 8.15   Vasculitic ulcer in a patient with rheumatoid arthritis.

should always be sought in the patient presenting with polyarthritis. Remember to examine the scalp. Psoriatic nail changes include pitting and onycholysis (separation of the nail from the nailplate). In reactive arthritis, a rash of the feet called 'keratoderma blennorrhagica' can occur (Fig. 8.16). This is clinically indistinguishable from the pustular variant of psoriasis, emphasising the overlap between different HLA-B27-related disorders. Other mucocutaneous features of reactive arthritis are mouth ulceration and balanitis.

Eye. Episcleritis and scleritis can occur in rheumatoid arthritis, and iritis in the

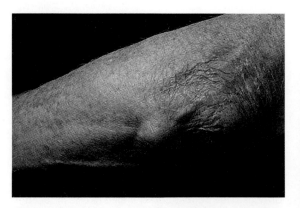

Figure 8.14   A rheumatoid nodule.

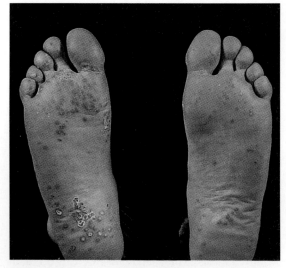

Figure 8.16   Keratoderma blenorrhagica.

spondyloarthropathies. Slit-lamp examination will confirm these diagnoses.

Investigations

Investigations are indicated in the patient with polyarthritis to:

- support a diagnosis suspected from the history and examination
- assess disease activity/severity and its response to treatment
- assess internal organ involvement
- identify/monitor drug toxicity.

Haematology

Chronic inflammation is associated with anaemia and a raised ESR, seen in patients with rheumatoid arthritis and the spondyloarthropathies when disease is active. These points have has already been mentioned in Chapter 4 but are worth repeating. The anaemia is usually normochromic and normocytic but can be hypochromic and microcytic, and reflects a failure of iron utilization. It is important to exclude iron deficiency. However, this can pose a diagnostic dilemma because ferritin is an acute-phase reactant and so serum ferritin (which is low in iron deficiency) may be 'falsely' elevated in patients with polyarthritis. Iron and serum iron binding capacity should be checked. Both are low in the anaemia of chronic inflammation, whereas in iron deficiency the serum iron is low but the iron binding capacity is raised. Bone marrow examination will show excessive iron in chronic inflammation, whereas iron will be absent in iron deficiency.

If a patient with polyarthritis is iron-deficient, this may be a result of NSAIDs, but other possible causes may require investigation.

Monitoring of the ESR is useful in assessing disease activity: as a patient's arthritis comes under control, so the ESR falls and the haemoglobin rises. Patients with chronic inflammation often have a raised platelet count.

Blood dyscrasias may occur as a result of treatment with 'disease-modifying' or immunosuppressive drugs. Regular full blood counts may detect bone marrow toxicity at an early stage.

Biochemistry

Patients with polyarthritis may demonstrate a polyclonal rise in immunoglobulins. The C-reactive protein (an acute-phase reactant) may be used to monitor disease activity in the same way as the ESR. Abnormalities of renal and liver function may denote renal or hepatic involvement of disease or drug toxicity.

Urinalysis

Proteinuria can occur as a result of drug toxicity (e.g. with gold or penicillamine), renal amyloidosis or (rarely) a glomerulonephitis, in which case the urinary sediment may be abnormal. It is worth mentioning amyloidosis in this chapter (Box 8.5), because although only a minority of patients with rheumatoid arthritis develop this complication of their disease, for those individuals it has a major effect on prognosis.

Serology

The rheumatoid factor and antinuclear factor should be checked in patients presenting with polyarthritis. Approximately 75% of patients with rheumatoid arthritis will at some point in their disease course be seropositive for rheumatoid factor. However, as discussed in Chapter 4, rheumatoid factor is not specific for rheumatoid arthritis. While a significant proportion of patients with rheumatoid arthritis are antinuclear antibody (ANA) positive, in an appropriate clinical setting (e.g. a young woman with photosensitivity and a symmetrical polyarthritis), a diagnosis of SLE should be considered.

HLA-typing

As already stated, there is an association between HLA-B27 and the spondyloarthropathies. Over 90% of patients with ankylosing spondylitis are HLA-B27-positive, but the association is weaker for the other spondyloarthropathies, and it should be remembered that around 10% of the healthy population are HLA-B27-positive.

There is much research currently ongoing into various HLA associations and the different types of polyarthritis. One recognised association is between HLA-DR4 and rheumatoid arthritis. However, HLA-DR typing is not currently used in

Box 8.5   Amyloidosis

Amyloidosis is a syndrome in which an insoluble protein complex is deposited extracellularly. Both hereditary and non-hereditary forms of amyloidosis occur. Non-hereditary forms may occur in association with a variety of chronic inflammatory diseases (in which case it is termed AA amyloid) or with monoclonal gammopathy (AL amyloid). Amyloid can be detected histologically by staining tissue with the dye Congo red: under polarising light amyloid shows apple-green birefringence (Fig. 8.17). If amyloidosis is suspected, then it can be looked for histologically on rectal biopsy or biopsy of, for example, kidney or any other organ suspected of being involved.

The most important point about amyloidosis with respect to rheumatic disease is that AA amyloidosis can occur as a complication of rheumatic disease associated with a marked acute phase response, especially rheumatoid arthritis and juvenile chronic arthritis. Those patients with long-standing, active disease are most at risk, although only a small proportion of these patients develop amyloidosis. The serum amyloid A precursor protein (produced during the acute-phase response) is processed into AA amyloid fibrils. The kidney is commonly involved, and patients usually present with proteinuria which can progress to renal failure. Prognosis is poor. Treatment is directed at suppressing the underlying acute-phase response.

AL amyloidosis, occurring in association with monoclonal gammopathy, including multiple myeloma, is also of relevance to rheumatologists because AL amyloid can be deposited periarticularly and cause arthropathy which can mimic rheumatoid arthritis.

A third form of amyloidosis, β_2-microglobulin amyloidosis, may occur in patients on haemodialysis (see Ch. 12). β_2-Microglobulin amyloid is deposited periarticularly. Carpal tunnel syndrome is a common feature.

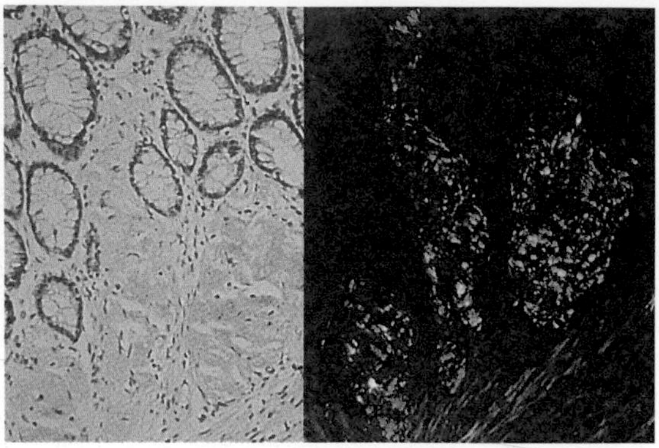

Figure 8.17   Bowel wall containing deposits of amyloid. These deposits stain pink with Congo red (left) and in polarized light (right) show typical yellow/green birefringence. Courtesy of Professor A J Freemont.

(Ch. 4). If there is any concern that a joint may be infected in a patient with polyarthritis, then that joint must be aspirated and the fluid sent for culture and an urgent Gram stain.

Imaging

X-rays may be useful in diagnosis and in staging of disease. In rheumatoid arthritis, the earliest X-ray change (as in other forms of inflammatory arthritis) is soft tissue swelling. This is followed by periarticular osteopenia, loss of joint space, bone erosion and, in some cases, eventual ankylosis. Figure 8.18 shows the hand X-ray of a patient with advanced rheumatoid arthritis. If X-rays of, for example, hands and feet are repeated after a certain time interval (e.g. 1 year), progression of disease may be evident.

In the spondyloarthropathies, X-rays of the sacroiliac joints may show sclerosis and erosions and later, in advanced disease, complete joint fusion (Fig. 8.19). Typical lumbar spine changes on lateral X-ray in ankylosing spondylitis are squaring of the lumbar vertebrae and syndesmophyte formation. In severe disease, the anterior longitudinal and interspinous ligaments may become ossified, resulting in the so-called 'bamboo spine' (Fig. 8.20). Lumbar spine changes may also be seen in the other spondyloarthropathies. Fusion of the apophyseal joints may be seen in the cervical spine (Fig. 8.21).

clinical practice and remains primarily a research tool.

Synovial fluid analysis

In polyarthritis, the synovial fluid is inflammatory

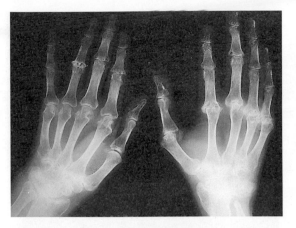

Figure 8.18 Hand X-ray of a patient with rheumatoid arthritis showing periarticular osteopenia, loss of joint space and erosions.

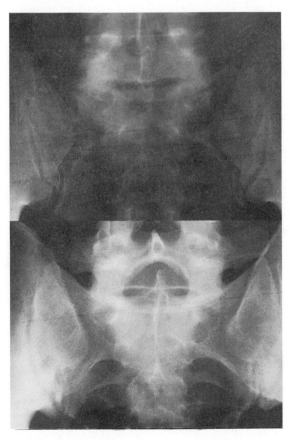

Figure 8.19 Sacroiliac X-rays showing normal appearances (top) and sacroiliitis (bottom) (with periarticular sclerosis and loss of distinction of the joint line bilaterally).

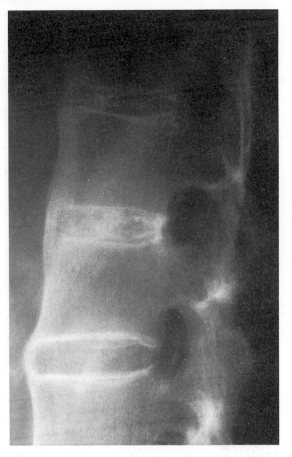

Figure 8.20 Typical lumbar spine X-ray appearances in advanced ankylosing spondylitis: 'bamboo spine' showing squaring of the vertebral bodies; calcification of the anterior ligaments and of the apophyseal joints posteriorly; and calcification of the intervertebral discs.

Other X-ray changes in the spondyloarthropathies include plantar spurs. In severe psoriatic arthritis with marked erosive disease, a 'pencil in cup' deformity may be seen, e.g. at the interphalangeal joints.

CT and MR scanning are useful in spinal assessment of polyarthritis, especially MR scanning in the assessment of the rheumatoid neck (Fig. 4.6).

Electrophysiology
The main indication is the assessment of entrapment neuropathy.

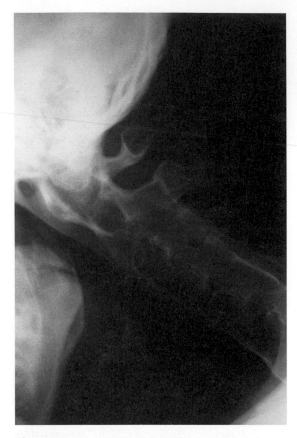

Figure 8.21 Cervical spine X-ray showing ankylosis of the apophyseal joints in a patient with ankylosing spondylitis. Calcification of the anterior spinal ligament is also evident.

Others

Other investigations may be required in the assessment of internal organ involvement. For example, in the patient in whom pulmonary fibrosis is suspected, chest X-ray and pulmonary function tests are indicated, and possibly high-resolution CT scanning (Fig. 8.22). Similarly, echocardiography is indicated in the patient with suspected pericardial or valvular heart disease.

MANAGEMENT

An approach to the management of polyarthritis is outlined in Box 8.6. There are two important concepts in the management of polyarthritis:

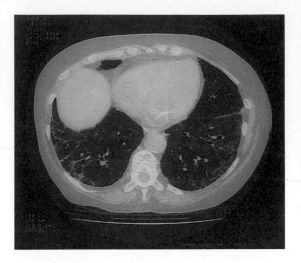

Figure 8.22 High-resolution CT scan of a patient with rheumatoid arthritis and interstitial fibrosis, in a mainly peripheral and basal distribution.

Box 8.6   Principles of management of polyarthritis

The management of polyarthritis is multidisciplinary.

- General measures
  — patient education
  — physiotherapy
  — occupational therapy (including splinting)
  — chiropody

- Drug treatment
  — symptomatic (analgesics and NSAIDs)
  — drugs with effects on disease activity ('disease-modifying' and immunosuppressants)
  — corticosteroids (including intra-articular)

- Surgery

- Treatment of acute flare
  — bed rest and joint aspiration/injection (once infection has been excluded)
  — review of drug treatment
  — graded exercise programme

- Effective management depends on a full assessment of disease activity and severity in each patient; what is appropriate in a patient with early, active inflammatory disease is inappropriate for a patient with 'end-stage' disease, with major joint destruction but little ongoing inflammation.

- The management of polyarthritis is multidisciplinary, delivered by a skilled multidisciplinary team (Ch. 5). Drug treatment is only one aspect of management.

In early disease, the emphasis is on suppressing inflammation, in order to suppress the underlying disease process and prevent joint destruction and deformity. Drug treatment with anti-inflammatory and 'disease-modifying' agents therefore plays a major role. In the patient at the other end of the spectrum, with 'burnt-out' disease (joint destruction but no inflammation), there is no place for potentially toxic 'disease-modifying' drugs: treatment should be with analgesics, occupational therapy (to provide home aids and appliances) and surgery as necessary. Physiotherapy is important at all stages of disease. Many patients fall midway between these two extremes: they have gone on to develop joint destruction and deformity but still have evidence of active inflammatory disease. These patients require disease-modifying therapy in addition to measures to minimise the effects of joint destruction.

Measurement of 'outcome'

One problem in the management of polyarthritis such as rheumatoid arthritis has been measurement of disease activity and severity. How do we know that treatment is effective? There are a number of measures which can be used, often in combination, e.g. duration of morning stiffness and the ESR. Changes on X-ray (e.g. the amount of joint space loss and the number of erosions on X-rays of the hands and feet) are also used to monitor disease progression. However, what is important to the patient is function, and a number of assessment methods based on function have been developed, e.g. the Health Assessment Questionnaire (HAQ). These can be used in the outpatient clinic.

General measures

Patient education

The majority of patients with rheumatoid arthritis and the spondyloarthropathies have chronic disease. Patient education is therefore important.

The disease, its therapy and the limitations of that therapy (including potential side-effects of drug treatment) must be discussed.

Drug treatment

While NSAIDs and analgesics could be included under the heading of 'general measures', as these are used to reduce symptoms without altering the course of the disease, we feel it best to discuss these below in the section on drug treatment.

Rest vs exercise

Acutely inflamed joints are usually rested and splinted in the position of optimum function. This may necessitate hospital admission for a patient with a severe flare. However, once the inflammation settles, a graded exercise programme should be commenced.

Physiotherapy

Physiotherapy is all-important in the management of patients with polyarthritis. Patients must be taught exercises to prevent joint deformity and strengthen muscles, which is important with respect to joint protection (Fig. 5.1). Many patients benefit from hydrotherapy if this is available (Fig. 5.2). Patients with ankylosing spondylitis must be taught a programme of home exercises to maintain their range of spinal movement.

Occupational therapy

The provision of simple and more complicated aids (Figs 8.23 and 8.24, and Fig. 5.4) minimises the effects of disability and may allow a patient who would not otherwise have done so to remain independent. The occupational therapist should visit the patient at home in order to assess their needs adequately. Many patients require advice regarding the suitability of their work. It may be possible for the workplace to be modified to allow a return to work.

Splinting

The use of splints may be recommended by the physiotherapist or occupational therapist. Resting splints (Fig. 8.25) allow the joint to be rested in a satisfactory position while acutely inflamed and 'working' wrist splints (Fig. 8.26) provide support while allowing some finger movement.

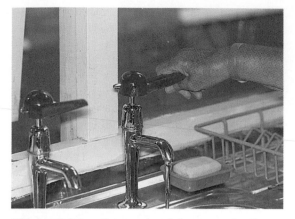

Figure 8.23 Occupational therapy aid: turning taps is difficult for many patients with hand problems.

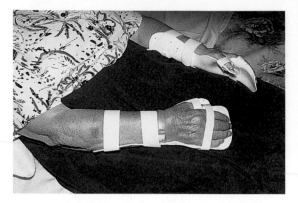

Figure 8.25 Resting wrist splint.

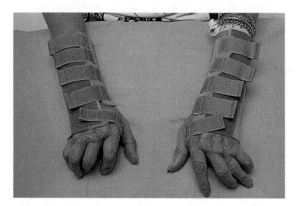

Figure 8.26 'Working' wrist splint.

Chiropody

Many patients with polyarthritis have foot problems. A chiropody assessment forms an important aspect of management. Treatment of callosities, prevention of foot ulcers and provision of suitable footwear, often with moulded insoles (Fig. 8.27), allow the patient to walk less painfully and therefore remain mobile.

Drug treatment of rheumatoid arthritis (Box 8.7)

The current approach to drug treatment is to commence with an NSAID. If NSAIDs fail to suppress the disease, then a 'disease-modifying' antirheumatic drug (DMARD) is added. These 'disease-modifying' drugs are sometimes termed 'slow-acting' anti-arthritic drugs (SAARDs) or

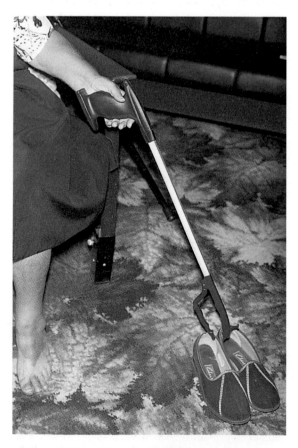

Figure 8.24 Occupational therapy aid.

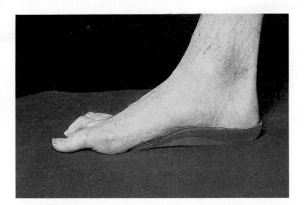

Figure 8.27 Provision of a moulded insole for a patient with rheumatoid arthritis and subluxation at the MTP joints. Courtesy of Mrs A Williams.

Box 8.7 Key points about drug treatment of rheumatoid arthritis

- There is no drug currently available which will 'cure' rheumatoid arthritis

- Some drugs control symptoms (e.g. NSAIDs), others modify disease activity ('disease-modifying' drugs, e.g. methotrexate)

- Most patients who have active rheumatoid arthritis require both a disease-modifying drug and an NSAID and/or analgesic

- Disease-modifying therapy should be commenced early, before irreversible joint damage has occurred

- All drugs used in the treatment of rheumatoid arthritis are potentially toxic: careful assessment of the risk–benefit ratio is therefore indicated for each patient

- Many of the disease-modifying drugs require safety monitoring, in order to identify toxicity at an early stage (e.g. monitoring of the blood count and urinalysis on gold)

- Oral corticosteroids are highly effective in controlling inflammation but their use is limited by their long-term toxicity (e.g. osteoporosis)

- Drug treatment is only one aspect of management

'second-line agents' (although the term 'second-line agent' is not usually taken to include immuno-suppressant drugs such as methotrexate). If the first disease-modifying agent is ineffective or not tolerated, then a second drug from this group is chosen, and if this second choice is ineffective or not tolerated, then a third is tried, and so on. Methotrexate, an immunosuppressant agent, is being used increasingly in the management of rheumatoid arthritis and also cyclosporin. Occasionally other immunosuppressants, e.g. cyclosporin, azathioprine or cyclophosphamide, are used in the patient refractory to other treatments.

Corticosteroids are used in a proportion of patients who have not responded to NSAIDs and 'disease-modifying' drugs. Some rheumatologists prescribe low-dose prednisolone in early disease. Corticosteroids (sometimes together with immunosuppressant drugs) may be indicated in patients with life-threatening internal organ involvement or vasculitis.

NSAIDs

These are the first-line treatment for inflammatory arthritis. NSAIDs are both anti-inflammatory and analgesic, but have no significant effect on modifying the underlying disease process. They are inhibitors of the enzyme cyclo-oxygenase and so have effects on prostaglandin synthesis. While inhibition of prostaglandin synthesis contributes to their mechanism of action, this is responsible also for many of the adverse effects of NSAIDs. Side-effects include: gastrointestinal toxicity (peptic ulceration, erosions, acute and occult gastrointestinal blood loss), fluid retention and reduced platelet aggregation. The potential toxicity of NSAIDs should not be overlooked, especially in the elderly, who often have comcomitant disease (e.g. cardiac failure, peptic ulceration) or who are on concomitant drug therapy (e.g. anticoagulants) which increase the risks of NSAID treatment.

There are many different NSAIDs and it is best to know a few well, e.g. aspirin (the prototype NSAID), ibuprofen, naproxen, indomethacin and diclofenac. Aspirin is seldom used as it is more toxic than other NSAIDs. Usually an NSAID is commenced in low dosage and increased if indicated and if tolerated. Before dismissing a particular NSAID as ineffective, it is important that the patient should have been on the maximum tolerated dose for at least 2 weeks. It is also worth noting that patients who find one NSAID ineffective may respond to another.

NSAIDs are usually given orally but many may also be given by suppository. Several NSAIDs are also available as sustained-release and enteric-coated preparations.

One recent exciting advance in the treatment of inflammatory joint disease with NSAIDs has been the development and introduction into clinical practice of what are termed 'selective COX-2 inhibitors'. These form a subgroup of NSAIDs. It is now well recognised that there are two isoforms of the enzyme cyclo-oxygenase (COX) – COX-1 and COX-2. It is believed that COX-1 is important in many homeostatic functions, such as maintenance of gastric mucosa integrity. In contrast, COX-2 expression is increased in inflamed tissues. It is hoped that selective inhibition of COX-2 will be effective at reducing inflammation, at the same time resulting in fewer side-effects (such as gastrointestinal toxicity) which are believed to be due mainly to inhibition of COX-1. Over the next few years, the place of these selective COX-2 inhibitors in the treatment of inflammatory joint disease should become apparent.

Simple analgesics

These are often required in addition to NSAIDs and disease-modifying agents, and in patients intolerant of NSAIDs. Examples include paracetamol, codeine, and various combination preparations such as coproxamol (paracetamol and dextropropoxyphene). Simple analgesics have no significant anti-inflammatory action.

Disease-modifying agents

Until we understand more fully the aetiopathogenesis of rheumatoid arthritis, it is unlikely that any drug treatment specific for the disease will become available. None of the currently used disease-modifying agents is effective in all patients, and their mechanisms of action in patients with rheumatoid arthritis are not well understood. These

drugs are often termed 'slow-acting' because none has an immediate effect in controlling inflammation, and they often take several weeks (sometimes months) to exert a beneficial effect. This must be explained to the patient, who should also be told to continue taking the NSAID.

All these drugs are potentially toxic and all therefore require some form of monitoring. This is especially true of immunosuppressant drugs. Before commencing disease-modifying therapy, therefore, the rheumatologist must weigh up the potential risks and benefits of that particular drug for that particular patient. Many patients stop disease-modifying therapy because of adverse effects (and others because of lack of efficacy), in which case an alternative drug is introduced.

With respect to safety monitoring, often this is shared between the patient's rheumatologist and GP. For example, most 'disease-modifying' drugs (with the exception of the antimalarials) require regular checking of the full blood count. In many hospitals the patient is issued with a drug monitoring booklet (Fig. 8.28) in which the GP enters the results of the blood monitoring; the patient can then bring this along to the rheumatology clinic. Safety monitoring is essential: if a drug cannot be monitored then it should not be prescribed.

The emphasis now is not to restrict disease-modifying therapy to patients with established, erosive disease but to prescribe this early in the course of the rheumatoid arthritis, in an attempt to prevent irreversible joint destruction. There is now an increasing tendency to prescribe disease-modifying drugs in combination.

Antimalarials. Hydroxychloroquine is the antimalarial most often used in rheumatoid

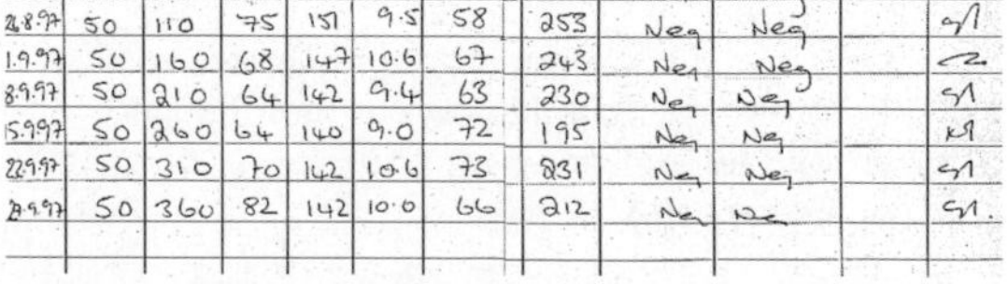

Date	Dose of Myocrisin mg.	Cumulative dose mg	BLOOD TESTS					URINE TESTS		Additional information	Signature
			ESR	Hb	WCC	% Neutrophils	Platelets	Proteinuria	Haematuria		
18.97	Test 10mg	10mg	95	147	10.3	65	257	Neg	Neg		CM
88.97	50	60	74	145	10.1	62	249	Neg	Neg		—
88.97	50	110	75	151	9.5	58	253	Neg	Neg		✓1
1.9.97	50	160	68	147	10.6	67	243	Neg	Neg		⊂2
8.9.97	50	210	64	142	9.4	63	230	Neg	Neg		✓1
5.9.97	50	260	64	140	9.0	72	195	Neg	Neg		✓1
22.9.97	50	310	70	142	10.6	73	831	Neg	Neg		✓1
29.97	50	360	82	142	10.0	66	212	Neg	Neg		✓1.

Figure 8.28 Monitoring booklet – the doctor or practice nurse writes in the blood results.

arthritis, although chloroquine is sometimes prescribed. Antimalarials are usually well tolerated, but rarely retinopathy can occur and it is usually recommended that patients prescribed antimalarials for rheumatoid arthritis should have regular eye checks. Antimalarials are also used in the treatment of SLE.

Sulphasalazine. Sulphasalazine comprises salicylic acid joined to sulphapyridine. A number of patients develop 'minor' side-effects, such as nausea or headache, which require discontinuation or dose reduction. Serious side-effects are rare, but occasionally blood dyscrasias or hepatotoxicity can occur and monitoring of the full blood count and liver function tests are required.

Penicillamine. Penicillamine may cause blood dyscrasias, nephrotoxicity, rashes and, rarely, autoimmune phenomena. The full blood count and urinalysis (looking for blood and protein) must be monitored regularly. Many patients experience altered taste on penicillamine; this side-effect usually resolves with continued use.

Gold. Gold is usually given by intramuscular (i.m.) injection although an oral preparation (auranofin) is available. Initially a 10 mg i.m. test dose is given, followed by 50 mg i.m. once weekly for 20 weeks, or until a response occurs, when the frequency of injections is reduced to fortnightly and then to monthly. If no response occurs after 1 g, gold is usually discontinued. As with penicillamine, blood dyscrasias, nephrotoxicity and rashes can occur and prior to each gold injection a full blood count and urinalysis should be checked (as in Scenario 1). Some patients on gold develop a pneumonitis.

Methotrexate. Methotrexate is a folic acid antagonist, and in recent years has become widely used in the treatment of rheumatoid arthritis. Methotrexate works more quickly than many of the other disease-modifying drugs: many patients experience benefit within 4–6 weeks. It is given orally once per week, although occasionally the intramuscular preparation is prescribed. Methotrexate can cause bone marrow suppression and therefore blood dyscrasias, gastrointestinal side-effects (including hepatotoxicity) and pulmonary toxicity, as well as increasing susceptibility to infection. Monitoring of the full blood count and of the plasma biochemistry, including liver function, is required. Folic acid is often co-prescribed with methotrexate, the rationale being that the addition of folic acid reduces the chance of methotrexate toxicity.

Other immunosuppressants. Cyclosporin is now being used to modify disease activity in rheumatoid arthritis. However, its use may be associated with hypertension and nephrotoxicity, and close monitoring of the blood pressure and renal function is required. Azathioprine (a purine analogue) and cyclophosphamide (an alkylating agent) are used in patients refractory to other treatments, or in patients with vasculitis. These immunosuppressants are all associated with an increased risk of infection and with blood dyscrasias, and so require blood monitoring. Cyclophosphamide may cause haemorrhagic cystitis and bladder malignancy, so regular checks for haematuria are also required.

Corticosteroids

Corticosteroids are potent anti-inflammatories, used in a wide number of conditions as well as in rheumatoid arthritis. However, their use (especially in the long term) is associated with a formidable range of adverse effects, including osteoporosis, myopathy, Cushing's syndrome, hypertension and increased susceptibility to infection. While the risk of adverse effects can be minimised by prescribing as low a dose as possible, nonetheless these remain a concern even at doses of below 10 mg daily. Corticosteroids are indicated when rheumatoid arthritis remains refractory to other treatment. In the elderly, it may be preferable to prescribe a small dose of prednisolone, rather than commence a 'slow-acting' drug necessitating frequent monitoring.

High-dose steroids are indicated for the treatment of vasculitis and internal organ involvement. *Intra-articular steroids* suppress inflammation in individual joints. For example, in a patient whose arthritis is under reasonable control apart from in one single joint, then that joint may be aspirated and injected with a long-acting steroid such as methylprednisolone acetate or triamcinolone hexacetonide, providing there is no possibility that the joint is infected.

Because patients prescribed prednisolone are at increased risk of osteoporosis, consideration should be given to measuring their bone density. If a patient is found to have osteoporosis then this should be treated appropriately (Ch. 11). The issue of prophylactic treatment (e.g. with bisphosphonates) for patients being prescribed steroids is currently a subject of much research and debate, but there is now an increasing trend to prescribe this. The rationale for prophylaxis is to prevent the bone loss that is likely to occur as a result of steroid treatment.

Possibilities for the future

As more is understood about the pathophysiology of rheumatoid arthritis, new treatments are being investigated. Examples include therapies directed against cytokines, T-cell receptors or class II major histocompatibility complex proteins, all of which are thought to be important in the pathogenesis of rheumatoid arthritis.

Specific therapies for extra-articular features

Sjögren's (sicca) syndrome. Artificial tears and artificial saliva preparations may provide some symptomatic relief.

Scleritis requires referral to an ophthalmologist. Systemic steroids and immunosuppressants may be required in severe cases.

Vasculitis, if severe or affecting internal organs, requires treatment with systemic corticosteroids and immunosuppressants.

Drug treatment of the spondyloarthopathies

This follows similar lines to the treatment of rheumatoid arthritis. Symptomatic treatment is with analgesics and NSAIDs. In ankylosing spondylitis, indomethacin may be more effective than other NSAIDs and is often used in high doses. Intra-articular steroids may be beneficial for single inflamed joints, as in rheumatoid arthritis.

Ankylosing spondylitis

The single most important aspect of treatment in patients with ankylosing spondylitis is to maintain an active exercise programme. NSAIDs help the patient to achieve this. Disease-modifying drugs are used in only a small proportion of patients: sulphasalazine is, in this situation, the drug of choice. Oral corticosteroids are best avoided.

Psoriatic arthritis

Disease-modifying therapy is indicated in patients whose disease is unresponsive to NSAIDs. The drugs most commonly used are sulphasalazine and methotrexate. Methotrexate suppresses both the psoriatic skin disease and the arthritis. Other options are gold and cyclosporin. Oral corticosteroids are very seldom used in the treatment of psoriatic arthritis.

Reactive arthritis

Antibiotic treatment is indicated if an organism is isolated. Sulphasalazine may be indicated for patients who, after their acute arthritis, go on to develop chronic joint inflammation.

Enteropathic arthritis

Care must be taken with NSAIDs in the patient with inflammatory bowel disease. If disease-modifying therapy is indicated, then sulphasalazine is generally considered drug of first choice.

Treatment of iritis

Iritis can occur in all forms of spondylo-arthropathy. The patient should be referred to an ophthalmologist: treatment is with topical corticosteroids and mydriatics.

Surgical management

Potential problems in the patient with polyarthritis

Specific care needs to be given to select the most appropriate surgical procedures for patients, to avoid surgery which may either be unsuccessful or not particularly helpful and to minimise the risk of complications. Some increased risk may be inevitable in rheumatoid surgery in some patients, but all such risks should be discussed with the patient prior to undertaking the operation.

Planning a sequence of operations. Patients with multiple joint arthritis pose particular problems of planning. Many of these patients require a sequence of operations and it is important that this sequence is carried out with both the minimum total number of in-patient stays and the correct order of operations (Scenario 8). Thus it is not helpful to perform a lower limb operation such as a hip replacement on a patient with rheumatoid arthritis, only to discover that they are completely unable to mobilise thereafter. This may be due to the severity of their upper limb arthritis rendering it impossible for them to use either crutches or a walking frame. The logical sequence of treatment in such a patient would be to improve upper limb function first and then perform the required lower limb surgery. Similar considerations arise if the patient has severely deformed feet, which may get infected either prior to corrective surgery or as a result of the surgery. If this patient also requires a joint replacement in the lower limb, it is logical to perform the foot surgery first both to allow the patient to mobilise well after the joint replacement and to minimise the risk of haematogenous spread from any infection on the foot to the joint replacement.

Scenario 8 – Rheumatoid arthritis – surgery

The patient, now aged 58 and with an 11-year history of rheumatoid arthritis, was seen at the combined rheumatology and orthopaedic clinic, complaining of severe pain in the right knee and in both elbows (especially the left). On examination there was very little in the way of joint inflammation of any of the peripheral joints. She had a 10° fixed flexion deformity of her right knee, with a 20° valgus deformity. She had normal peroneal nerve function. There was a rheumatoid nodule on her elbow and she was mostly tender around the radial head. Although there was a 15° block to full extension, flexion and extension of the elbow were not all that painful. Rotation of the forearm, however, was severely painful on the lateral side of the elbow.

The possibilities for surgery were discussed with patient. Although she would have preferred to have a knee replacement done first, the consultant explained that it would be difficult for her to use crutches with the elbow remaining as painful as it was, and accordingly surgery to the elbow was planned first: a synovectomy of the elbow and a radial head excision. A total knee replacement was proposed for the painful knee. Prior to her leaving the clinic, the surgeon arranged for her neck to be X-rayed, explaining that this was essential for patients with rheumatoid arthritis prior to anaesthetic. He also mentioned that she would need some extra steroids to 'cover' the operation (her drug treatment included prednisolone 7.5 mg daily).

The patient underwent the surgery as planned, first having the elbow operation and then the knee. Following the radial head excision and synovectomy, she had substantial pain relief in the elbow and found it easier to use the arm for activities such as cooking and dressing. She found the use of crutches important as, unfortunately, she developed a foot drop after her total knee replacement. The surgery was otherwise successful and she had a much straighter knee with a good range of movement of up to 90° of flexion and excellent pain relief. The foot drop recovered within 2 months, and she was then able to discard the crutches.

Skin problems and infection risk. Patients with polyarthropathy, particularly those with rheumatoid disease, are at relatively high risk of wound complications and infections after surgery, due to the rheumatoid disease itself or to the patient's drug treatment which, if including immunosuppressant drugs or corticosteroids, increases the risks of infection. These risks are further increased in a patient with rheumatoid disease due to the skin problems (thinning of skin and fragility) which frequently occur. Vasculitis may also complicate wound healing. There is some evidence that bone healing in rheumatoid arthritis is abnormally slow, and the severe osteoporosis which may accompany rheumatoid arthritis may cause difficulty in many bony operations including joint replacement and joint fusion.

Reconstruction of severe deformities. Rheumatoid arthritis affects most tissues in the body and may be associated with a remarkable degree of joint deformity. Such deformity, which is particularly noted in the feet, hands and knees, may pose severe technical problems during surgery. Thus, obtaining adequate correction of a severe valgus deformity of the knee may require the surgeon to accept the risk to the common peroneal nerve, which will inevitably be stretched to some degree, as occurred in Scenario 8.

Cervical spine instability.   An additional risk in rheumatoid arthritis is that posed by cervical spine instability. All patients with rheumatoid arthritis should have an assessment of neck stability prior to (general) anaesthetic, almost always including a flexion and extension lateral X-ray of the neck. All levels should be examined for the possibility of instability, although the atlanto-axial joint at C1/2 is the commonest site of severe instability (Fig. 8.11). Evidence of instability, including variation in the gap between the dens of the axis and the arch of the atlas (normal maximum measurement on lateral X-ray of 3 mm), should prompt assessment of the safety of surgery and consideration of cervical spine stabilisation prior to proceeding to other surgery. Otherwise gross instability may ensue, with a consequent risk of severe and permanent damage to the spinal cord; neck flexion during anaesthetic induction and intubation poses a particular risk. Surgery may be required both to decompress the spinal cord and to fuse the spine to minimise further instability.

Operations in patients with polyarthritis

Hands and wrist.   There are several operations which are almost specific to patients with polyarthritis. These include metacarpophalangeal (MCP) joint replacement in the hand and forefoot arthroplasty in the foot. The MCP joint arthroplasty is principally for patients who have severe ulnar drift of this joint consequent to rheumatoid arthritis. The surgery aims to correct the ulnar drift, improving hand function by permitting apposition of the thumb to finger tip. The commonly used prosthesis is the silastic Swanson replacement which acts as a spacer between the metacarpal head and the base of the proximal phalanx of the finger. Although it is possible to replace individual MCP joints, many

patients have disease affecting all of the fingers and consequently have multiple replacements.

Rheumatoid arthritis may affect extrasynovial structures around the hand, and a tendon rupture is particularly common on the ulnar side of the wrist in this disease. The extensor tendons are particularly affected. It is sometimes possible to restore function by tendon transfer, but

---

Box 8.9   Key points: polyarthritis

Rheumatoid arthritis
- **Rheumatoid arthritis is a common disease. It is the most common of the inflammatory arthritides.**
- **Women are more often affected than men.**
- **Although synovial inflammation is the major clinical feature, rheumatoid arthritis is a systemic disease, often with extra-articular features. Internal organ involvement can be life-threatening.**
- **Arthritis is symmetrical, with early involvement of the small joints of the hands and feet. No synovial joint is exempt.**
- **The disease course is characterised by relapses and remissions.**
- **Because synovitis erodes cartilage and articular bone, rheumatoid arthritis is often a destructive, deforming disease.**
- **Management is multidisciplinary.**

Spondyloarthropathies
- **There are four main forms of spondyloarthropathy:**
  - **ankylosing spondylitis**
  - **psoriatic arthritis**
  - **reactive arthritis (Reiter's syndrome)**
  - **enteropathic arthritis.**
- **All are HLA-B27 associated. There may be a family history of B27 related disease, e.g. ulcerative colitis.**
- **Enthesopathy is the pathological hallmark, but synovitis also occurs.**
- **Patients may present with involvement of the axial skeleton (spondylitis and/or sacroiliitis), the peripheral skeleton, or both.**
- **Peripheral joint involvement is usually assymmetrical, lower limb and large joint (except in psoriatic arthritis)**
- **All forms of spondyloarthropathy can be associated with extra-articular features**
- **Management is multidisciplinary.**

development of any tendon ruptures should provoke consideration of early surgery to minimise the risk of further ruptures. Such surgery includes protecting the remaining extensor tendons by placing them superficial to the extensor retinaculum, and removing sharp areas of bone which will commonly include the head of the ulna and the tubercle of Lister.

Foot and ankle. Many foot and ankle deformities occur in rheumatoid arthritis, resulting in ankle arthritis, valgus deformities in the hindfoot with flat feet (pes planus) and forefoot deformities which include clawing of the lesser toes with subluxation and dislocation of the MTP joints. The great toe is also affected, characteristically resulting in either a very stiff first MTP joint or marked hallux valgus. Surgical treatment includes shoes and corrective splints and callipers, fusions (arthrodesis) around the hindfoot and ankle to both correct deformity and hold this corrective position, and operations to treat the dislocated MTP joints. A common operation in these circumstances is excision of the lesser metatarsal heads which have adopted a prominent position in the sole of the foot and resulted in callosities and a sensation of walking on pebbles. This is known as forefoot arthroplasty, and although it may appear to be somewhat mutilating, it generally offers good and reliable results in patients with severe foot deformities.

Other joints. Knee, hip, elbow and shoulder replacements are commonly carried out in patients with polyarthritis. Pain relief is usually good, but functional benefits may be limited by arthritis in other joints. It is therefore important to be realistic about the likely outcome. Long-term results of total joint replacements in patients with rheumatoid arthritis generally compare well with those in osteoarthritis. This might appear surprising at first sight, due to the extremely osteoporotic bone into which such joint replacements are often implanted. However, these patients often place low demands on their joint replacements which may partly explain the low rate of loosening of the joint prostheses.

Many of these joints may also be treated by synovectomy. It is not possible to perform a complete synovectomy in any joint, and such surgery is not thought to prevent progression of rheumatoid arthritis. However, it may be helpful in patients with severe swelling in one or two joints (particularly the knees) and in whom it is felt that substantial increases or changes in medical treatment are not merited.

9 | Connective tissue diseases

Case history

A 35-year-old female was admitted with breathlessness and pleuritic pain. She had a temperature of 38°C. Air entry was poor at both lung bases and she had some basal crepltations. Her haemoglobin was 112 g/L, white blood count 3.1×10^9/L and platelets 115×10^9/L. ESR was 50 mm/h. Chest X-ray showed widespread patchy shadowing.

Despite broad-spectrum intravenous antibiotics (the presumptive diagnosis was pneumonia, possibly atypical pheumonia) her condition deteriorated, with falling Po_2. She was transferred to the intensive care unit. Because of her failure to respond to antibiotic treatment, and because the senior house officer reported that over the past 6 months she had been experiencing Raynaud's pheno-menon, a connective tissue disorder was queried and serum immunology checked. She was strongly positive for ANA (1/10 000 IgG), C3 and C4 were low, and she had antibodies to U1 RNP.

The most likely diagnosis was thought to be some form of connective tissue disease. After treatment with intravenous methylpredniso-lone, her clinical condltion improved and the infiltrates on the chest X-ray resolved. She was later commenced on oral prednisolone.

The connective tissue diseases (sometimes termed 'collagen vascular diseases') are a heterogenous group of diseases which affect connective tissues and blood vessels. At an undergraduate level, it is helpful to consider each as a distinct entity with its own characteristic features, recognising that in reality distinctions are less clear-cut. Certain important points with respect to both diagnosis and management are common to most of the connective tissue diseases. Most can be associated with circulating autoantibodies and are therefore often termed 'autoimmune' diseases.

These are complex diseases which are often difficult to diagnose and treat. Patients with connective tissue disease require specialist referral. It would be inappropriate in this textbook to include detailed descriptions of each individual disease. These can be found in larger texts. The main objective of this chapter is to make you aware of the importance of diagnosing these

---

Key points

- Connective tissue diseases are multisystem diseases, affecting connective tissue and blood vessels

- They are important to recognise because they can be life-threatening, but they are often difficult to diagnose

- Most are inflammatory (an exception is systemic sclerosis), with systemic features

- Usually the aetiology is unknown

- They are associated with abnormalities of the immune system

- Overlap between pathological and clinical features can occur between diseases

- Drug treatment for severe disease is usually with corticosteroids and/or immunosuppressant therapy

- All age groups (including children) can be affected

conditions, and when to suspect the diagnosis. You need to recognise the clinical features which make you think: 'Could this patient have connective tissue disease?' It is important to make the diagnosis early, because these conditions can be life-threatening and early treatment can be life-saving.

The connective tissue disorders which you are most likely to meet and of which you should have some knowledge are listed in Box 9.1. An important clinical point is that some patients have overlap syndromes in which features of more than one connective tissue disease may coexist. However, at this stage in your careers, you should concentrate on the typical case (if patients with connective tissue disease are ever typical!). This will give you the necessary framework from which you can then learn to recognise which features in individual patients are suggestive of an overlap syndrome. Some of these overlap syndromes are defined by a specific serological test, the best example of which is mixed connective tissue disease, which is defined by the presence of antibodies to an antigen termed U1 ribonucleoprotein (U1 RNP, as in the case described above).

All age groups (including children) can be affected by connective tissue disease. Classification criteria have now been established for most of the connective tissue diseases, details of which can be found in larger texts.

This chapter is divided into two main sections:

- A brief account of the aetiology and immunopathology of the connective tissue

---

Box 9.1   Connective tissue diseases

- Systemic lupus erythematosus (SLE) and antiphospholipid syndrome
- Systemic sclerosis
- Inflammatory muscle disease (polymyositis and dermatomyositis)
- Sjögren's syndrome and overlap conditions
- The vasculitides, including polymyalgia rheumatica

---

diseases, followed by the general approach to the patient with connective tissue disease, or in whom connective tissue disease is suspected. Important points in the history-taking and examination are outlined, and the approach to investigation and management. We are aware that this first section introduces diseases which you have not previously encountered. When this happens it may be useful to refer to the relevant section of the 'atlas' of connective tissue diseases which forms the second part of this chapter.

- An atlas of connective tissue diseases. This is essentially a series of 'disease-based' subsections, each comprising a case history, a set of key points and a diagram summarising the main clinical features. Note that all the connective tissue diseases are potentially systemic diseases associated with internal organ involvement and that by no means are all of the possible clinical manifestations of each disease covered in the diagrams.

Both these sections should be read together. Some of you may prefer to read the case histories in the atlas first of all, to give you an insight into the spectrum of clinical problems with which patients with connective tissue disease present.

AETIOLOGY AND PATHOGENESIS

In most connective tissue diseases the aetiology and pathogenesis are unknown. However, we now know far more than we did 10 years ago about the molecular and cellular biology of these diseases, and much research is currently underway to elucidate how these different molecular and cellular mechanisms interact to produce characteristic patterns of tissue damage.

In most connective tissue diseases the aetiology is likely to be multifactorial, involving a combination of genetic and environmental factors. As with rheumatoid arthritis and many other rheumatic diseases, it is likely that some environmental agent, acting via a cascade of interrelated events, triggers disease in a genetically predisposed host. The relative importance of genetic and environmental factors may vary

Musculoskeletal medicine and surgery
137
Connective tissue diseases

between patients. Specific examples of environmental agents being important in aetiology are as follows:

- Certain drugs can induce systemic lupus erythematosus (SLE), e.g. hydralazine and procainamide. Usually drug-induced lupus is less severe than idiopathic disease.
- Systemic sclerosis can occur after exposure to certain toxins, such as vinyl chloride.
- Hepatitis B has been associated with certain forms of vasculitis, such as polyarteritis nodosa.

Both cellular and humoral immunological mechanisms are involved in the pathogenesis of connective tissue diseases, most of which are associated with circulating autoantibodies. For example, in SLE, excessive B-lymphocyte activity results in hypergammaglobulinaemia, production of a variety of non-organ-specific antibodies, and immune complex formation. It is not known what drives this B-cell activity. In SLE, abnormalities of T-cell and accessory (antigen-presenting) cell function occur in addition to abnormalities of B-cell function. It is likely that in SLE these abnormalities interrelate, and that there is a loss of the normal T-cell control over B-cell function. This is an area of much research, including research into animal models of lupus (several strains of mice spontaneously develop clinical and serological abnormalities similar to SLE). One clinical consequence of this autoantibody excess is that, in SLE, circulating immune complexes (antigen–antibody complexes) are deposited in the microvasculature, where they may trigger complement activation and an inflammatory response. This complement activation reduces the ability of the patient to clear immune complexes from the circulation, allowing further deposition in the tissues. This induces further inflammation and more complement consumption, thereby perpetuating a vicious cycle. Some patients with SLE have genetic deficiencies of the complement pathway, further exacerbating the process in this subgroup of patients. As well as causing tissue injury via immune complex-mediated mechanisms, autoantibodies can cause disease by direct binding to cell surfaces, e.g. in autoimmune thrombocytopenia.

Therefore, by taking SLE as an example, it can be seen that the pathogenesis of the connective tissue diseases is complex and incompletely understood. Theories regarding the important mechanisms vary between diseases, but abnormalities of the immune system are always likely to play a key role. In systemic sclerosis, abnormalites of the microvasculature and of collagen production also play a key role.

PATHOLOGY

An important point to make here is that, in the connective tissue diseases, pathology (from a biopsy specimen) may make/confirm a diagnosis or may influence treatment decisions. Pathology varies between diseases.

SLE

Two sites where immunopathological changes are classically seen in SLE are the skin and kidney. In the skin, deposits of immunoglobulin and complement components are observed along the dermal–epidermal junction, not only at the site of cutaneous lesions but also in 'normal skin' of many patients with SLE. These deposits are detected by their characteristic immunofluorescence (the 'lupus band' test). Renal biopsies from patients with renal involvement of SLE may demonstrate a variety of changes. There may be mild mesangial changes only, or conversely, especially in proliferative glomerulonephritis, there may be a marked inflammatory response with necrosis, going on eventually to scarring with sclerosis and fibrosis (Fig. 9.1).

Systemic sclerosis

Excessive fibrosis (typically seen in the skin, which is thickened, but also occurring in internal organs) and characteristic vascular changes occur. These vascular changes can result in marked arterial narrowing (Fig. 9.2).

Inflammatory muscle disease

Histology of muscle from a patient with polymyositis shows injured, dying and regenerating muscle cells, with an inflammatory cell infiltrate (Fig. 9.3). In later stages of the

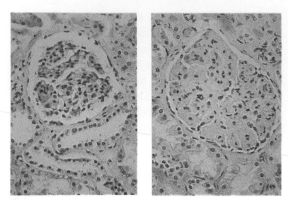

Figure 9.1 By comparison with the normal glomerulus on the left, that on the right is expanded and shows an increase in the number of cells and gross thickening of the basement membrane. Courtesy of Professor A J Freemont.

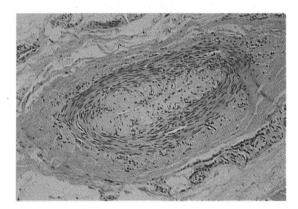

Figure 9.2 A digital artery from a patient with systemic sclerosis. There is gross thickening of the intima with an amorphous, as yet uncharacterised, material. Courtesy of Professor A J Freemont.

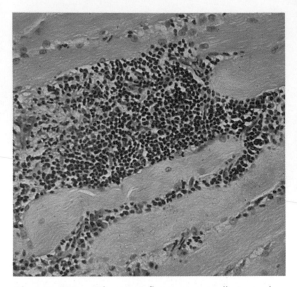

Figure 9.3 Chronic inflammatory cells typical of polymyositis. Courtesy of Professor A J Freemont.

blood vessel is the characteristic feature, often accompanied by necrosis (necrotising vasculitis). When the whole of the blood vessel wall is affected, vessel stenosis/occlusion can occur, leading to infarction (Fig. 9.4). If only part of the vessel wall is affected, then an aneurysm may

disease, muscle may be replaced by fibrosis and fat.

Vasculitides

These are a group of diseases characterised by inflammation of the blood vessel wall (vasculitis). Their classification is usually based on the size of the blood vessel wall affected by the inflammatory process (Table 9.1, p. 156). The diagnosis of vasculitis is often made on the basis of histological change on biopsy. An inflammatory infiltrate of the

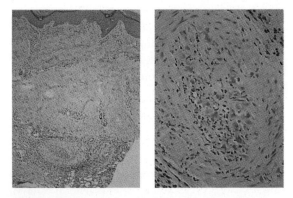

Figure 9.4 Section of skin with epidermis uppermost (left). In the subcutaneous tissue is a small artery showing the changes of a vasculitis (right). The artery has been enlarged and shows inflammation of the intima and occlusion of the lumen. Courtesy of Professor A J Freemont.

form. Aneuryms may rupture. Granulomas are seen in several of the vasculitides:

- Giant cell arteritis
- Takayasu's arteritis
- Churg–Strauss arteritis
- Wegener's granulomatosis.

CLINICAL FEATURES

Careful clinical assessment is required to establish the diagnosis or, in the patient known to have connective tissue disease, to establish disease activity and severity.

History

When a diagnosis of connective tissue disease is suspected, it is essential to take a full history: these are multisystem diseases. For example, in the patient with unspecified vasculitis, no tissue/organ is exempt. An immediate question might be: 'But how do I know to suspect connective tissue disease?' Features pointing to a possible diagnosis of connective tissue disease are listed in Box 9.2. *Always* suspect connective tissue

---

> **Box 9.2 Features consistent with a diagnosis of connective tissue disease**
>
> - Tiredness, non-specific malaise, often weight loss
> - Unexplained fever
> - Multisystem disease which is usually inflammatory
> - Joint or muscle inflammation
> - Splinter haemorrhages or a vasculitic rash
> - Raynaud's phenomenon – episodic digital ischaemia usually in response to temperature change
> - Features consistent with internal organ ischaemia
> - Anaemia (usually normochromic, normocytic) and an acute-phase response, e.g. raised ESR or C-reactive protein

---

disease (including vasculitis) in a patient who presents with multisystem inflammatory disease. Because clinical features are often non-specific, especially in the early stages of disease, a patient may have been unwell for some time without a diagnosis being made. The principles of history-taking are described in Chapter 2. Only relevant points in the systemic enquiry and drug history are mentioned here.

Presenting complaint

There is a wide range of possible presenting complaints reflecting the multisystem nature of the disease. Some examples are given in the case histories.

Systemic enquiry

General. Ask about tiredness and weight loss. Patients may report feeling feverish and while this may be part of a generalised inflammatory process (e.g. SLE), always follow this up by asking about symptoms of infection, to which patients may be predisposed either as a result of their disease or as a result of its treatment. Note also that there are associations between some of the connective tissue diseases and malignancy (see below), and so always consider the possibility (albeit usually unlikely) that some symptoms or signs may be a result of neoplasia rather than of the connective tissue disease itself.

Skin, mucous membranes and Raynaud's phenomenon. Ask about rashes: SLE, derma-tomyositis and the vasculitides can all be associated with rashes. Hair loss (which may be patchy or diffuse) is a distressing and common complaint in patients with SLE. Ask also about mouth ulcers, which occur in SLE and also in Behçet's syndrome (which is also associated with genital ulceration). Mouth dryness is a feature of Sjögren's syndrome.

Raynaud's phenomenon is the term used to describe episodic colour changes of the hands in cold weather, due to digital vasospasm. The fingers classically turn white (reflecting ischaemia) then blue/purple (reflecting deoxygenation of the blood), then red (reflecting reperfusion hyperaemia). Raynaud's phenomenon can be primary (idiopathic) or secondary (the differential diagnosis of Raynaud's phenomenon is given in Box 9.3. The significance of Raynaud's phenomenon to the rheumatologist is that it can be a feature of several of the connective tissue diseases. 'Alarm bells' indicating that Raynaud's is unlikely to be primary are as follows:

- The patient developed Raynaud's phenomenon when middle aged or elderly. Primary Raynaud's is most common in young women, occurring in as many as 20%.
- The Raynaud's is so severe that irreversible tissue loss has occurred, such as loss of the finger pulp (digital pitting).
- There are clinical features of connective tissue disease, such as skin thickening (scleroderma).
- Serological testing is suggestive of connective tissue disease, e.g. a high titre of antinuclear antibody (ANA).

Musculoskeletal. Ask about joint pain, swelling and stiffness: arthralgias and arthritis are common features of connective tissue disease. Proximal muscle pain and weakness may reflect polymyositis. Therefore, ask: 'Do you have difficulty in getting out of a chair?' Always remember the possibility of myopathy due to chronic use of corticosteroids.

Cardiorespiratory. As with all rheumatic diseases which may be multisystem, ask about cardiorespiratory symptoms such as breathlessness and/or pleuritic chest pain, which may reflect anaemia, cardiac or pulmonary involvement including infection or pulmonary embolism, especially in patients with an antiphospholipid syndrome, which is discussed later.

Gastrointestinal. Swallowing difficulty is characteristic of systemic sclerosis; note that the gastrointestinal dysmotility of systemic sclerosis can affect the small and large bowel as well as the oesophagus, but oesophageal dysmotility is most commonly recognised. If a patient with connective tissue disease has abdominal pain, consider intestinal ischaemia due to, for example, mesenteric artery vasculitis.

Renal. Remember that ankle swelling can be a sign of nephrotic syndrome (occurring especially in SLE, as in Case history, p. 150), as well as of cardiorespiratory pathology.

Neuropsychiatric. SLE is the connective tissue disease most likely to be associated with neuropsychiatric manifestations (see Fig. 9.12, p. 151). Involvement of central, peripheral or autonomic nervous systems may occur in SLE, as well as cognitive dysfunction and psychiatric disturbance, and so a wide variety of clinical presentations is possible, including headaches and seizures. An important clinical point is that neuropsychiatric features may occur not only as a primary manifestation of connective tissue disease but also as a result of drug treatment (e.g. corticosteroids), infection, hypertension, metabolic imbalance (e.g. uraemia) or coagulation problems (e.g. in the antiphospholipid syndrome; see below).

Remember that patients with connective tissue disease often become depressed in reaction to having a chronic disease.

Eyes. Patients with Sjögren's complain of dry, gritty eyes.

Drug history
This is important because:

Box 9.3   Main differential diagnosis of Raynaud's phenomenon

Primary Raynaud's phenomenon (Raynaud's disease)

Secondary Raynaud's phenomenon (Raynaud's syndrome)
- **Secondary to connective tissue disease**
  - **systemic sclerosis**
  - **inflammatory muscle disease**
  - **systemic lupus erythematosus**
  - **overlap syndromes**
- **Secondary to mechanical vascular obstruction**
  - **cervical rib**
- **Secondary to use of vibratory tools**
  - **vibration white finger**
- **Secondary to drug treatment**
  - **beta-blockers**
  - **ergotamine**
- **Secondary to increased blood viscosity**
  - **paraproteinaemia**
  - **cryoglobulinaemia**

- connective tissue disease (e.g. SLE and small vessel vasculitis) and muscle weakness can all be related to drug treatment – always take a careful drug history and ask yourself: 'Could this illness possibly be a result of the drug treatment?'
- drugs used to treat the patient's connective tissue disease may cause adverse effects.

One diagnostic challenge is when a patient being treated with prednisolone for polymyositis develops progression of muscle weakness. Is this active disease requiring an increase in therapy, or is it a corticosteroid-related myopathy requiring a reduction in prednisolone?

Examination

Only specific points will be highlighted. A full clinical examination is required for the same reason as a detailed history: these are multisystem diseases. Therefore, look for signs of the clinical manifestations outlined in Figures 9.13–9.16 and 9.18–9.24 (in the 'atlas' below).

General examination

Fever can occur in active connective tissue disease. However, as patients with connective tissue disease (especially SLE) may be predisposed to infection, both as a result of their disease (with abnormalities of immune function and complement deficiency) and as a result of its treatment (with corticosteroids or immuno-suppressants), a source of infection should be actively sought.

Skin and mucous membranes

The following lesions are suspicious of a connective tissue disorder. While for the purposes of this chapter these have been grouped by disease (and summarised in Box 9.4), the main point always is to examine the skin and mucous membranes carefully in any patient in whom you suspect connective tissue disease.

SLE. Certain characteristic rashes occur. A photosensitive skin rash (typically a 'butterfly' facial rash) is one of the cardinal clinical features of SLE (Fig. 9.5). More chronic cutaneous lesions in

---

Box 9.4   Typical skin manifestations in connective tissue disease

- **SLE**
  — photosensitive ('butterfly' rash)
  — alopecia
  — mouth ulcers

- **Antiphospholipid syndrome**
  — livido reticularis

- **Systemic sclerosis**
  — scleroderma (skin thickening)
  — digital pitting/digital ulceration
  — telangiectasiae
  — calcinosis

- **Dermatomyositis**
  — facial rash ('heliotrope') with periorbital oedema
  — Gottron's papules

- **Vasculitis**
  — splinter haemorrhages and nailfold infarcts
  — palpable purpura
  — oral and genital ulcers in Behçet's syndrome

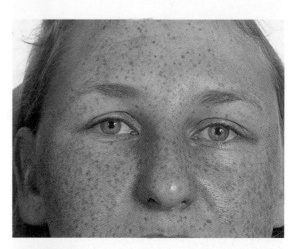

Figure 9.5   'Butterfly' rash of SLE. Courtesy of Dr J Yell.

sun-exposed areas may be a manifestation of a related condition termed discoid lupus. This condition is confined to the skin: lesions are initially erythematous but then develop thick

Connective tissue diseases

scale. A livido rash (Fig. 9.6) should make you think of an antiphospholipid syndrome (discussed below), which may occur in association with SLE.

Alopecia occurs in SLE (and scarring alopecia in discoid lupus). It may also occur as a side-effect of immunosuppressant treatment. Patients with SLE often develop mouth ulcers.

Systemic sclerosis. The most characteristic clinical feature is skin tightening (scleroderma). Usually, the hands, feet and face are affected first. The typical facial appearance, with loss of skin folds, a pinched nose and small mouth (Fig. 9.7), often allows an immediate diagnosis. Scleroderma of the fingers is termed 'sclerodactyly'. Systemic sclerosis is divided into two main subtypes:

- limited cutaneous systemic sclerosis, when skin involvement is confined to the extremities and face

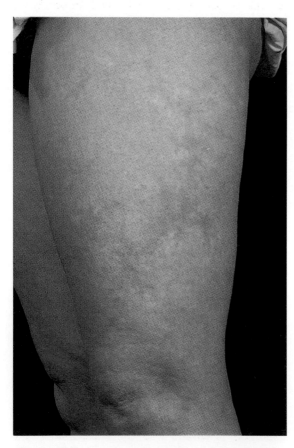

Figure 9.6 Livido reticularis.

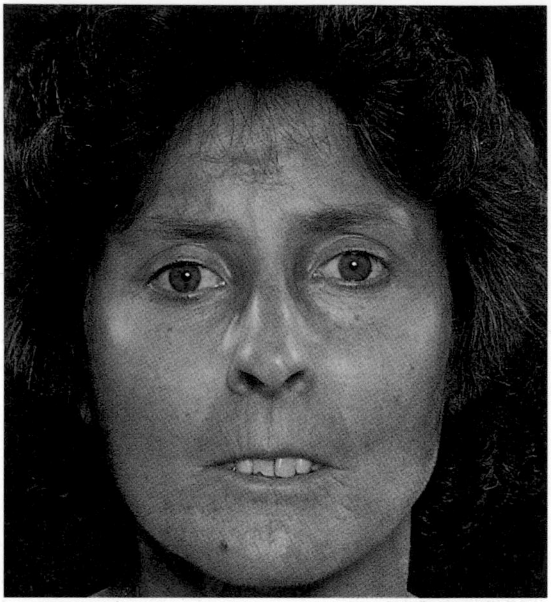

Figure 9.7 Typical facies in a patient with systemic sclerosis.

- diffuse cutaneous disease, when at its worst the skin of the whole body may become sclerodermatous.

The limited cutaneous variant of systemic sclerosis is sometimes termed the CREST variant of systemic sclerosis (**C**alcinosis, **R**aynaud's, o**E**sophageal dysmotility, **S**clerodactyly, **T**elangiectasiae).

Skin thickening can result in reduced range of movement and contractures, which can be very marked in the fingers, leading to loss of function and predisposing to finger ulcers over the proximal and distal interphalangeal joints (Fig. 9.8). However, the fingertip is the most common site of digital ulceration, and loss of tissue of the finger pad ('digital pitting') is a well recognised feature of systemic sclerosis. This appearance may be associated with bony resorption of the tuft of the distal phalanx on hand X-ray. In a minority of patients with systemic sclerosis, digital ulceration and/or ischaemia can be so severe that irreversible tissue damage can occur, with gangrene, and amputation may be required.

Calcinosis and telangiectasiae (Figs 9.9 and 9.10) may occur especially in the limited cutaneous

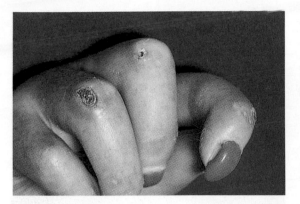

Figure 9.8   Scleroderma of the fingers (sclerodactyly) with ulceration. Note the tight, shiny skin.

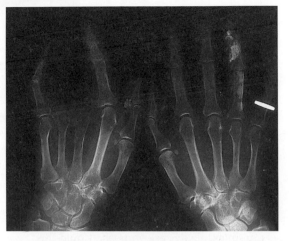

Figure 9.10   Hand X-ray showing calcinosis in a patient with systemic sclerosis. Note the amputations.

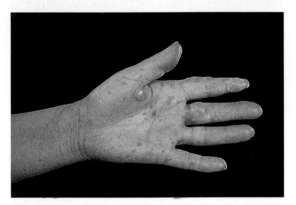

Figure 9.9   The hand of a patient with limited cutaneous systemic sclerosis, showing marked calcinosis and telangiectasiae. Note the loss of finger pulp.

(CREST) variant of systemic sclerosis. Calcinosis occurs most commonly in the finger pads and forearms, and telangiectasiae on the face and hands.

Scleroderma (skin thickening) can occur in a small number of conditions other than systemic sclerosis, such as porphyria cutanea tarda, and scleroderma can be 'localised' (occurring without internal organ involvement). Localised scleroderma can be divided into linear scleroderma (seen in children, although rare) and morphoea (discrete plaques of skin thickening).

Dermatomyositis.   The rash of dermatomyositis most commonly affects the face (sometimes with periorbital oedema, with heliotrope discoloration of the upper eyelids), neck and upper back, extensor aspects of the hands, elbows and knees and the periungal areas. Erythematous plaques over the dorsal aspects of the small joints of the hands are termed Gottron's papules.

Vasculitis.   Typical lesions include splinter haemorrhages (Fig. 3.6, p. 19), nailfold infarcts (Fig. 8.6, p. 116) and palpable purpura. If you see any of these always query a diagnosis of vasculitis and search for evidence of vasculitis elsewhere. Digital cyanosis progressing to gangrene can occur in patients with vasculitis as well as in systemic sclerosis. Mucous membrane ulcers (oral and genital) are characteristic features of Behçet's syndrome. Remember that vasculitis can occur in association with most connective tissue diseases (e.g. SLE) and in rheumatoid arthritis.

Musculoskeletal

SLE.   Look for evidence of arthritis and/or tenosynovitis. Hands, wrists and knees are commonly affected. Unlike in rheumatoid arthritis, the arthritis is seldom erosive but can be deforming. This can be seen in the fingers when 'swan-necking' occurs. Unlike in rheumatoid, this swan-necking is usually reversible (can be passively corrected). This deforming, non-erosive arthritis is termed 'Jaccoud's arthritis',

Systemic sclerosis. Marked fixed flexion deformities can occur, especially at the fingers and elbows.

Inflammatory muscle disease. Test muscle power and check for muscle tenderness. Proximal muscle weakness and tenderness are suggestive of inflammatory muscle disease.

Nervous system

While a range of neurological signs may be elicited depending upon the underlying pathology, important points are as follows:

- If a patient has a mononeuritis, or mononeuritis multiplex, always ask yourself: 'Could this patient have vasculitis?'
- Peripheral neuropathy occurs in a variety of connective tissue diseases.
- Always have a high index of suspicion of meningitis in an unwell patient with SLE, drowsiness and possibly fever. Aseptic meningitis in SLE has been reported, but bacterial meningitis is always of concern in this clinical context.

Investigations

As these are complex multisystem diseases which may be difficult to diagnose, have variable clinical courses and which may be treated with potentially toxic drugs, a number of investigations are often indicated in any one patient. The exact investigations indicated will vary from patient to patient but some broad generalisations can be made. It would be true to say that most patients with connective tissue disease (or in whom connective tissue disease is suspected) will, on presentation, require the following investigative 'work-up':

- a full blood count
- a plasma biochemical profile
- assay of an acute-phase reactant, usually the ESR or C-reactive protein
- Dipstix testing of urine, and microscopy of urine
- immunology tests, including antinuclear antibody (ANA)

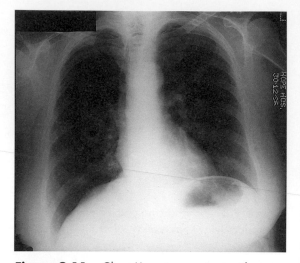

Figure 9.11 Chest X-ray in a patient with Wegener's granulomatosis, showing multiple ill-defined opacities with probable cavitation of the lesion of the right mid zone. Courtesy of Dr R Chisholm.

- a chest X-ray (Fig. 9.11)
- other tests as clinically indicated.

Only the broad principles will be discussed here.

Haematology

Patients with active connective tissue disease often have a normochromic normocytic anaemia ('anaemia of chronic disease'), a high ESR and a slightly raised platelet count. However, this is not true of systemic sclerosis or primary antiphospholipid syndrome, which unlike the others are not inflammatory diseases. If the ESR is high in a patient with systemic sclerosis you should suspect an overlap syndrome or some additional pathology.

Active SLE is associated with a fall in the haemoglobin, white cell and platelet count. A lymphopenia is characteristic. Autoimmune haemolytic anaemia can occur (as in Case history on p. 149). An eosinophilia occurs in patients with Churg–Strauss syndrome.

The full blood count must be monitored in patients on immunosuppressive treatment. One clinical dilemma is what to do when a patient with SLE on, for example, azathioprine develops a pancytopenia. Is this a result of active SLE (necessitating an increase in treatment) or is this azathioprine toxicity (necessitating reduction or discontinuation of azathioprine)? If there is no other evidence of active disease (with normal ESR and negative double-stranded DNA antibodies; see below) then the pancytopenia is probably drug-induced. Bone marrow examination may be helpful.

Blood biochemistry

Plasma biochemical profile. Always check the plasma biochemical profile. Abnormalities may suggest internal organ involvement (renal, hepatic) which was not clinically suspected.

C-reactive protein. This is typically raised in active inflammatory disease, although it is not usually raised in active SLE unless serositis (inflammation of the serosal linings, e.g. peritonitis, pleuritis) is present: a raised CRP level in an unwell patient with SLE should prompt a search for concomitant infection.

Muscle enzymes. Certain enzymes which leak from damaged skeletal muscle are useful diagnostically and in monitoring disease activity and response to treatment; therefore, if inflammatory muscle disease is suspected check the muscle enzymes. Creatine phosphokinase is the most sensitive: blood levels may be very high in the patient presenting with polymyositis. Raised levels of aldolase, transaminases and lactate dehydrogenase may also be a result of muscle inflammation.

Urine

An abnormal Dipstix may be the first clue to renal involvement of connective tissue disease. A glomerulonephritis can occur in association with either SLE or the vasculitides; Dipstix may show proteinuria and/or haematuria, with microscopy showing an 'active sediment' with white and red blood cells and casts. Haematuria alone can occur in renal vasculitis.

In a patient with renal involvement of connective tissue disease, a 24-hour urine collection allows quantitation of proteinuria and estimation of creatinine clearance.

Immunology

The connective tissue diseases are associated with circulating autoantibodies, some of which are fairly disease-specific and so are useful diagnostically. As well as being disease-specific, certain antibodies to specific antigenic components tend to be associated with certain clinical disease subtypes.

In a patient who presents with what may be a connective tissue disease (e.g. fever, a few splinter haemorrhages, a normochromic anaemia and a raised ESR), the following 'immunological screen' is indicated:

- *Antinuclear antibody (ANA).* This is a non-specific test (Ch. 4). Over 95% of patients with SLE are ANA-positive.
- *Antibodies to double-stranded DNA (dsDNA).* These are highly specific for SLE, and the level of these antibodies can be a useful measure of disease activity. However, not all patients with active SLE have raised circulating levels of dsDNA antibodies.
- *Antibodies to specific antigens.* These are more disease-specific than the ANA. Detailed descriptions are outwith the scope of this textbook but some useful disease/antibody associations are listed in Box 9.5. Which antibodies are requested depends on the clinical scenario, but *always remember to check for ANCA (see below) if vasculitis is a possibility.*

   It is important to note that not all patients with the disease have these 'disease-specific' antibodies. For example, only around 30% of patients with the diffuse cutaneous variant of systemic sclerosis have antibodies to Scl-70.
- *Complement* (Ch. 4). Low levels of circulating complement (C3, C4 and CH_{50}) may be found in some forms of active vasculitis (e.g. in patients with circulating cryoglobulins see below) and in SLE.

While the above immunological tests are the main 'screening' immunological tests, two others need to be highlighted.

Cryoglobulins. Cryoglobulins are immunoglobulins which precipitate when cold, and can occur in association with connective tissue disease (e.g. SLE), infections (particularly hepatitis C) or

Box 9.5   Associations between connective tissue diseases and serum autoantibodies

SLE
This is associated with anti-Sm, anti-Ro (SS-A), anti-La (SS-B) and antihistone antibodies. Anti-Ro and anti-La tend to be associated with Sjögren's syndrome which may be secondary to SLE. Antihistone antibodies are characteristic of drug-induced SLE. Neonatal lupus syndrome consists of a transient rash in the newborn period and/or complete heart block. It occurs in a minority of infants whose mothers have antibodies to either anti-Ro or anti-La.

Systemic sclerosis
Anticentromere antibodies are associated with limited cutaneous systemic sclerosis and antibodies to the extractable nuclear antigen Scl-70 with diffuse systemic sclerosis.

Inflammatory muscle disease
In recent years, a number of antibodies specific to inflammatory muscle disease have been described, and these may be associated with specific disease subsets. The most frequently identified muscle-specific antibody is anti Jo-1, and patients with this antibody frequently have interstitial lung disease.

Sjögren's syndrome
This is associated with anti-Ro and anti-La antibodies. Patients with Sjögren's syndrome often have hypergammaglobulinaemia.

Overlap syndromes
Antibodies to U1 RNP (ribonucleoprotein) must, by definition, be present for the diagnosis of the overlap syndrome 'mixed connective tissue disease'.

Vasculitis
The description of antineutrophil cytoplasmic antibodies (ANCAs) has been a major step forward in the identification and classification of the vasculitides. ANCAs are found in the systemic vasculitides, especially in Wegener's granulomatosis. Staining for ANCA can be either diffuse cytoplasmic (cANCA) or perinuclear (pANCA). cANCA is highly specific for Wegener's granulomatosis. While pANCA also occurs in Wegener's, it can also be associated with other forms of vasculitis.

Box 9.6   Antiphospholipid syndrome

Antiphospholipid syndrome can be either primary or secondary to connective tissue disease e.g. SLE. It is characterised by antibodies to phospholipids (although recent research suggests that the antibodies may be primarily directed against cofactors, such as B_2-glycoprotein I).

Main clinical features
• Thromboses (either arterial or venous)
• Pregnancy loss
• Thrombocytopenia

Laboratory features
• Anticardiolipin antibodies (moderate or high titre)
• Lupus anticoagulant

malignancy. Circulating cryoglobulins may also be associated with a vasculitis. Therefore always check cryoglobulin levels if features of vasculitis are present. Cryoglobulins may be monoclonal (in which case underlying myeloma should be suspected) or mixed.

Testing for antiphospholipid syndrome. If a patient is suspected of having an antiphospholipid syndrome (Box 9.6), there are two main types of test to detect antiphospholipid antibodies:

• anticardiolipin test – although many patients have low circulating levels of anticardiolipin antibodies, moderate or high titres in a patient with thrombosis should suggest a diagnosis of antiphospholipid syndrome
• lupus anticoagulant test – this is a functional assay which measures the ability of a patient's serum to prolong in-vitro measures of clotting.

These tests do not always give the same result. In other words, a patient with a high titre of anti-cardiolipin antibodies may be lupus anticoagulant negative, and vice versa.

Other investigations
These will be dictated by the clinical picture. Certain general points are described below.

Investigation of suspected muscle inflammation. In addition to measuring muscle enzymes (see above), arrange an EMG (electromyography) and muscle biopsy. The majority of patients with inflammatory muscle disease demonstrate abnormal EMG patterns. An important clinical point is that a normal muscle biopsy does not exclude the diagnosis of inflammatory muscle disease as the histological change accompanying the myositic process is patchy and may therefore be 'missed' on biopsy.

Investigation of suspected vasculitis. Histological appearances on biopsy may be diagnostic. Sometimes the histological appearances will point to a specific type of vasculitis. For example, a necrotising vasculitis affecting small and medium arteries, with a mainly polymorpho-nuclear infiltrate and no granulomas, is highly suggestive of polyarteritis nodosa. The site of biopsy will depend upon the clinical scenario. Renal biopsy was performed in the patient with Wegener's granulomatosis described in the Case history on page 158 because he had renal impairment and (although not explicitly stated) an active urinary sediment. Other possible biopsy sites include skin, sural nerve, temporal artery (if giant cell arteritis is suspected) or muscle. Angiography should be considered in a patient in whom a diagnosis of vasculitis is suspected but in whom biopsy is either not feasible or less likely to be diagnostic than angiography. Characteristic angiographic features of polyarteritis nodosa are aneurysms and/or occlusions of visceral arteries. Arch aortography may allow a diagnosis of Takayasu's arteritis to be made.

Further investigation to identify the presence and degree of internal organ involvement. A comprehensive list cannot be included here but three examples are:

- *Investigation of breathlessness in a patient with SLE.* This could have a variety of causes, but a chest X-ray, pulmonary function tests, and perhaps a high-resolution CT (computed tomography) scan will be required.
- *Investigation of diarrhoea in a patient with systemic sclerosis.* This may be due to malabsorption, caused by small bowel overgrowth secondary to gastrointestinal dysmotility. Investigations will include

hydrogen and $[^{14}C]$-labelled breath test to look for bacterial overgrowth.
- *Suspected cerebral SLE.* This is a difficult one. Suffice it to say that cerebral lupus is difficult to diagnose. MR scanning is capable of detecting areas of increased signal corresponding to active inflammation, but no MRI findings are specific for active cerebral lupus. Remember to have a high index of suspicion of meningitis in the unwell patient with SLE.

MANAGEMENT

A detailed discussion of treatment of connective tissue disorders is outwith the scope of this book. Here we outline the broad principles of management and then highlight some important points specific to the different diseases.

The principles of management are as follows:

- The connective tissue diseases are complex chronic disorders. Patients should be under regular specialist review.
- Patient education is important as in all chronic diseases.
- Management is multidisciplinary, often involving several medical specialists.
- Patients with active, severe inflammatory disease will usually require corticosteroids, often given in conjunction with an immuno-suppressive drug such as azathioprine or cyclophosphamide. These drugs are potentially toxic and so careful assessment of the risk–benefit ratio must be made for each patient.
- New treatments are being currently researched.

SLE

Avoidance of precipitating factors. Patients should be advised to wear strong sun-block when appropriate. Any drug which might be exacerbating or causing the SLE should be withdrawn. Infections must be promptly treated as these may precipitate a flare of disease activity. Therefore, always have a high index of suspicion of infection in an unwell patient with SLE, although it can be difficult to differentiate between a flare of SLE and infection.

Non-drug treatment. Patients with joint and/or muscle involvement should be assessed by a physiotherapist

Drug treatment. Control of blood pressure is an essential part of management: poor blood pressure control will cause further renal impairment. NSAIDs are used in patients with arthritis. A significant proportion of patients benefit from antimalarials, which are especially useful for the treatment of skin and joint disease. For patients with severe nephritis, there is now good evidence that treatment with cyclophosphamide, given in combination with corticosteroids, significantly improves outcome. A major problem is that cyclophosphamide adversely affects ovarian function and so this must be explained to the patient. Cyclophosphamide may cause other serious side-effects including haemorrhagic cystitis. Steroids and/or immunosuppressants may be indicated for aspects of the disease other than nephritis.

Pre-pregnancy counselling is an important part of the management of young women with SLE.

Antiphospholipid syndrome

If a patient has suffered a thrombosis, they should be anticoagulated, and consideration given to long-term warfarin and/or aspirin.

Systemic sclerosis

There is no place for corticosteroids (unless there is an inflammatory component or overlap syndrome, e.g. with polymyositis). At present there is no effective disease-modifying drug for systemic sclerosis, but a number of treatments are available for specific manifestations of the disease.

Remember to advise the patient with Raynaud's phenomenon to keep warm (including warm gloves and hat and keeping the torso warm). Patients who smoke should be strongly discouraged from continuing. Vasodilators should be tried for Raynaud's phenomenon, and in a patient with severe digital ischaemia, hospitalisation for intravenous vasodilators such as prostacyclin (or a prostacyclin analogue) is required. Hypertension should be controlled, usually with angiotensin-converting enzyme

(ACE) inhibitors, together with other antihypertensives if required. Treatment of scleroderma renal crisis/accelerated hypertension is a medical emergency, and should include ACE inhibition. Gastrointestinal involvement is treated symptomatically, e.g. with proton pump inhibitors for upper gastrointestinal symptoms, and cyclical antibiotics are used to eradicate bacterial overgrowth.

Inflammatory muscle disease

Physiotherapy is important, as well as prednisolone and/or immunosuppressant treatment. The aim of treatment is to suppress muscle inflammation in order to regain/prevent further loss of muscle function and strength, and to prevent fibrosis. In the older patient, look for an underlying malignancy.

Sjögren's syndrome

Treatment of dry eyes and a dry mouth is essentially symptomatic and unsatisfactory. A number of articificial tear preparations are available, as are saliva substitutes. Watch specifically for any suggestion of development of lymphoid malignancy.

Vasculitides

Most patients require corticosteroids, although mild cases of cutaneous vasculitis may not require therapy. Immunosuppressants are required in severe disease, especially in patients with Wegener's granulomatosis (see Case history on p. 156), polyarteritis nodosa, Churg–Strauss syndrome and rheumatoid vasculitis; the introduction of cyclophosphamide has dramatically improved the prognosis of patients with systemic necrotising vasculitis. Patients with polymyalgia rheumatica experience a dramatic response to small or moderate doses of corticosteroids.

Kawasaki disease is treated with intravenous immunoglobulin and aspirin. It is an acute febrile illness of children under the age of 5 years. Its most feared feature is coronary vasculitis. A detailed description of this disease will be found in textbooks of paediatrics and so it is not discussed further in this book.

AN ATLAS OF CONNECTIVE TISSUE DISEASES

A key point about connective tissue diseases is that they are multisystem, involving connective tissue and blood vessels in internal organs, the musculoskeletal system, the skin and mucous membranes. Different connective tissue diseases and vasculitides tend to be associated with different constellations of clinical features: this helps to differentiate them from each other. However, as earlier discussed, many patients have overlapping features of more than one disease.

The aim of the following section is to summarise the major 'typical' features of each of the connective tissue diseases and vasculitides. For each connective tissue disease the format comprises a case history, a key points box, brief notes on epidemiology and a diagram highlighting the main clinical features. Other clinical features can occur, but less frequently.

For the different vasculitides, only two case histories are given. These exemplify the multisystem involvement and accompanying constitutional upset which should lead to the question: 'could this patient have a vasculitis?' Firstly, vasculitides affecting medium and small vessels are outlined, then small vessel vasculitides, and lastly large vessel vasculitis.

SYSTEMIC LUPUS ERYTHEMATOSUS (SLE)

Case history – SLE

A 24-year-old woman presented to her GP with a 6-week history of tiredness, with the more recent development of breathlessness and ankle swelling. A blood sample was taken and she was telephoned the following day to be told that she was very anaemic and that further tests at the hospital would be required.

On arrival at the hospital she was questioned further. When specifically asked, she reported that recently she had been having mouth ulcers. Two doctors asked if she was sensitive to the sun, but she had never been troubled by this, although because it was February she had not been out in the sun much recently.

On examination she was pale, with a tachycardia of 110/min. There was no fever. The other significant points on examination were that she was dull to percussion at both lung bases and had bilateral pitting ankle oedema.

She was admitted and underwent a large number of tests. A Dipstix test showed that she had proteinuria, and this was confirmed by the 24 h urine collection (urinary protein 3.5 g/24 h). Haemoglobin was low at 70 g/L, white blood count was also low at 3.4×10^9/L (with a lymphopenia 0.7×10^9/L) and platelets 130×10^9/L. The reticulocyte count was raised. ESR was high at 75 mm/h. Plasma biochemistry was normal other than the albumin being low at 28 g/L. Chest X-ray showed bilateral small pleural effusions and an echocardiogram a small pericardial effusion. Immunology testing included ANA titre 1/1000 IgG, and double-stranded DNA antibodies were present in high titre. Subsequent renal biopsy showed diffuse proliferative glomerulonephritis.

After discussion with the patient, treatment with pulsed intravenous cyclophosphamide and oral prednisolone was commenced and she was subsequently regularly reviewed by both the nephrologist and the rheumatologist. Three months later she felt much better, although she was concerned that her illness and its treatment might make it difficult for her to have a family. She had become engaged to be married the month before she became unwell.

Epidemiology

Female:male ratio = 9:1
Peak age of onset: 15–40 years
Commoner in Afro-Caribeans and Asians than in Caucasians

Main differential diagnosis

- Rheumatoid arthritis, especially in a young woman with symmetrical polyarthritis (SLE often presents with arthralgia or mild arthritis)
- Bacterial endocarditis (especially in patients with pyrexia, splinter haemorrhages and microscopic haematuria)

Key points

- SLE is a multisystem inflammatory disease, which can be life-threatening if associated with major internal organ involvement.

- Young women are predominantly affected, but SLE can occur at any age.

- Constitutional upset (e.g. tiredness, malaise) is often a prominent feature.

- Immunological abnormalities are a feature of the disease, with excessive autoantibody production. Almost all patients (>95%) are ANA-positive. Antibodies to double-stranded DNA are relatively disease-specific, but are not always present even in patients with active disease.

- Corticosteroids are used in treatment of severe, active disease, sometimes in combination with immunosuppressant treatment.

- Pregnancy may adversely affect SLE, and SLE may adversely affect pregnancy.

Clinical course

This is variable and unpredictable. The 5-year survival for patients with a diagnosis of SLE has improved from 50% in the 1950s to over 90% today. Severe nephritis and CNS disease are associated with a poorer prognosis.

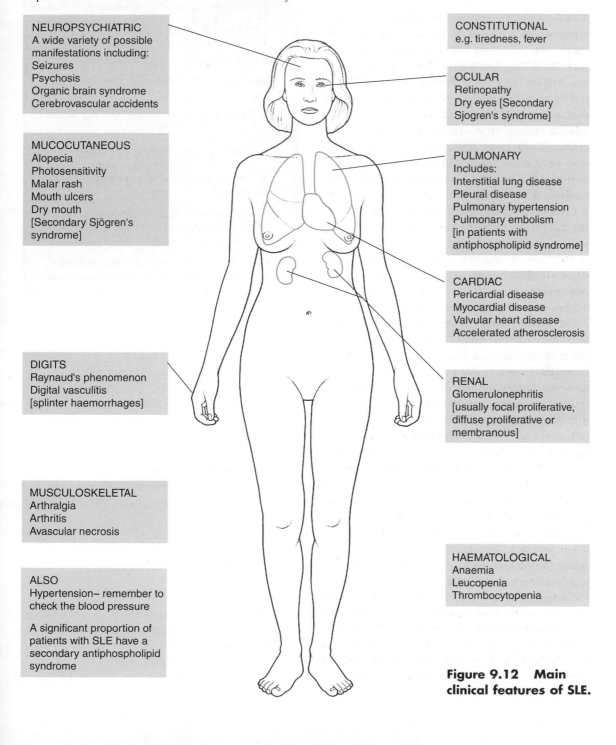

NEUROPSYCHIATRIC
A wide variety of possible manifestations including:
Seizures
Psychosis
Organic brain syndrome
Cerebrovascular accidents

MUCOCUTANEOUS
Alopecia
Photosensitivity
Malar rash
Mouth ulcers
Dry mouth
[Secondary Sjögren's syndrome]

DIGITS
Raynaud's phenomenon
Digital vasculitis
[splinter haemorrhages]

MUSCULOSKELETAL
Arthralgia
Arthritis
Avascular necrosis

ALSO
Hypertension– remember to check the blood pressure

A significant proportion of patients with SLE have a secondary antiphospholipid syndrome

CONSTITUTIONAL
e.g. tiredness, fever

OCULAR
Retinopathy
Dry eyes [Secondary Sjogren's syndrome]

PULMONARY
Includes:
Interstitial lung disease
Pleural disease
Pulmonary hypertension
Pulmonary embolism
[in patients with antiphospholipid syndrome]

CARDIAC
Pericardial disease
Myocardial disease
Valvular heart disease
Accelerated atherosclerosis

RENAL
Glomerulonephritis
[usually focal proliferative, diffuse proliferative or membranous]

HAEMATOLOGICAL
Anaemia
Leucopenia
Thrombocytopenia

Figure 9.12   Main clinical features of SLE.

SYSTEMIC SCLEROSIS

Case history – Systemic sclerosis (limited cutaneous disease)

A 45-year-old woman attended her GP's surgery with a 2-week history of a painful finger ulcer. The pain had become so severe that it was disturbing her sleep at night. For 3 years her fingers had been turning white and then purple in cold weather, then red as they were rewarming, but she had not sought medical advice about this. Recently these colour changes had been occurring more frequently, and were associated with pain and a tingling sensation. Another new symptom was heartburn.

On examination, there was a small ulcer of the tip of the right index finger. The fingertip was extremely tender, and there was thickening of the skin of the fingers (sclerodactyly). An urgent appointment was made to attend the hospital the next day.

She was fully assessed by a doctor at the rheumatology clinic. A blood sample was taken and her hands were X-rayed. The doctor prescribed flucloxacillin and nifedipine, and arranged to see her the following week. There was no improvement at this follow-up: the fingertip was blue and very tender. She was admitted for an intravenous infusion of prostacyclin and intravenous antibiotics. Prostacyclin helped her pain and the finger became less blue, but the fingertip remained very tender and she was seen by a surgeon who told her that she required an operation to remove some pus beneath the nail. After the operation she felt much better.

Investigation results included a normal full blood count and an ESR of 20 mm/h. Immunology testing showed that she was ANA-positive (1/100 IgG) and anticentromere antibody-positive. A barium swallow showed impaired peristalsis of the lower oesophagus.

Key points

- Systemic sclerosis is a multisystem disease characterised by excessive production of collagen (which is deposited in the skin and viscera) and microvascular occlusion: the clinical features are a result of fibrosis and ischaemia. There is seldom a major inflammatory component.

- Raynaud's phenomenon is often the presenting symptom.

- Scleroderma (skin thickening) is the most characteristic feature.

- There are two main subtypes (limited cutaneous and diffuse cutaneous) separated on the basis of the extent of skin involvement.

- The highest incidence of life-threatening internal organ involvement is in patients with widespread skin disease.

- Steroids are seldom used in management.

Subtypes

There are two main subtypes:

- Limited cutaneous systemic sclerosis (sometimes termed CREST syndrome: Calcinosis, Raynaud's, oEsophageal dysmotility, Sclerodactyly, Telangiectasiae). Skin thickening is confined to face and extremities.
- Diffuse cutaneous disease.

Epidemiology

Female:male ratio = 3:1
Peak age of onset: 30–50 years

Clinical course

Prognosis is dependent upon the degree of internal organ involvement. Patients with diffuse disease have a higher incidence of life-threatening major internal organ involvement (heart, lung and renal disease), and this often occurs in the first 5 years of disease. However, in patients with the limited cutaneous variant of the disease, there is a late mortality from pulmonary vascular disease ('primary-type' pulmonary hypertension).

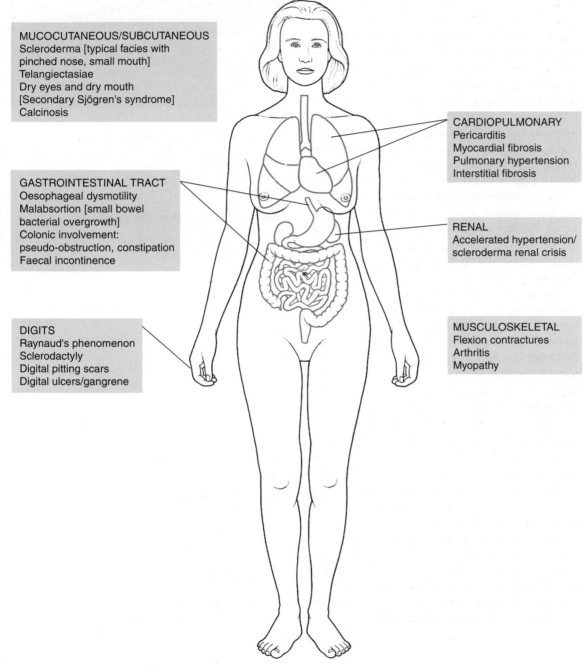

MUCOCUTANEOUS/SUBCUTANEOUS
Scleroderma [typical facies with pinched nose, small mouth]
Telangiectasiae
Dry eyes and dry mouth
[Secondary Sjögren's syndrome]
Calcinosis

GASTROINTESTINAL TRACT
Oesophageal dysmotility
Malabsortion [small bowel bacterial overgrowth]
Colonic involvement:
pseudo-obstruction, constipation
Faecal incontinence

DIGITS
Raynaud's phenomenon
Sclerodactyly
Digital pitting scars
Digital ulcers/gangrene

CARDIOPULMONARY
Pericarditis
Myocardial fibrosis
Pulmonary hypertension
Interstitial fibrosis

RENAL
Accelerated hypertension/
scleroderma renal crisis

MUSCULOSKELETAL
Flexion contractures
Arthritis
Myopathy

Figure 9.13   Main clinical features of systemic sclerosis.

INFLAMMATORY MUSCLE DISEASE (POLYMYOSITIS AND DERMATOMYOSITIS)

Case history – dermatomyositis

A 50-year-old male presented to his GP with a 3-week history of feeling tired and weak. For the past 2 days he had had difficulty even getting out of a chair. Recently he had been aware of a facial rash.

On examination his face and neck were erythematous. He had marked proximal muscle weakness, with proximal muscle tenderness.

His ESR was raised at 45 mm/h and his creatine phosphokinase (CPK) was very high at 3400 u/L. He was referred to hospital where his peak expiratory flow rate was checked and an ECG performed. Both were normal. He had some further tests, including electromyography (EMG) and muscle biopsy. High-dose prednisolone (60 mg/day) was commenced and after 1 week he felt much improved.

He went on to have a number of other tests, including gastroscopy and colonoscopy. This seemed very strange to him, because he had no other health problems. The doctor explained that he was a little anaemic and there had been a trace of blood in his bowel motions, and that he just wanted to check that nothing important was being missed.

Key points

- There is inflammation of striated muscle ('polymyositis'). If this occurs in association with inflammation of the skin it is termed 'dermatomyositis'.

- The main clinical feature is proximal muscle weakness.

- The peak age of onset is in childhood (Box 9.7) and middle/late adulthood.

- In older patients, there is a probable association between dermatomyositis and malignancy.

Box 9.7　Inflammatory muscle disease in children (juvenile dermatomyositis)

Specific points to highlight in children include:
- Polymyositis in the absence of skin involvement is rare in childhood
- There is no association between juvenile dermatomyositis and malignancy
- Calcinosis is common late in disease and can result in severe disability.

Epidemiology

Female:male ratio = 2–3:1

Peak age of onset: childhood and middle/late adulthood

Main differential diagnosis

Non-inflammatory myopathies
- Motor neurone disease
- Myasthenia gravis
- Muscular dystrophies
- Disease of glycogen storage or lipid storage. Standard histochemical staining of the muscle biopsy will reveal glycogen or fat. In McArdle's disease there is an inability to degrade glycogen under anaerobic conditions. Hence the patient complains of weakness, pain and muscle swelling after prolonged exercise.
- Endocrine myopathies/metabolic. These include myopathies associated with hyper- and hypothyroidism, Cushing's disease and vitamin D deficiency.
- Drug-induced. A variety of drugs can induce myopathy, including corticosteroids (and alcohol).

Other inflammatory myopathies
- Inclusion body myositis. Weakness is insidious (often over years), characteristic inclusions are seen in the muscle biopsy, and there is no response to steroids.
- Infectious myositis. Rarely a septic myositis can occur.

Polymyalgia rheumatica
This is described later in this chapter.

Clinical course

While some patients with inflammatory muscle disease have a short self-limiting illness, most have persistent disease in which exacerbations and remissions occur. Over 90% of patients without associated malignancy survive more than 5 years.

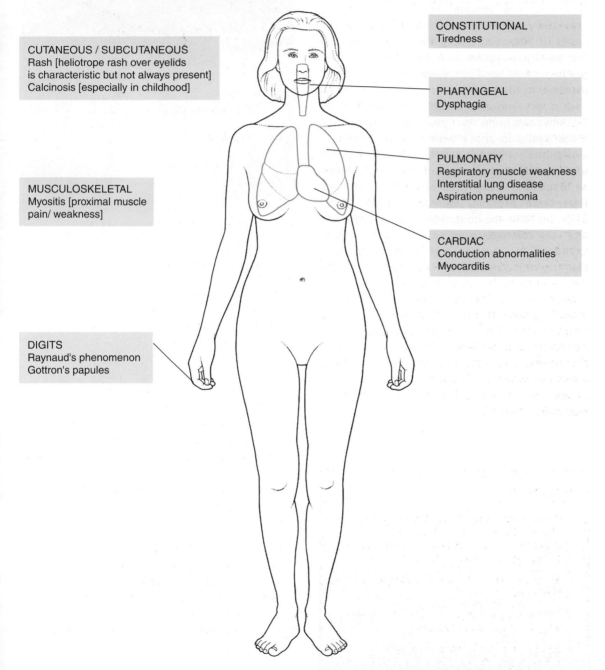

CONSTITUTIONAL
Tiredness

PHARYNGEAL
Dysphagia

PULMONARY
Respiratory muscle weakness
Interstitial lung disease
Aspiration pneumonia

CARDIAC
Conduction abnormalities
Myocarditis

CUTANEOUS / SUBCUTANEOUS
Rash [heliotrope rash over eyelids
is characteristic but not always present]
Calcinosis [especially in childhood]

MUSCULOSKELETAL
Myositis [proximal muscle
pain/ weakness]

DIGITS
Raynaud's phenomenon
Gottron's papules

Figure 9.14   Main clinical features of inflammatory muscle disease (polymyositis and dermatomyositis).

SJÖGREN'S SYNDROME

Case history – Sjögren's syndrome (secondary to systemic sclerosis)

A 55-year-old female, diagnosed 3 years previously as having systemic sclerosis (on the basis of Raynaud's, calcinosis, oesophageal dysmotility and telangiectasiae), began to have problems with her eyes. They felt gritty much of the time. At the hospital her doctor asked if she had a dry mouth (which she had noticed recently) and hung filter paper strips from each lower eyelid to check what he called the tear secretion (Schirmer's tear test: Fig. 9.15). This test confirmed that she had 'dry eyes', which he explained were part of her disease. He prescribed artificial tears, but while these helped a little she continued to have problems and was referred to an ophthalmologist, who examined her eyes through a slit lamp, after staining with a dye called Rose Bengal. He told her she had a small corneal ulcer.

Over the next 2 years she went on to develop more and more problems with her mouth. She found dry food very difficult to swallow, and her teeth started to give her a lot of problems. She became depressed about her eye and mouth problems, which she felt had become more of a problem to her than the other features of systemic sclerosis.

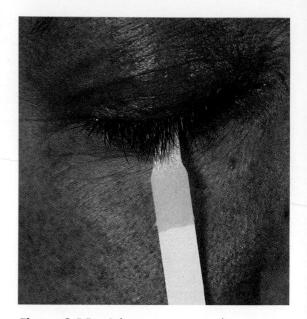

Figure 9.15 Schirmer's test — in this case demonstrating normal wetting of the filter paper.

Epidemiology

Female:male ratio = 9:1
Peak age of onset: 30–50 years

Key points

- Sjögren's syndrome can be primary (occurring in the absence of other autoimmune diseases) or secondary (associated with other autoimmune diseases).

- It affects predominantly the exocrine glands and its most characteristic features are dry eyes (keratoconjunctivitis sicca) and a dry mouth (xerostomia).

- It is distressing, and difficult to treat.

- Patients with Sjögren's syndrome are at increased risk of lymphoid malignancy.

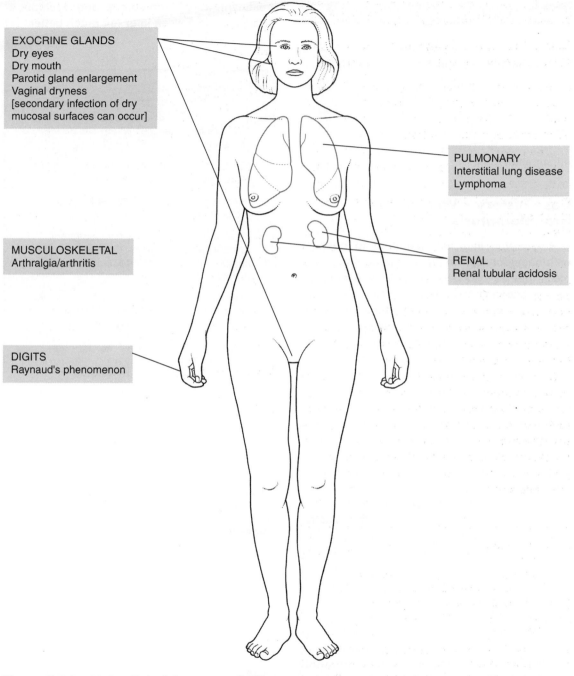

EXOCRINE GLANDS
Dry eyes
Dry mouth
Parotid gland enlargement
Vaginal dryness
[secondary infection of dry
mucosal surfaces can occur]

PULMONARY
Interstitial lung disease
Lymphoma

MUSCULOSKELETAL
Arthralgia/arthritis

RENAL
Renal tubular acidosis

DIGITS
Raynaud's phenomenon

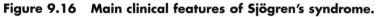

Figure 9.16   Main clinical features of Sjögren's syndrome.

THE VASCULITIDES

Two case histories are given, to give some insight into the broad spectrum of complaints with which patients with vasculitis may present. The main clinical features of several of the vasculitides are summarised in the figures. Remember always to ask yourself 'Could this patient have vasculitis?' when a patient presents with multisystem inflammatory disease.

Case history – Wegener's granulomatosis

A 48-year-old man was admitted to hospital with haemoptysis. On close questioning it was clear that he had been unwell for 6 months. Things began with a sinusitis, which had never really cleared up despite antibiotic therapy. He felt tired and had lost 5 kg in weight. Another point of concern to him was that 3 months prior to admission, at a routine health check, he was found to have some blood in his urine. A cystoscopy had been normal.

On examination he was pale, and his heart rate was 110/min. Blood pressure was 150/90 mmHg and he had some ankle oedema. Otherwise there were no abnormalities.

Investigations included a haemoglobin of 77 g/L, white blood count 10.5×10^9/L, platelet count 540×10^9/L and ESR very high at 110 mm/h. He had renal impairment, with a plasma urea of 15.0 mmol/L and a creatinine of 210 µmol/L. His plasma albumin was low at 27 g/L. Dipstix testing of the urine showed blood and protein. A chest X-ray showed some shadowing in the right upper zone and mid-zone, with a small cavity in the right upper zone.

Blood was sent to the immunology laboratory and results were available 3 days later. He had antibodies to antineutrophil cytoplasmic antigens (ANCA) and the staining was in a cytoplasmic distribution (cANCA). A repeat biochemical profile at this stage showed that the creatinine had risen to 310 µmol/L. A renal biopsy was performed, which showed a lot of inflammation. He was commenced on treatment with prednisolone and cyclophosphamide, and 1 week later felt much better.

Key points

- The vasculitides are multisystem inflammatory diseases which can be life-threatening.

- They are characterised by inflammation of blood vessel walls (vasculitis).

- Infarction and haemorrhage of internal organs are the most feared features of disease.

- Most of the vasculitides are uncommon (exceptions are Henoch–Schönlein purpura in children and giant cell [temporal] arteritis in the elderly).

- Their classification is usually based on the size of the blood vessel wall affected by the inflammatory process (Table 9.1).

- Diagnosis can be difficult. Suspect the diagnosis in an unwell patient with multisystem inflammatory disease.

- Treatment of active disease is usually with steroids and/or immunosuppressants.

Table 9.1
Size of blood vessels mainly involved in the major vasculitic syndromes

Syndrome	Size of vessel involved
Takaysu's arteritis	Large (including aorta)
Giant cell arteritis	Large arteries
Polyarteritis nodosa	Medium and small
Churg–Strauss syndrome	Medium and small
Wegener's granulomatosis	Medium and small
Behçet's syndrome	Medium and small
Kawasaki disease	Medium and small
Vasculitis associated with SLE and rheumatoid arthritis	Medium and small
Small vessel/cutaneous vasculitis (leucocytoclastic vasculitis)	Small vessels

WEGENENER'S GRANULOMATOSIS
Epidemiology

This is an uncommon disease   Males and females are equally affected   Peak age of onset: 40s

UPPER RESPIRATORY TRACT
e.g. Otitis media; nasal ulcers;
saddle nose deformity, sinusitis,
subglottic stenosis

OCULAR
e.g. Proptosis, scleritis

MUSCULOSKELETAL
Myalgias
Arthralgia/arthritis

CONSTITUTIONAL
Fever
Weight loss

PULMONARY
Pulmonary infiltrates
Pulmonary nodules
[radiographic abnormalities
may be asymptomatic]
Pulmonary haemorrhage
Always remember
possibility of infection

RENAL
Glomerulonephritis

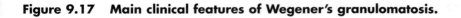

Figure 9.17   Main clinical features of Wegener's granulomatosis.

POLYARTERITIS NODOSA
Epidemiology

This is an uncommon disease

Male:female ratio = 1–2: 1
Peak age of onset: 40–65 years
Polyarteritis nodosa can occur in children
Polyarteritis nodosa can be associated with hepatitis B infection.

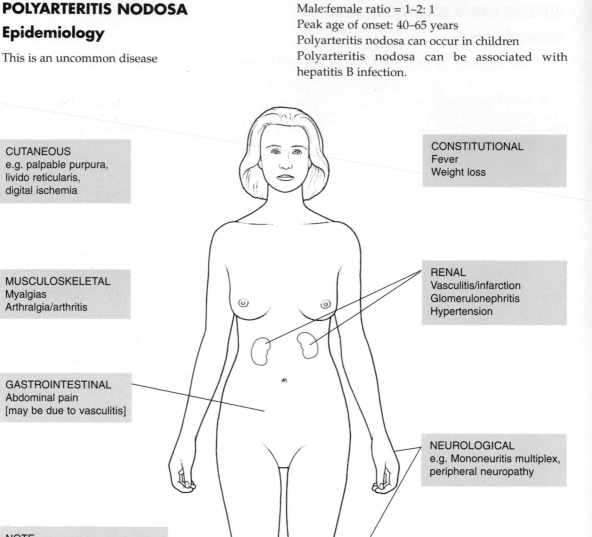

CUTANEOUS
e.g. palpable purpura,
livido reticularis,
digital ischemia

CONSTITUTIONAL
Fever
Weight loss

MUSCULOSKELETAL
Myalgias
Arthralgia/arthritis

RENAL
Vasculitis/infarction
Glomerulonephritis
Hypertension

GASTROINTESTINAL
Abdominal pain
[may be due to vasculitis]

NEUROLOGICAL
e.g. Mononeuritis multiplex,
peripheral neuropathy

NOTE
Biopsy or angiography may
confirm the diagnosis. Typically
angiography shows aneuryms
and stenoses of medium-sized
vessels.

Figure 9.18   Main clinical features of polyarteritis nodosa.

CHURG–STRAUSS SYNDROME

Epidemiology

This is an uncommon disease   Male:female ratio = 2:1   Adults of all ages may be affected

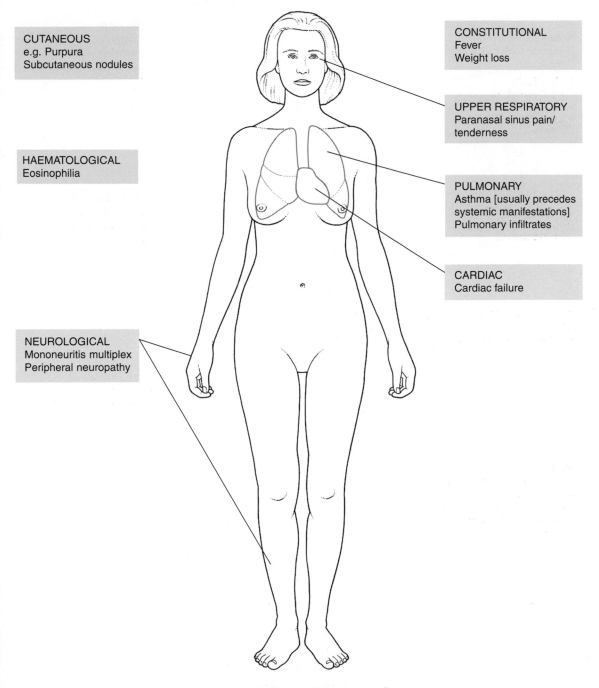

CUTANEOUS
e.g. Purpura
Subcutaneous nodules

HAEMATOLOGICAL
Eosinophilia

NEUROLOGICAL
Mononeuritis multiplex
Peripheral neuropathy

CONSTITUTIONAL
Fever
Weight loss

UPPER RESPIRATORY
Paranasal sinus pain/
tenderness

PULMONARY
Asthma [usually precedes
systemic manifestations]
Pulmonary infiltrates

CARDIAC
Cardiac failure

Figure 9.19   Main clinical features of Churg–Strauss syndrome.

BEHÇET'S SYNDROME

Epidemiology

This is an uncommon disease

Female:Male ratio = 1
Young adults mainly affected
Commonest in Japan and around the Mediterranean

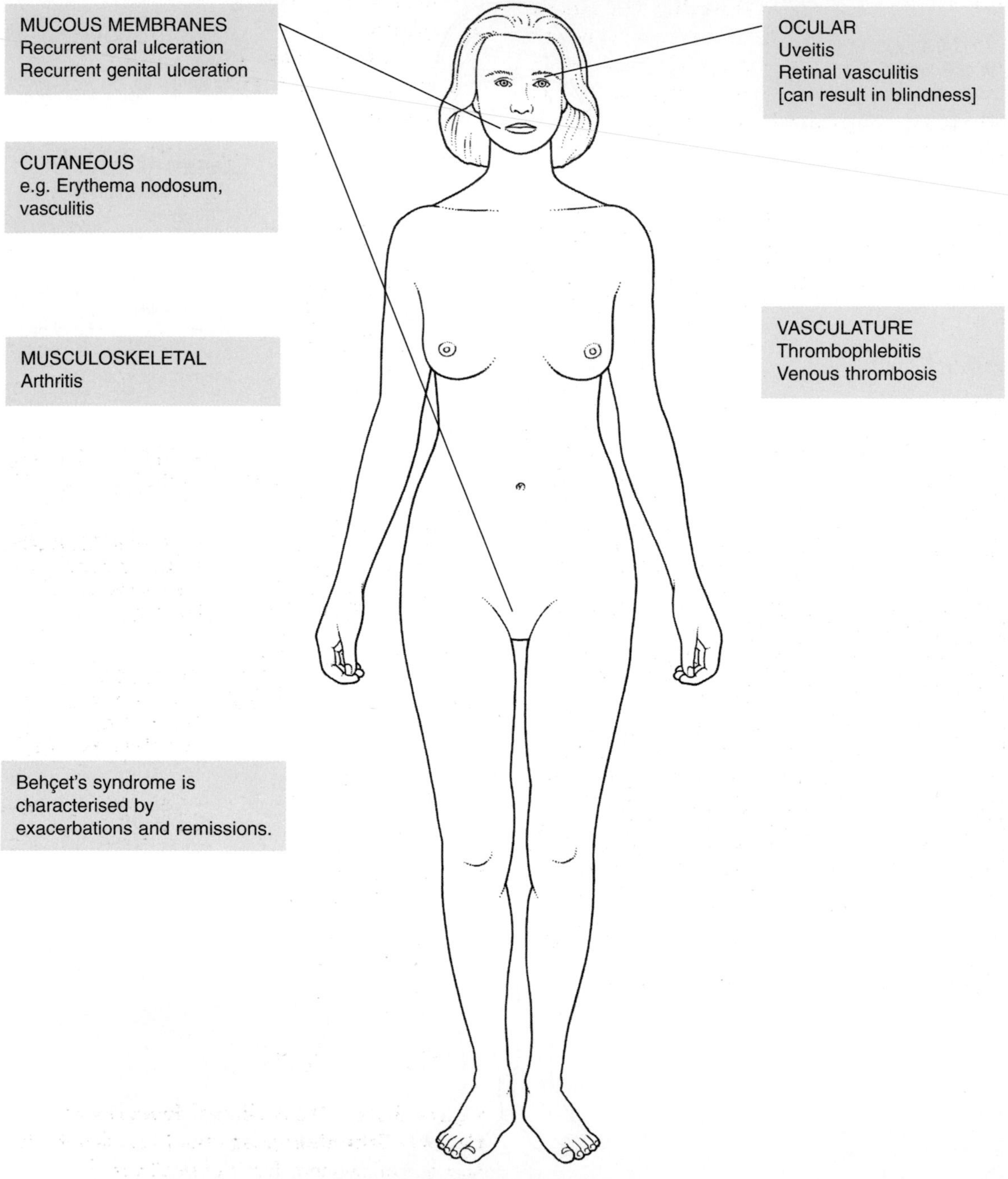

MUCOUS MEMBRANES
Recurrent oral ulceration
Recurrent genital ulceration

OCULAR
Uveitis
Retinal vasculitis
[can result in blindness]

CUTANEOUS
e.g. Erythema nodosum,
vasculitis

VASCULATURE
Thrombophlebitis
Venous thrombosis

MUSCULOSKELETAL
Arthritis

Behçet's syndrome is
characterised by
exacerbations and remissions.

Figure 9.20   Main clinical features of Behçet's syndrome.

SMALL VESSEL VASCULITIS

Small vessel vasculitis affects mainly the skin (cutaneous vasculitis, Fig. 9.21). However, other microvessels may be involved, e.g. in the joints and kidney. 'Leucocytoclastic vasculitis' is, strictly speaking, a pathological term (it should not be regarded as a clinical syndrome). There is an inflammatory infiltrate with neutrophils, some of which are fragmented (leucocytoclasis), with fibrinoid necrosis.

Small vessel vasculitis occurs in association with a variety of disease processes:

- Henoch–Schönlein purpura (Fig. 9.22) (this is predominantly a disease of childhood)
- drug hypersensitivity
- malignancy
- mixed cryoglobulinaemia
- connective tissue diseases
- infections

Note. Small vessel vasculitis is often self-limiting.

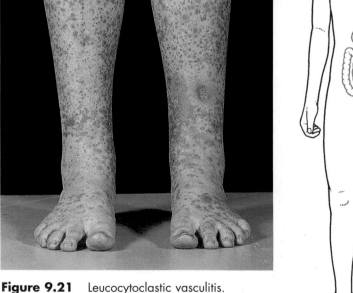

Figure 9.21 Leucocytoclastic vasculitis.

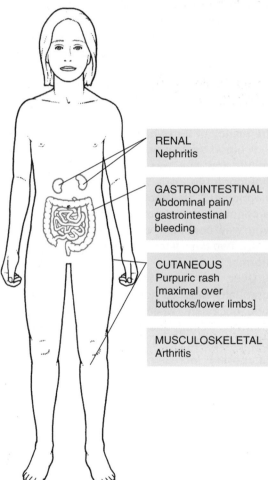

RENAL
Nephritis

GASTROINTESTINAL
Abdominal pain/
gastrointestinal
bleeding

CUTANEOUS
Purpuric rash
[maximal over
buttocks/lower limbs]

MUSCULOSKELETAL
Arthritis

Figure 9.22   Main clinical features of Henoch–Schönlein purpura. (Note that this is only one of the many forms of small vessel vasculitis)

POLYMYALGIA RHEUMATICA AND GIANT CELL ARTERITIS

Case history – polymyalgia rheumatica

A 70-year-old female who was previously quite independent reported that for the past 6 weeks she had been having considerable pain and stiffness, especially of her upper arms and the tops of her legs. Things had become so bad that for 1 week she had hardly been able to get out of bed in the morning. Later in the day she generally felt a little better.

When she went to the doctor she was asked a lot of questions, including whether she had had any headaches or any problems with her vision. She had suffered from headaches intermittently for many years, but was able to reassure her doctor that there had been no recent change in the character, severity or frequency of these headaches.

A blood sample was taken. Her ESR was 80 mm/h and she was slightly anaemic with a haemoglobin of 105 g/L (normochromic, normocytic). Her doctor explained that she had a condition called polymyalgia rheumatica and she was commenced on prednisolone 15 mg daily. Two days later she felt completely back to normal.

Over the next few months her doctor gradually reduced her dosage of steroids. On one occasion (when the dose was dropped down to 7.5 mg) she experienced some of her old aches and pains, but these responded to a temporary increase in steroid dosage. The prednisolone dosage was then reduced very slowly and 2 years after diagnosis she was off treatment.

Although there is a clear association between polymyalgia rheumatica and temporal arteritis (both can occur together, or myalgic symptoms can precede or follow those of giant cell arteritis), each can occur without clinical features of the other being present.

Key points

- Polymyalgia rheumatica is a disease of the elderly, characterised by pain and stiffness of the shoulder and pelvic girdles. The ESR is usually high.

- There is an association between polymyalgia rheumatica and giant cell arteritis.

- Giant cell arteritis is an arteritis of large vessels, sometimes termed 'cranial arteritis' because there is a high incidence of head and neck vessel involvement, or 'temporal arteritis' because the temporal arteries are often involved.

- In polymyalgia rheumatica, there is a dramatic response to moderate-dose prednisolone. High-dose prednisolone is not required for polymyalgia rheumatica alone.

- Characteristic features of giant cell arteritis include headaches and visual loss.

- Giant cell arteritis is a medical emergency. High-dose corticosteroids may prevent permanent blindness.

Epidemiology

Females more commonly affected
Rare below the age of 50 years

Differential diagnosis of polymyalgia rheumatica

- Malignancy, including multiple myeloma
- Rheumatoid arthritis
- Connective tissue disease (especially SLE or polymyositis)
- Osteoarthritis, spondylosis and/or soft tissue rheumatism, particularly of the neck and shoulders (note that in these conditions the ESR should be normal)
- Hypothyroidism
- Infections (e.g. tuberculosis, bacterial endocarditis)

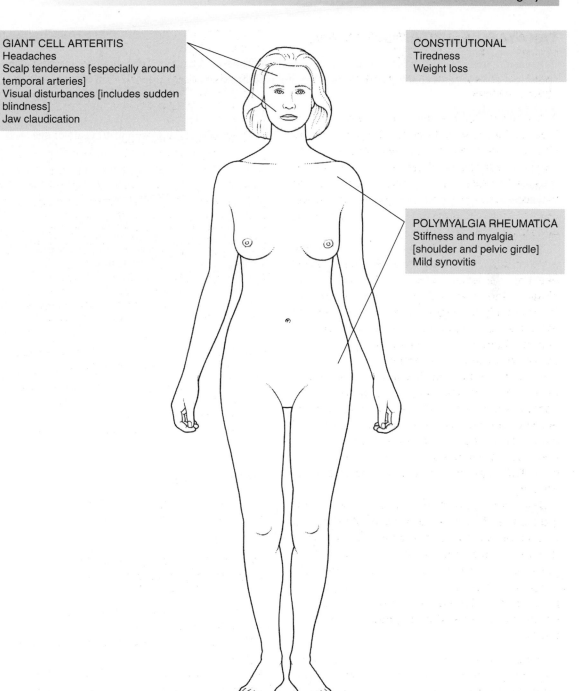

GIANT CELL ARTERITIS
Headaches
Scalp tenderness [especially around temporal arteries]
Visual disturbances [includes sudden blindness]
Jaw claudication

CONSTITUTIONAL
Tiredness
Weight loss

POLYMYALGIA RHEUMATICA
Stiffness and myalgia [shoulder and pelvic girdle]
Mild synovitis

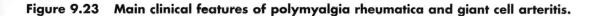

Figure 9.23   Main clinical features of polymyalgia rheumatica and giant cell arteritis.

TAKAYASU'S ARTERITIS

Takayasu's arteritis (Fig. 9.24) affects principally the aorta and its major branches. It was first named 'pulseless disease', as a characteristic clinical finding is reduced or absent upper or lower limb pulses.

Epidemiology

This is an uncommon disease   Female:male ratio = 9:1   Onset usually at less than 40 years of age

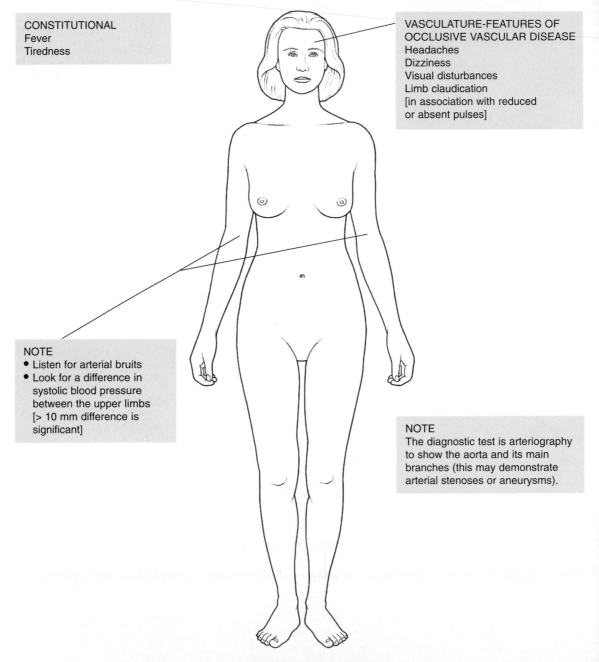

CONSTITUTIONAL
Fever
Tiredness

VASCULATURE-FEATURES OF
OCCLUSIVE VASCULAR DISEASE
Headaches
Dizziness
Visual disturbances
Limb claudication
[in association with reduced
or absent pulses]

NOTE
• Listen for arterial bruits
• Look for a difference in
  systolic blood pressure
  between the upper limbs
  [> 10 mm difference is
  significant]

NOTE
The diagnostic test is arteriography
to show the aorta and its main
branches (this may demonstrate
arterial stenoses or aneurysms).

Figure 9.24   Main clinical features of Takayasu's arteritis.

10 | Osteoarthritis

Case history

A 60-year-old primary school teacher had a 2-year history of aching legs, especially towards the end of the day. She no longer enjoyed the 1 mile walk home at the end of the afternoon and she had started to take the bus. To make matters worse, she had begun to suffer pain in her back as well, and even her neck had been aching recently. While she felt stiff in the mornings, this was only for around 5 minutes.

As her pains became worse she attended her GP, who noticed that she had bony swelling of the distal interphalangeal joints of her hands (Heberden's nodes). She remembered that her mother also had them. Internal rotation of both hips was limited (more so on the right) and all hip movements were painful. The knees flexed painfully, with crepitus; flexion and extension of the lumbar spine were limited. The GP arranged for X-rays of her pelvis and knees, and took a blood sample. The following week he explained to her that she had osteoarthritis, which was very common. She was reassured to hear that the blood test results were normal. He arranged for physiotherapy and recommended paracetamol for the pain. He said that if the pain in the hip became worse then at some stage she might require an operation.

The physiotherapist taught her a programme of exercises and recommended using a walking stick in her left hand. The situation remained acceptable for 3 years, but then the pain in the right groin and hip deteriorated; she was woken by the pain on most nights. She was referred to the local orthopaedic surgery department, where a total hip replacement was subsequently performed. She obtained excellent pain relief, but found that the stiffness of her hip was not improved very much. She was told that she would have to remain under follow-up for her hip replacement indefinitely as 'she was quite young for this operation, and the joint might wear out'.

Osteoarthritis used to be considered a 'degenerative' or 'wear and tear' process, usually related to ageing. However, it is now recognised that joints affected by osteoarthritis are involved in a dynamic process comprising not only degeneration but also attempts at repair.

Osteoarthritis may be considered as structural 'failure' of a joint, the end result of biochemical and biomechanical events which have progressed to irreversible joint damage. Traditionally, osteoarthritis has been divided into primary (idiopathic) and secondary forms (Box 10.1).

Key points

- Osteoarthritis is common and is age-related.

- The pathology does not represent 'simple wear and tear'.

- Most patients can be managed with conservative measures, including physiotherapy and analgesic treatment.

- Simple analgesics should be tried before NSAIDs.

- Total joint replacement can provide excellent symptom relief for some patients with osteoarthritis, but severe complications occur in a small proportion of cases and selection of patients should take this into account.

Box 10.1   Causes of secondary osteoarthritis

Congenital or developmental
- **Congenital hip dislocation (developmental hip dysplasia)**
- **Slipped femoral epiphysis**
- **Perthe's disease**
- **Leg length inequality**
- **Hypermobility**

Metabolic
- **Calcium pyrophosphate deposition disease**
- **Ochronosis**

Traumatic
- **Fracture**
- **Internal derangement, e.g. meniscal injury**
- **Joint instability (e.g. anterior cruciate ligament injury)**
- **Joint surgery, e.g. meniscectomy**
- **Neuropathic joint (Charcot's joint)**
- **Repetitive use (e.g. occupational)**

Inflammatory
- **Rheumatoid arthritis**
- **Septic arthritis**
- **Other inflammatory arthritis associated with joint damage, e.g. gout**

Secondary osteoarthritis can be monoarticular or polyarticular, the site(s) involved depending upon the nature of the initial joint disease or insult. However, this distinction into primary and secondary forms is not absolute: there may be genetic susceptibility to 'secondary' osteoarthritis. 'Primary generalised osteoarthritis' is a term used to describe a variant of osteoarthritis which typically strikes at middle-aged women, predominantly affecting hands (characteristically with Heberden's nodes and involvement of the carpometacarpal joints of the thumbs), knees, hips and apophyseal (facet) joints of the spine. 'Degenerative' disease affecting the spine is termed 'spondylosis' (e.g. cervical and lumbar spondylosis); this term usually includes disease both of the apophyseal joints and around the intervertebral disc.

EPIDEMIOLOGY

Osteoarthritis is a common disorder: most people over the age of 65 will have radiographic evidence of the disease. Prevalence rises with age. While both men and women are commonly affected, overall the prevalence is higher in women; this is especially true for polyarticular osteoarthritis.

PATHOLOGY
Aetiology

A number of 'susceptibility' factors predispose to development of osteoarthritis, including genetic susceptibility, age and hypermobility (hypermobility is discussed in Ch. 13). In addition, local biomechanical factors, including those occurring as a result of the conditions listed in Box 10.1, play a major role. Whether or not an individual develops osteoarthritis will depend upon the interaction between these factors and their relative importance. For example, osteoarthritis may develop after a major knee injury without any 'systemic' predisposing factor, and similarly primary generalised osteoarthritis will develop without any obvious mechanical precipitant. On the other hand, whether an individual develops osteoarthritis after a minor knee injury may depend upon general predisposing factors.

Occupational causes are important; for example, heavy physical work is associated with an increased incidence of osteoarthritis, the distribution of the joint disease depending upon the exact nature of the work involved.

The neuropathic joint (Charcot's joint) is worth special mention but is rare. A sensory neuropathy (most commonly now related to diabetes, discussed in Ch. 12) leads to very florid joint destruction.

Pathogenesis

While the pathogenesis of osteoarthritis is not fully understood, the disease is now considered to be the result of complex biochemical and biomechanical processes which lead to loss of cartilage integrity. Calcium-containing crystals may be found in synovial fluid and tissues from osteoarthritic joints, but the significance of these with respect to pathogenesis is not known.

The extracellular matrix of articular cartilage comprises mainly collagen molecules (which provide the framework) and proteoglycans. The proteoglycans, which are complex macromole-cules, are hydrophilic, and articular cartilage has a high water content. This extracellular matrix is synthesised and degraded by the chondrocytes, which are embedded in the extracellular matrix and which are metabolically very active cells. In normal cartilage, there is a 'steady state' between anabolic and catabolic processes. This steady state is disrupted in osteoarthritis, when several changes occur, including:

- an increase in activity of degradative enzymes such as collagenase
- an increase in water content
- a decrease in the proteoglycan content,
- damage to the collagen framework.

Pathology

Osteoarthritis can affect any synovial joint, but those most commonly affected are the distal interphalangeal (IP) and thumb carpometacarpal (CMC) joints in the hand, the hips, knees, the great toe metatarsophalangeal (MTP) joint and apophyseal joints of the spine.

Osteoarthritis, as its name suggests, is a process affecting both bone and joint. Cartilage is destroyed. Initially there is fibrillation (disruption of the surface collagen) and softening of the cartilage, which results from an increase in its water content. Then there is loss of volume and eventually destruction with loss of joint space. This means that there is bone to bone apposition in the joint, instead of the normal situation when cartilage keeps the bone surfaces apart. However, osteoarthritis is a dynamic process involving cartilage repair as well as degradation. Histologi-cally, clumps of proliferating chondrocytes may be seen.

In subchondral bone, osteoblasts proliferate and new bone is formed. The subchondral bone becomes sclerotic, often with cysts (Fig. 10.1). When there is complete loss of cartilage the subchondral bone, now the articulating surface, has a polished appearance (eburnation). Overgrowth of bone at the joint margins results in formation of the osteophytes (Fig. 10.2). A secondary synovitis can occur: breakdown products of bone and cartilage are removed by the phagocytic cells of the synovial membrane, which becomes hyperplastic.

Although the 'wear and tear' theory of causation of osteoarthritis is now largely superseded, it is nevertheless true that excessive loading of an area of cartilage may precipitate the condition. Further, the fibrillation and softening of cartilage reduce its resistance to mechanical overload. The loss of joint space means that deformity may develop, and any pre-existing deformity may be increased by the disease. Such

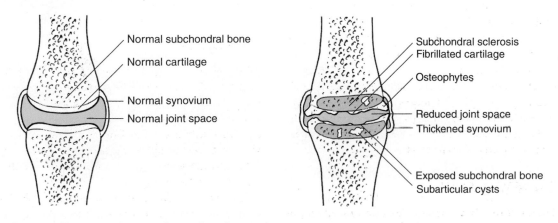

A Normal synovial joint

Normal subchondral bone
Normal cartilage
Normal synovium
Normal joint space

B Osteoarthritic synovial joint

Subchondral sclerosis
Fibrillated cartilage
Osteophytes
Reduced joint space
Thickened synovium
Exposed subchondral bone
Subarticular cysts

Figure 10.1   Cartilage and articular abnormalities occurring in osteoarthritis.

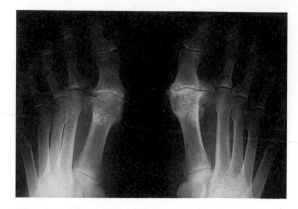

Figure 10.2 Osteoarthritis of great toe, hip joints with florid osteophyte formation on the right.

deformities may cause an increase in local overloading of cartilage. This is particularly true of the medial compartment of the knee, where a varus deformity may be followed by chronic overloading of the medial side of the knee and early osteoarthritis. The medial arthritis in the knee causes increased varus and increases the overloading.

The changes of loss of joint space, subchondral bone sclerosis and cyst formation, and osteophytosis are mirrored in X-ray appearances (Fig. 10.3), which are, however, insensitive to early changes of osteoarthritis.

Diagnostic features of osteoarthritis are given in Box 10.2.

CLINICAL FEATURES

Osteoarthritis is a process solely affecting joints; internal organ involvement does not occur. It is, however, important when assessing patients with osteoarthritis to take into account their general health, as this may influence management. Also, if a patient is systemically unwell, e.g. with fever and/or weight loss, this indicates that another cause must be sought.

History

Musculoskeletal

Symptoms often correlate poorly with severity of disease as judged by radiographic appearances: some patients have severe osteoarthritis on X-ray, but no, or minimal, symptoms; others have severe pain but only minor radiographic changes.

The key points to ask about are:

- *Is pain related to activity or 'use'?* The pain from an osteoarthritic joint is generally worse after use of that joint. For example, an osteoarthritic hip is especially painful after walking or standing. Similarly, pain from lumbar spondylosis (Ch. 17) is worse after activity. This is in contrast to the pain from inflammatory arthritis such as ankylosing spondylitis, which is worse after inactivity and is relieved by exercise. Therefore, pain from osteoarthritis is often worse later on in the day, and while there may be an element of morning stiffness and 'gelling' after periods of

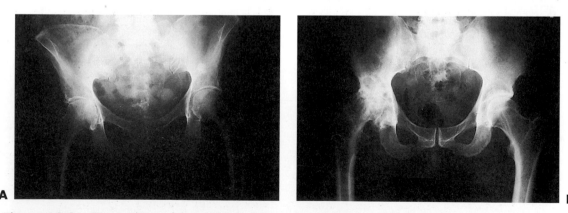

Figure 10.3 Osteoarthritis of the right hip. Changes can be slight (A) with mild loss of joint space, or severe (B) with complete loss of joint space, sclerosis and an acetabular cyst. An osteophyte is seen at the acetabulum.

inactivity, this is usually only for a few minutes (in contrast to inflammatory arthritis when morning stiffness usually lasts much longer). The onset of osteoarthritic pain is usually slow and insidious.

- *What is the pattern of joint involvement?* In 'primary' osteoarthritis, the typical joints involved are in the hand (IP joints, and the CMC joint of the thumb), the hip, the knee, the first MTP joint, and the apophyseal (facet) joints of the cervical and lumbar spine. Therefore, symptoms at these sites may suggest osteoarthritis. When there is only one joint involved, e.g. the knee, there may be a history of a previous knee problem such as a football injury.

- *How severe are the symptoms?* Most people develop osteoarthritis in one or more joints. However, only a minority will ever require surgical treatment. The principal factor determining whether surgery is required, once the diagnosis is established, is the severity of the symptoms. Night pain severe enough to disturb sleep and pain which severely limits walking ability are commonly used yardsticks. The decision to opt for surgery in cases of osteoarthritis involves balancing the risks (sometimes considerable) against the possible benefits. The risks are unlikely to be worth taking if the symptoms are not severe. The symptom of stiffness may be prominent; most forms of surgery do not improve this very reliably and it should generally not be used as the principal indication for operation.

- *How is the patient limited by the joint problems?* Patients may find that their movement and activities are limited. The importance of this will depend upon each patient's circumstances. For example, knee osteoarthritis in an 80-year-old man whose walking is limited by breathlessness from severe chest problems may be perceived as being associated with very little disability. However, knee osteoarthritis in a middle-aged man who is employed in heavy manual work would be perceived very differently.

Other medical conditions

A number of medical conditions have been associated with osteoarthritis, e.g. diabetes and obesity. Therefore, it is necessary to consider whether any other medical problems the patient might have may be associated with osteoarthritis.

Diabetes is associated with a condition termed 'DISH' (diffuse idiopathic skeletal hyperostosis, sometimes termed Forestier's disease). Like osteoarthritis this is a non-inflammatory age-related condition, characterised by excessive new bone formation, especially at entheses. The thoracolumbar spine is particularly involved. DISH may be asymptomatic, diagnosed as an incidental finding on X-ray.

Family history

There is a hereditary component to polyarticular osteoarthritis, although a positive family history of osteoarthritis is usually of less diagnostic importance than in the inflammatory arthritides.

Social

Ask about occupation and about leisure activities, both of which may predispose to osteoarthritis. As always in patients with musculoskeletal disease, it is important to know about support at home, especially if the patient is significantly disabled.

Musculoskeletal examination

The main signs of osteoarthritis are bony swelling, with pain and crepitus on movement, restriction of movement and muscle wasting. In addition, there may be tenderness and signs of a secondary synovitis. Bony deformity may also occur.

Take note as to whether the patient is overweight. Some specific and characteristic features of osteoarthritis are described below.

Hands

The characteristic features are:

- Heberden's nodes (Fig. 10.4) – these are bony swellings of the distal IP joints; they are usually non-tender but may be tender early on in the natural history of the disease, when they may be associated with mucinous cysts
- Bouchard's nodes – these are bony swellings of the proximal IP joints (Fig. 10.5)
- 'squaring' of the hand due to involvement of the thumb CMC joint, which is often tender (this can result in severe pain in power grip, e.g. opening jars; Fig. 10.6).

These finger and thumb deformities can lead to difficulty especially with fine finger movement. Osteoarthritis may rarely occur in the wrist: this most commonly follows trauma.

Remember that rheumatoid arthritis does not involve the distal IP joints. Therefore, rheumatoid arthritis and osteoarthritis in the hand should not be confused.

Elbow

Osteoarthritis of the elbow was previously thought to be very rare, but has recently been shown to be fairly common with ageing in those previously engaged in heavy manual work.

Shoulder region

Osteoarthritis of the glenohumeral joint is uncommon. Pain in the shoulder region is commonly caused by acromioclavicular arthritis, where the pain is generally well localised at this joint, or by rotator cuff problems (e.g. 'painful arc' syndromes, cuff tears – Ch. 15), when the pain is diffuse and occurs in the deltoid area. Distinguishing between the two may be difficult.

Hip

Passive movements are reduced (especially internal rotation) and painful at the end of the range. There may be an antalgic gait (an asymmetric gait where the patient hurries on the painful side and is slower on the normal side). There is frequently a fixed flexion deformity (Thomas' test) and often a leg length discrepancy due to shortening on the affected side.

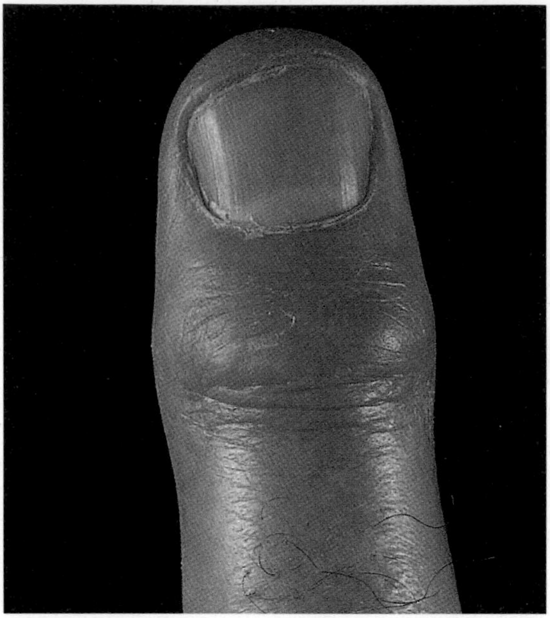

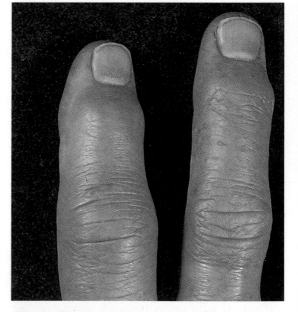

Figure 10.4   Heberden's nodes.

Figure 10.5   Bouchard's nodes (PIP joints) and Heberden's nodes (DIP joints).

It is worth mentioning at this point two relatively common conditions which can also cause 'pain in the hip', as these are not covered elsewhere in the textbook.

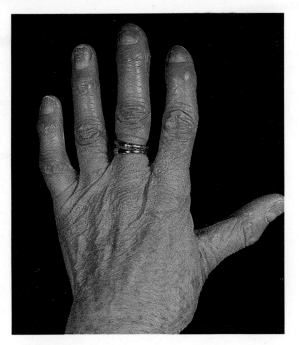

Figure 10.6   'Squaring' of the hand in osteoarthritis.

Avascular necrosis. Like osteoarthritis, this is not so much a single disease process as an end result of a number of different conditions, which lead to bone necrosis or 'osteonecrosis' through impairment of the blood supply to bone. Most commonly it is the blood supply of the femoral head which is affected, although other areas can be involved, e.g. the humeral head and the second metatarsal head (Freiberg's disease). A large number of factors predispose to avascular necrosis, e.g. corticosteroids, excessive alcohol intake, a number of diseases (including SLE and sickle cell disease) and trauma (e.g. femoral neck fracture). At an early stage X-rays may be normal, and it is important to think of this diagnosis in young patients with hip pain but normal X-rays. MR scanning will pick up early changes of avascular necrosis. Later on, an area of subchondral lucency may be seen on plain X-ray ('crescent sign'). This represents a subchondral fracture and presages collapse of the femoral head and osteoarthritis.

Trochanteric bursitis. This is a very common cause of 'hip' pain, felt laterally over the area of the greater trochanter. The pain tends to be worse with activity or with lying on the affected side at night.

On examination, there is tenderness over the area of the greater trochanter.

Knee

Osteoarthritis may affect the medial tibiofemoral joint, the lateral tibiofemoral joint, the patellofemoral joint, or a combination of these. Loss of articular cartilage is often most marked in the medial tibiofemoral compartment, leading to a varus (bow-legged) deformity. Look for quadriceps wasting, bony swelling (due to osteophytes), joint line tenderness, limitation of flexion, pain on flexion, and crepitus (felt during passive flexion and extension of the knee). In patellofemoral osteoarthritis, there may be tenderness on pressing over the patella. The patient often complains of pain going up and down stairs, and after sitting for long periods.

Foot

Osteoarthritis very often occurs in the first MTP joint. This may occur as a primary problem (hallux rigidus), which is common in young men, and it may also be secondary to a hallux valgus deformity.

Spine

Cervical and lumbar spine movements may be reduced. Pain exacerbated by extension suggests facet joint disease. Two types of joints may be affected in the spine. First, the intervertebral discs; these are not synovial joints, and therefore strictly speaking are not affected by osteoarthritis. However, they are affected by spondylosis, which may lead to large osteophytes at the joint margins. Secondly, the apophyseal or posterior facet joints, which are synovial, are frequently affected by osteoarthritis. Osteoarthritis of the apophyseal joints can lead directly to pain, and furthermore, osteophytes in this site may lead to nerve root impingement and associated nerve root pain. The facet joints are less obvious on initial inspection of standard X-rays than the discal joints. Spondylosis is discussed further in Chapter 17.

Investigations

As osteoarthritis is not a systemic disease, the full blood count, biochemical profile and immuno-

Osteoarthritis

logical tests should all be normal and there should be no elevation of the ESR or of other acute-phase reactants.

Plain radiographs

These are the mainstay of assessment of the osteoarthritic joint (Figs 10.2 and 10.3). Remember, however, that many patients have radiographic evidence of osteoarthritis and that minor change on X-ray does not mean that this is the cause of the patient's problems. Therefore, the X-rays always must be interpreted in light of the clinical situation. Box 10.3 lists the principal radiographic features of osteoarthritis compared to those of rheumatoid arthritis.

Box 10.3   Principal radiographic features of osteoarthritis and rheumatoid arthritis

Osteoarthritis
- Subchondral sclerosis
- Narrowing of the joint space
- Osteophytes (periarticular new bone)
- Subchondral cysts

Rheumatoid arthritis
- Juxta-articular osteoporosis
- Narrowing of the joint space
- Periarticular erosions

Magnetic resonance imaging

MRI is now increasingly being used in the assessment of patients with musculoskeletal problems and is particularly useful in the assessment of those suspected to have another coexisting pathology, such as osteoarthritis, bone or joint sepsis, avascular necrosis or internal joint derangement (e.g. a meniscal tear in the knee). However, it is currently of limited value in establishing the severity of osteoarthritis in a joint. Occasionally, arthroscopy is required to assess the degree of arthritis in a joint. For example, in the knee, it is not unusual to find that a patient who complains of severe pain may have relatively normal X-rays, but severe changes on arthroscopy.

MANAGEMENT

At present there is no 'specific' treatment for osteoarthritis. However, much can be done to relieve the symptoms and minimise the disability associated with the disease (Box 10.4). The large number of patients with osteoarthritis has meant that a wide variety of surgical techniques have been employed, including osteotomy, arthrodesis, excision arthroplasty and total joint replacement. For those patients with advanced osteoarthritis, the development of joint replacement techniques over the last 30 years has revolutionised management, especially with respect to relieving severe pain.

Many patients with osteoarthritis have minimal symptoms and are cared for in the community. This is entirely appropriate, but care should be taken to exclude other causes of joint pain, such as rheumatoid arthritis, which require specific measures to attempt to control the underlying disease process. Most patients with inflammatory arthritis should be assessed by a rheumatologist.

Box 10.4   Treatment modalities used in osteoarthritis

- Patient education
  - weight reduction
  - avoidance of aggravating activities
  - remaining reasonably active

- Physiotherapy
  - joint protection
  - exercises
  - walking aids

- Occupational therapy
  - joint protection
  - splinting
  - aids and appliances

- Chiropody (footwear)

- Drugs
  - analgesics
  - NSAIDs (sometimes)

- Surgery
  - osteotomy
  - excision arthroplasty
  - arthrodesis
  - total joint replacement

However, most patients with osteoarthritis are treated by general practitioners and community services such as physiotherapy, with referral to orthopaedic or rheumatology services when required.

Once the diagnosis of osteoarthritis is established, for patients with other than mild symptoms, treatment is multidisciplinary and includes:

- patient education
- identification and removal of factors which may contribute to disease progression
- physiotherapy and occupational therapy
- drug treatment (analgesics, sometimes an NSAID)
- surgery in selected patients.

General measures

Patient education

Patients may be reassured by the knowledge that they do not have a systemic inflammatory process which is likely to progress rapidly. Although in a proportion of patients osteoarthritis can worsen rapidly, e.g. at the hip, in most any progression is slow. The importance of joint protection and of remaining reasonably active should be emphasised.

Identification and removal of aggravating factors

The overweight patient should be given dietary advice and it should be explained that excessive loading of weight-bearing joints may lead to progression of osteoarthritis. Patients may need to modify their lifestyle. For example, heavy lifting should be avoided. In practice, however, attempts at weight loss and lifestyle modification are often unsuccessful.

Physiotherapy, occupational therapy and other rehabilitative measures

The aims of physiotherapy include preservation and improvement of range of motion and muscle strengthening. For example, quadriceps exercises are usually recommended in early knee osteoarthritis. The physiotherapist may also identify ways in which to avoid excessive joint loading, e.g. with various types of walking aid. A cane or stick should usually be held in the hand opposite to the side of the weight-bearing joint problem; for example, a patient with a painful left hip holds the walking aid in the right hand.

The occupational therapist also plays an important role in advising on joint protection. Splints and orthoses may be required for the patient with an unstable joint (instability may accelerate the osteoarthritic process). Disabled patients may need to be assessed at home by the occupational therapist, who can recommend necessary adaptations, such as raising the height of a toilet seat. Good footwear (with cushioning) is essential – 'trainers' are often helpful.

Drug treatment

A conservative approach should be adopted. Many patients with osteoarthritis are elderly, with an increased risk of adverse drug effects. A simple analgesic such as paracetamol should be tried in the first instance. Only if simple analgesics fail should an NSAID be used: osteoarthritis is not usually associated with a significant inflammatory component and elderly patients are particularly at risk of NSAID side-effects (Ch. 8). However, NSAIDs do benefit a proportion of patients.

Systemic steroids are not used in the treatment of osteoarthritis. While intra-articular steroids may be helpful, as in patients with osteoarthritis of the CMC joint of the thumb or with an exacerbation of osteoarthritis in the knee with an effusion, they are much less frequently used than in inflammatory arthritis. However, they can be very successful in some patients; this is of interest as these injections work by decreasing inflammation, emphasising that inflammation due to a secondary synovitis plays an important part in osteoarthritic symptoms in some patients.

Surgical treatment of osteoarthritis

Operations on osteoarthritic joints form a major part of the workload of most orthopaedic departments. The mainstay of operative treatment is total joint replacement, but other types of

Osteoarthritis

procedure are also used. Remember that surgery is only one part of the treatment, and patients undergoing it also need analgesia and rehabilitation. Most patients with osteoarthritis never need surgical treatment; only those in whom initial conservative treatment has failed, and for whom an appropriate operation is possible, should be considered for surgery.

Goals of surgical treatment

Most surgery for osteoarthritis is undertaken for pain, which may be very severe, disturbing sleep and preventing mobility to the stage that patients become chair-bound (occasionally) or house-bound (frequently). As with all surgery, the balance of risks and benefits should be discussed with the patient pre-operatively, and generally the final decision about whether to proceed rests with the patient, as they are the best judge of the severity of pain and disability which they are suffering. However, the surgeon has the duty to inform the patient fully about the risks, both short- and long-term, and may not offer surgery if these are considered unacceptable.

Surgical methods

Total joint replacement. This procedure has transformed the outlook for patients with large joint osteoarthritis over the last 30 years. Attempts at total joint replacement were started in the early years of this century, but an inadequate knowledge of biomechanics and inadequate materials prevented progress. In the 1960s, Charnley developed the low friction arthroplasty (of the hip), introducing the basic form of joint replacements which are in current use.

Charnley's total hip replacement had several features which remain in widespread use. First, the replacement uses one soft bearing surface and one hard bearing surface. The most widely used surfaces are ultra-high molecular weight polyethylene (UHMWPE) for the concave part of the joint (acetabulum, tibial plateau) and stainless steel for the convex part (femoral head, femoral condyles) (Fig. 10.7). Second, the implants are attached to bone using a micro-interlock system with a grout of polymethylmethacrylate. This is a fast-setting polymer which hardens over about 10

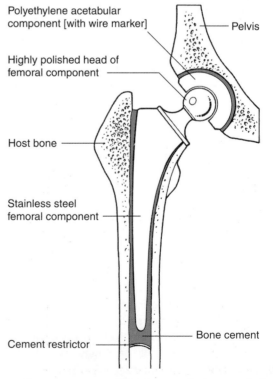

Figure 10.7   Bilateral total hip replacements. The femoral components are stainless steel; the acetabular component is polyethylene (which is radiolucent) so only the marker wires attached to the prothesis can be seen.

minutes after insertion of the prosthetic components at operation. Success and improvement of total joint replacements are critically dependent on development and improvement of the materials employed.

Total joint replacements often give spectacular pain relief for both inflammatory arthritis and osteoarthritis. The pain relief is rarely absolute, as some wound site pain is frequent, but for many patients the procedure gives a dramatic improvement in pain, and consequently in joint and limb function. In straightforward osteoarthritic hips and knees, approximately 90–95% of patients obtain satisfactory results. Joint replacements in the upper limb also yield good results, although their use in osteoarthritis is less widespread. The improvement in the range of motion may be less marked than that of pain.

Osteotomy. Realignment osteotomy is used to reduce local overloading in a joint. Thus, in the knee, a varus joint is realigned into valgus by a proximal tibial osteotomy (Fig. 10.8). Similar operations are also carried out at the proximal

femur and pelvis (for early osteoarthritis of the hip joint) and at the distal femur (principally for a valgus arthritic knee). The reduction in overloading is followed, if all goes well, by local cartilage repair; this is of fibrocartilage rather than hyaline cartilage (the normal cartilage type in a healthy joint). The fibrocartilage is less resilient than hyaline cartilage, having a tendency to degenerate even under the reduced loading conditions, but may give many years of satisfactory pain relief before further intervention is required.

There is an ill understood effect of osteotomy to produce pain relief even when the mechanical misalignment of the joint is not corrected. It is thought that this is related to reduction in local venous hypertension associated with osteoarthritis.

Osteotomies are less widely used than formerly in the treatment of osteoarthritis. Currently, they are reserved for young patients who would wear out a total joint replacement in a relatively short time. They have always had an element of unpredictability, so that a technically satisfactory operation may (in about 20% of cases in most series) give little or no pain relief. Similarly, some operations may only be followed by short-lived pain relief, giving a 60–70% rate of good outcomes after most series of osteotomies for osteoarthritis. There are at least two reasons why a significant proportion of patients have a poor outcome:

- The indications for operation may not have been closely followed. These include an almost normal range of motion of the affected joint.
- The ability of individuals to repair cartilage may vary.

Excision arthroplasty. This procedure consists of excision of one surface of a joint, together with some underlying bone. The excised surface is then held apart for a period, permitting fibrous tissue to form in the resulting gap. This fibrous joint should then be less painful than the previous arthritic joint. A satisfactory outcome depends on an adequate amount of fibrous tissue forming to prevent the bone end on one side merely rubbing on the residual cartilage surface on the other. The natural tendency of muscle forces to shorten

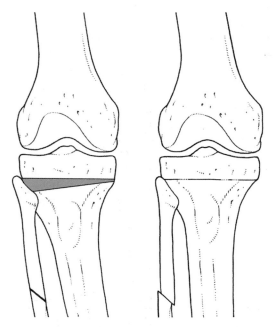

Figure 10.8 Closing wedge osteotomy of upper tibia for a varus knee deformity. A wedge of bone (based laterally) is removed. The fibula is also divided to allow it to shorten slightly.

this gap may limit the effectiveness of the operation. Thus, in the hip, excision arthroplasty (Girdlestone's procedure) is now rarely carried out for pain relief, as the strong muscles around the hip make it very difficult to maintain an adequate gap while fibrosis occurs.

Excision arthroplasty is still undertaken for osteoarthritis at some sites, including several in the upper limb. This method remains the standard surgical treatment of osteoarthritis of the acromioclavicular joint. A variant of this method is used for osteoarthritis at the scaphotrapeziometacarpal joint in the hand. In this procedure, the entire trapezium is excised and replaced with a rolled-up piece of fibrous tissue (frequently half of the flexor carpi radialis tendon), which forms a ready-made fibrous interposition.

Arthrodesis. This consists of excision of sufficient cartilage and bone from the opposing surfaces of the joint to obtain joint fusion. The resulting bone surfaces must be held in apposition until bone healing has occurred; internal fixation devices (screws or plates) are often used to achieve this. The advantage of arthrodesis is that excellent pain control is usually achieved. Against this there are disadvantages, including an understandable reluctance on the part of the patient to forego the normal mobility of the joint. First, arthrodesis may not be easy to achieve, and most series have a failure rate, at least of the initial operation. Second, the lack of movement in the arthrodesed joint places additional stresses on adjacent normal joints. Thus, after hip joint arthrodesis (previously widely used for osteoarthritis of the hip), good pain relief may be obtained, but later secondary degenerative changes in the knee and lumbar spine may eventually lead to unacceptable symptoms in these areas. In this particular example, it may be possible to relieve these secondary symptoms by conversion of the arthrodesis to a hip replacement at a later date. However, the presence of pre-existing osteoarthritis in these adjacent joints is a contraindication to arthrodesis.

Arthrodesis is still employed as the procedure of choice in some arthritic joints, e.g. the ankle joint where total joint replacement gives very poor results in osteoarthritis. The joints of the foot are also often treated by fusion, e.g. the subtalar joint

in post-traumatic osteoarthritis after fractures of the calcaneum.

Complications of joint surgery

Operations on joints are fairly major procedures, liable to be complicated by the consequences of long anaesthetics and prolonged recumbency:

- chest and urinary infections
- venous thromboembolism
- cardiovascular or cerebrovascular events
- pressure sores.

These are the same as for any surgery; however, thromboembolism is a particular problem after lower limb arthroplasty. There are also specific complications which must be mentioned in advance to the patient and guarded against during the operation and postoperative period.

The complications which cause most problems after total joint replacements are infection, usually presenting within the first few years after the operation, and aseptic loosening, which usually presents relatively late, commonly between 10 and 15 years after surgery.

Infection. This is a serious problem, which may lead to osteomyelitis, sinus formation and great difficulty in treatment. It may be necessary to remove the prosthesis and cement for a period before reimplantation in order to eradicate the infection. The most commonly incriminated organisms are *Staphylococcus aureus* and *Staphylococcus epidermidis*. Efforts to reduce the risk of infection include avoiding surgery until pre-existing infection (e.g. dental caries, urinary infection) has been eradicated, meticulous surgical technique, prophylactic antibiotics and the use of ultra-clean air enclosures in the operating theatre.

Aseptic loosening of the prosthesis in the bone is a complex problem, which is probably initiated by biomechanical factors. Revision of the joint replacement is frequently complicated by severe bone loss caused by a foreign body giant cell reaction to small (1–50 μm) particles of debris from the joint. Typically, these consist of fragments of UHMWPE from the joint prosthesis. Such particles are inevitable with most current implant designs, given the expected 1 million gait cycles/year which are experienced by a lower limb joint.

Venous thromboembolism. This is particularly frequent in patients with lower limb trauma or after lower limb surgery. The thrombi may form in the venous sinuses of the calf, around valve cusps or in areas of direct venous damage. Most deep venous thromboses (DVTs) are clinically silent, and it is clear from various investigations that high-risk patients (see Ch. 5) may have a risk of up to 75% of having a DVT. Distal (calf) DVTs may have a relatively low risk of embolism (although this is controversial), but thrombi proximal to the knee have a high risk of embolising to the pulmonary circulation. This is a common cause of death and serious morbidity in at-risk patients.

All patients should be assessed for their risk of DVT and pulmonary embolus. Low-risk patients may be managed by early mobilisation and by graduated compression stockings. Medium- and high-risk patients should receive specific anti-embolic precautions. These may include low-dose heparin (either fractionated or unfractionated), adjusted dose warfarin or treatment with one of several mechanical devices which mimic the calf muscle pump.

11 | Disorders of bone

Case history

A 50-year-old Asian woman presented with a femoral fracture. This had arisen after an apparently trivial fall on a garden path. It was treated successfully by internal fixation, but her history included two other fractures, albeit minor, in the last 5 years. She had no other serious illnesses. Possible causes for the fracture are explored later in other scenarios of this case history, any of which could have resulted in this presentation with fracture.

Key points

- **Bone has two principal functions: mechanical support and mineral (calcium and phosphate) homeostasis**

- **Bone diseases may be focal or general**

- **Most bone diseases predispose to fractures**

- **The prevalence of osteoporosis in the population is already high and is rising**

- **The commonest focal diseases of bone (metastases and infection) usually arise from haematogenous spread**

FUNCTIONS OF BONE

Bone has several functions. First, it acts as the principal mechanical support of the body structure. Second, it is the main calcium store of the body. Serum calcium regulation is vital, as ionic calcium is important in intracellular and extracellular signalling and homeostasis (key features of metabolism are covered in Box 11.1). Third, the skeleton is the site of the bone

marrow, which in postnatal life is the site of haematopoiesis.

Most of the subjects covered in this book relate to joint and (non-mineralised) connective tissue disorders, and mechanical injuries to bones and joints. Bone may also suffer from a variety of intrinsic disorders (Box 11.2); these include the various metabolic bone diseases, congenital disorders, primary and secondary tumours and infection. Apart from osteoporosis, these conditions are relatively uncommon. However, it is important to recognise them on presentation as many of them can be effectively treated.

OSTEOPOROSIS
Scenario 1

The patient was advised to have a scan to 'measure the strength of her bones'. A DEXA scan was arranged, and this showed that her bone mineral density was more than 2.5 standard deviations below the peak bone mass of young women at both lumbar spine and femoral neck.

Subsequent taking of her history revealed that she had undergone a bilateral oophorectomy as part of gynaecological surgery some 10 years earlier. After the results of the DEXA scan were available, she was advised to start hormone replacement therapy (HRT). She was not enthusiastic about the prospect of taking tablets, but acceded to the suggestion after explanation of the importance of controlling her osteoporosis.

Five years later she was scanned again. This showed that there had been no reduction in bone mass since her previous scan. She continued on HRT.

Box 11.1   Notes on bone metabolism

Bone metabolism can be viewed at several levels of detail. There is a whole-body view, relating calcium intake and excretion, together with hormonal influences on these. At higher magnification, local features of bone metabolism, particularly the coupling between bone formation and breakdown, are important. The central role of calcium in the control of cellular processes must be recalled in making sense of the body's metabolism of calcium; priority is given to serum and intracellular ionised calcium homeostasis, rather than to maintenance of the mechanical integrity of the skeleton.

Key players
Parathyroid hormone (PTH)
This is the peptide from parathyroid glands. It tends to increase serum calcium by (1) increasing bone resorption (effect on osteoclasts), and (2) decreasing urinary excretion of calcium by action on the kidney (but it increases excretion of phosphate – phosphaturic effect). Normally the control of release from parathyroids is sensitive to [Ca] – but not if an adenoma develops in the parathyroid glands. A related protein (PTHRP) with similar effects is released from some tumours.

Vitamin D (calciferol)
This vitamin is active in its double hydroxylated form (dihydroxy-cholecalciferol). There are two hydroxylation steps, first in the liver (generating 25-hydroxy vitamin D) and then in the kidney (generating 1,25-dihydroxy vitamin D). Thus, severe disease of either of these organs will affect bone metabolism. Its principal role is to permit calcium absorption in the gut (which is an active process, and may be affected by any form of malabsorption). Vitamin D also has a direct effect on osteoblasts and osteoclasts, tending to promote bone formation and mineralization and bone resorption.

Calcitonin
This is produced by C-cells of the thyroid. It inhibits osteoclasts and reduces serum calcium levels. The real extent of its physiological importance is unclear.

Box 11.2   Intrinsic disorders of bone

Focal conditions of bone
- Osteomyelitis
- Metastases
- Primary bone tumours (benign or malignant)
- Paget's disease (but often affects more than one bone)

Generalised conditions of bone
- Osteoporosis
- Osteomalacia
- Rickets
- Hyperparathyroidism
- Osteogenesis imperfecta

Osteoporosis is characterised by loss of bone, and is associated with an increase in the risk of fracture. The prevalence and incidence of osteoporosis have recently become clearer, as the World Health Organization has issued definitions relating the diagnosis of osteoporosis and osteopenia to bone mineral density (measured by techniques such as DEXA — dual energy X-ray absorptiometry).

Epidemiology

The condition is commonest in elderly women, over 30% of whom will experience an osteoporotic fracture at some stage in their lives. The incidence of osteoporosis has increased dramatically over the past 40 years. The effect is illustrated by data for hip fractures, the majority of which are related to osteoporosis. While the rise in hip fracture incidence over the years is mostly due to the change in age structure of the population (with an increase in the elderly population) the age specific incidence of hip fracture has also increased.

Pathology

Bone remodelling occurs throughout life. During this process, bone is removed by osteoclasts from the surface of bone trabeculae. Bone removal is normally tightly coupled to bone replacement, which is carried out by osteoblasts. The mechanisms of this coupling are the subject of a great deal of current research. Osteoporosis develops when bone remodelling is insufficiently tightly coupled to ensure that as much bone is replaced as is removed (Fig. 11.1). The factors controlling the development of osteoporosis are therefore the peak bone mass attained and the rate

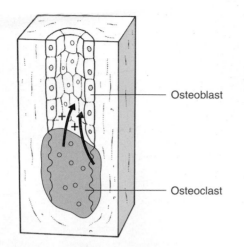

Figure 11.1 Schematic diagram demonstrating the coupling between bone replacement and removal. In normal bone remodelling, osteoclasts both produce factors (growth factors, prostaglandins) and release them from the bone matrix. These factors result in activation of osteoblasts to produce new bone, and coupling of resorption and formation.

Osteoblast

Osteoclast

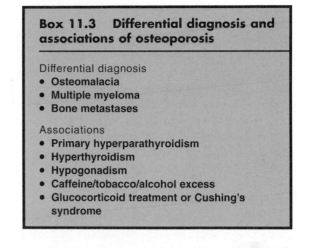

Box 11.3 **Differential diagnosis and associations of osteoporosis**

Differential diagnosis
- **Osteomalacia**
- **Multiple myeloma**
- **Bone metastases**

Associations
- **Primary hyperparathyroidism**
- **Hyperthyroidism**
- **Hypogonadism**
- **Caffeine/tobacco/alcohol excess**
- **Glucocorticoid treatment or Cushing's syndrome**

of loss of bone. Peak bone mass is generally attained at approximately age 25, and is determined by adequate nutrition throughout childhood and early adulthood, the presence of a normal hormonal environment and, importantly, by mechanical loading of the skeleton. Adequate mechanical loading is vital to ensure that a satisfactorily high peak bone mass is attained.

After attaining peak bone mass, most people will slowly lose bone. However, bone may be lost rapidly after the menopause in women. This is believed to be due to the loss of hormonal (oestrogen) control of the osteoclasts. It is this hormonal effect which accounts for the dramatic difference in osteoporosis between men and women. There are several established risk factors in addition to sex, including race (with osteoporosis being commoner in Caucasians), early menopause (whether constitutional or due to therapeutic intervention such as hysterectomy/oophorectomy) and chronic smoking.

A variety of diseases and medications are associated with osteoporosis (Box 11.3), including hyperthyroidism, hyperparathyroidism, hypogonadism and glucocorticoid administration.

Further, immobility results in disuse osteoporosis. This may be generalised (e.g. in bedridden patients) or localised (e.g. during disuse of a limb after fracture). Localised osteoporosis may also be a striking feature of conditions with altered blood flow, particularly algodystrophy/reflex sympathetic dystrophy (see Ch. 6).

Clinical features

Previous fractures

Most people with osteoporosis are asymptomatic, but it is important to ask about previous fractures. The commonest presentation of osteoporosis is with a fracture. This may affect any bone, but common sites include thoracic and lumbar vertebrae, proximal femur, distal radius and proximal humerus. All of these sites may present with fracture following minimal trauma. Some patients present with progressive vertebral deformity due to gradual collapse of several vertebrae leading to kyphosis (Dowager's hump). Interestingly, many such patients do not recall a specific episode associated with past fracture leading to deformity.

Fractures of the peripheral skeleton are described elsewhere. Vertebral fractures due to osteoporosis may cause prolonged pain and disability. They are a common cause of persisting backache in elderly patients. It is important to consider the possibility of other causes of vertebral collapse in patients thought to have osteoporotic vertebral disease, as the vertebrae are common sites of metastatic deposits. Examination of the breasts (a common primary site in female patients) and chest is therefore mandatory. Evidence of bone destruction should be sought on X-rays, and if necessary, additional investigations including blood tests (full blood count and ESR, bone profile and possibly myeloma screen — plasma electrophoresis) and bone scintigraphy should be carried out as described below. It is important to realise that osteoporosis *per se* is not a cause of back pain, but the related fractures and their sequelae are.

Menstrual history and lifestyle

Female patients should be asked about their menstrual history, as early menopause (whether natural or induced) is associated with osteoporosis. Other endocrine abnormalities to be sought include hyperthyroidism. Also ask about the patient's lifestyle – does the patient have a sedentary job, take regular weight-bearing exercise or smoke?

Investigations

The diagnosis of osteoporosis may be made on radiographic, bone densitometry or histological grounds. Plain X-rays are inaccurate for diagnosis; they are both insensitive and non-specific. The characteristic features of osteoporosis may possibly be seen in the vertebrae, where reduction in bone density together with a characteristic vertical striation of the bone trabeculae in the vertebral body is seen. Vertebral collapse is seen in patients with advanced disease (Fig. 11.2).

Bone density measurement. The unreliability of plain X-rays in diagnosis has led to a variety of techniques to measure bone mineral density (BMD). These rely on the attenuation of a waveform by calcified tissue, which is related to the mineral density of the bone. Algorithms are developed to correct for soft tissue absorption of the signal, or alternatively a site such as the calcaneum is used which has minimal soft tissue cover. Current widely used techniques include dual energy X-ray absorptiometry (DEXA), quantitative computed topography (QCT) and broad-band ultrasound attenuation. Further details of these are given in Table 11.1. Reduced bone densities are expressed in relation to a young adult mean; individuals with

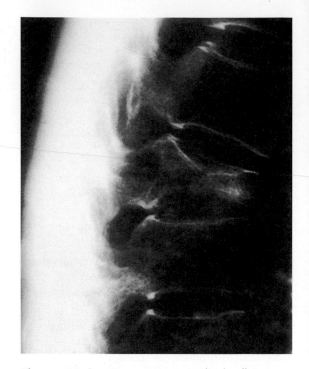

Figure 11.2   Osteoporotic vertebral collapse.

values reduced by more than 2.5 standard deviations are defined as having osteoporosis. Bone densities may also be considered compared with an age- and sex-matched population.

There is a reasonable correlation between bone mineral densities in different sites within a particular patient. The site of interest should ideally be screened directly to assess the risk of a particular bone becoming fractured. Thus, in order to assess the risk of femoral neck fracture, the femoral neck bone mineral density should be measured, or alternatively to assess the risk of a wrist fracture the distal radius needs to be measured. However, this is not always possible and some screening systems rely on measurement of bones which do not *per se* constitute a major fracture risk (e.g. calcaneum). Measurements of bone mineral density are used both to screen patients for osteoporosis and to follow the results of treatment.

Other tests (Table 11.2).   Simple blood tests are normal in primary osteoporosis. Investigations such as FBC, ESR and biochemical screen are nonetheless useful to exclude other conditions, notably osteomalacia which is usually associated

Table 11.1
Methods of investigation of bone mineral density. (Bone mineral density is strongly related to the strength of bone, and hence its resistance to fracture; it is also related to the degree of osteoporosis measured histologically.)

Method	Technique	Advantage	Disadvantage
Single photon absorptiometry (SPA) (also single X-ray, SXA)	Uses beam from single source of photons and measurement device on the other side of the patient	Economical; simple; quick; low-radiation dose	Rather inaccurate (difficult to correct for soft tissues)
Dual energy X-ray absorptiometry (DEXA)	Uses beams from two photon (X-ray) sources of different energies, and measurement device on the other side of the patient	Low-radiation dose; fairly cheap; much more accurate than SPA; possible to measure multiple sites with modern equipment	Capital cost of machine; slower to use (and hence more expensive for staff time) than SPA
Quantitative computed tomography (QCT)	Conventional computed tomography hardware; uses 'phantoms' of known density to calibrate machine output	Almost as accurate as DEXA; widespread availability of CT scanners; can scan most bones	High-radiation dose; scanning time long, therefore costly; accuracy is operator-dependent
Broad-band ultrasound attenuation	Ultrasound beam is passed through the heel (calcaneum) in a fluid bath; receiver detects amount of ultrasound removed by bone	Very cheap; portable; quick; no radiation; recent machines will also scan tibia or finger	Less accurate; relationship of calcaneum BMD to other bones is not very reliable

with a raised alkaline phosphatase and a low phosphate. Also requiring investigation are multiple myeloma (serum electrophoresis and urinary Bence–Jones' protein) and thyroid function. Serum testosterone should be measured in male patients. Histological evaluation of bone to confirm metabolic bone disease is occasionally required; it is also a reproducible way of quantifying the amount of osteoporosis for research. Measurement of rates of bone formation may be aided by giving the patient two doses of tetracycline prior to biopsy; this is visible as two fluorescent lines in the bone which is being laid down at the time of the tetracycline dosing. The distance between the lines reflects the amount of bone formation occurring.

Prevention and management

There are a variety of strategies available to both prevent and manage osteoporosis. Until recently, prevention was the only effective strategy

available, but there is now evidence that some treatments can both restore bone mineral density and reduce the risk of fracture in patients with osteoporosis. Simultaneously, any underlying cause should be treated vigorously.

Prevention

Prevention of eventual osteoporosis, which usually manifests itself in patients aged over 70, should begin in adolescence and be continued indefinitely. An adequate diet (including sufficient calcium) and development of a lifestyle involving sufficient amounts of exercise are important. These are both strategies which will result in patients achieving a high peak bone mass. Subsequently, continuation of both of these factors will maintain this peak bone mass. Hormone replacement therapy (HRT) is discussed below. Measures to prevent falls, especially in older patients, will reduce the risk of fracture. Consideration should be given to prophylactic treatment (e.g. with the bisphosphonate etidronate) in patients on

Table 11.2
Blood tests used in the investigation of bone disease

Blood test	Associated condition(s)	Comments
Alkaline phosphatase (AlkP) (high)	Metastases; osteomalacia; Paget's disease; normal children (slight); fractures; multiple myeloma; hyperparathyroidism	Bone-specific AlkP may be measured, but usually total AlkP is reported. Liver is another important source of the enzyme
Acid phosphatase (high)	Metastatic prostatic cancer	Prostate-specific antigen should also be measured
Calcium (high)	Hyperparathyroidism; multiple myeloma; metastases; sarcoid; vitamin D intoxication	Calcium is bound to serum proteins, hence it is important to measure corrected (available) calcium
Calcium (low)	Hypoparathyroidism (usually postoperative); may be marginally low in osteomalacia	Associated with nerve conduction abnormalities (e.g. Chvostek's sign)
Phosphate (high)	Hyperphosphataemia in metastases; multiple myeloma	Usually associated with hypercalcaemia
Phosphate (low)	Hypophosphataemia in hyperparathyroidism (due to phosphaturic effect of PTH); osteomalacia	Product of [corrected calcium] and [phosphate] should be > 2; if less, patient may have osteomalacia
Urinary hydroxyproline	Increased with increased bone formation—Paget's disease; fracture healing	Requires 24-h urine collection. Represents total body collagen turnover, therefore not particularly sensitive or specific
Parathyroid hormone (PTH)	Hyperparathyroidism; hypoparathyroidism; renal bone disease	Useful test in patients found to have hypercalcaemia; PTH related peptide (PTHRP) may be produced by lesions such as lung tumours
Vitamin D	Rickets; osteomalacia; renal disease; malabsorption	

corticosteroids, especially if these are given in high dosage and/or are likely to be prescribed for a prolonged period. This area is still, however, a subject of much research.

Management of established osteoporosis

HRT. Female patients may lose bone rapidly after menopause, and the risk of rapid bone loss at this stage may be countered by hormone (principally oestrogen) replacement therapy. There is controversy about whether the bone maintained by HRT is subsequently lost when HRT is stopped. As a minimum, it appears that HRT should be maintained for a period of approximately 5 years in order to be worthwhile in terms of osteoporosis prevention, although its use may be justified for shorter periods for other indications. HRT is also used in the treatment of established osteoporosis.

There is a risk of developing endometrial carcinoma on long term unopposed (by progestogens) oestrogen treatment, so women who have not had a hysterectomy should have combined oestrogen and progesterone treatment supplied. The risk of breast cancer appears to be marginally increased by HRT; this is a cause of great concern to many women and is the subject of ongoing research. It is important to set the other benefits of HRT against this, such as reductions in the risk of myocardial infarction, stroke and dementia (and of fractures!).

Bisphosphonates, calcium and vitamin D. Recently, a variety of bisphosphonates have become available for the management of osteoporosis. These can be given intravenously or orally. The latter is more convenient, but results in poor absorption relative to parenteral administration, and doses are higher by the oral route. Oral administration is also associated with oesophageal ulceration with some preparations. Bisphosphonates work by inhibiting osteoclast action, allowing bone formation to predominate over bone resorption, and can increase bone mineral density with associated reductions in fracture rates. The role of bisphosphonates in osteoporosis treatment is currently undergoing intensive investigation, and the optimal usage of these drugs is currently unclear. Indications for use, including the degree of osteoporosis at which they should be employed, are currently controversial. However, most specialists in osteoporosis now employ these medications for patients with proven disease in middle age for whom hormone replacement therapy is inappropriate or unacceptable.

Finally, it has been shown that protracted treatment with calcium and vitamin D can reduce fracture risk. This is true even in elderly patients, some of whom are likely to have established osteoporosis. The relative merits of treatment with vitamin D/calcium and bisphosphonates in elderly patients with osteoporosis are currently the subject of both scientific and commercial controversy.

Screening

The strategy for containment of the current epidemic of osteoporosis in Western countries is evolving rapidly. As effective treatments have become available, it is no longer tenable to argue that screening is of no value because no treatment is available. The current position of bone density screening programmes is not clear, but it must be recognised that the social and health care costs of established osteoporosis, with consequent hospital treatment for fractures, is considerable. The development of understanding about both prevention and management of osteoporosis makes an expansion of bone mineral density screening over the next few years highly likely.

OSTEOMALACIA AND RICKETS
Scenario 2

The patient had a history of multiple aches and pains as well as her previous fractures. Serum biochemistry was performed as part of the standard work-up prior to her surgery, and the alert house officer noted that both corrected calcium (2.20 mM) and phosphate (0.65 mM) levels were low. A bone biopsy was taken at surgery; histology confirmed the diagnosis of osteomalacia. No underlying cause (such as renal disease) was detected for her osteomalacia, although serum vitamin D levels were low. Her pain symptoms improved dramatically after treatment with dihydroxycholecalciferol, and she had no further fractures.

Epidemiology

Rickets and osteomalacia are uncommon diseases in the West at present, largely due to adequate diet. The condition is commonest in those with renal disease, and is also commoner in some ethnic groups (especially Asian females).

Pathology

Reduction in vitamin D levels results in rickets (in children) or osteomalacia (after skeletal maturity). The role of vitamin D, parathyroid hormone and calcitonin in controlling bone metabolism is discussed in Box 11.1. Disorders of such hormones may profoundly alter bone metabolism and frequently lead to bone weakness. The effects of these hormones are closely related to maintenance of serum calcium concentrations, and these concentrations will be maintained even at the cost of an adverse effect on bone strength. Lack of vitamin D leads to defective calcium absorption in the gut and causes decreased bone formation by osteoblasts. Rickets and osteomalacia are both uncommon, but are associated with a diet poor in vitamin D and a lack of exposure to sunlight. Malabsorption due to gut disease may also lead to osteomalacia, due to the inability of the gut to absorb calcium. Certain, drugs (notably anti-epileptics) may cause osteomalacia.

The principal metabolic feature of osteomalacia is an attempt by the body to maintain serum calcium in the face of reduced vitamin D levels. Because absorption of calcium from the gut is markedly reduced, calcium is released from

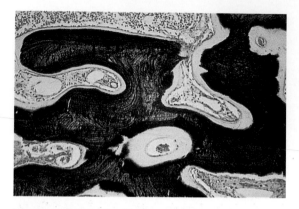

Figure 11.3   Von Kossa stained section showing all the mineralised bone (black) surfaces covered by thick seams of blue osteoid. Courtesy of Professor A J Freemont.

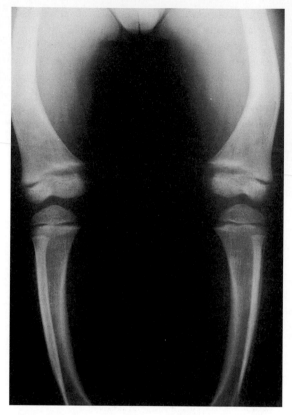

Figure 11.4   Deformity of rickets. The child has vitamin D resistant rickets.

skeletal stores into the circulation. As vitamin D has a direct effect on osteoblast action, and because of a lack of calcium, large amounts of unmineralised osteoid are laid down by osteoblasts (Fig. 11.3). Thus, the amount of bone substance present may be normal, but the degree of mineralisation of the bone is markedly reduced. This results in the bone becoming much weaker than normal.

Renal disease
The commonest current cause of rickets/ osteomalacia is renal disease. This arises because of failure of the hydroxylation stage of vitamin D which occurs in the kidneys.

Clinical features

The clinical features of early osteomalacia are vague, and diagnosis may be delayed. This is regrettable, as the condition is eminently treatable and later features include fractures and severe deformity (Fig. 11.4). Initial features include anorexia, weakness, lethargy and aching pains in any site in the skeleton. Some patients are first seen with fractures, and the possibility of the condition should be borne in mind in patients with low-energy fractures or a history of repeated fractures. There are often clinical features of associated diseases, particularly renal disease.

Childhood rickets has a characteristic set of features. It results in the development of deformities during growth, with marked genu varum (bowing of the femur and tibia) being particularly common. Chest deformities also occur; ricketty rosary is the name given to bossing of the costochondral junctions. A transverse sulcus (Harrison's sulcus) may occur in the lower chest due to deformity caused by the pull of the diaphragm on the softened ribs. Wrist swelling is also a feature of the condition.

Investigations
Diagnosis of osteomalacia may be inferred from blood tests, with a low calcium (sometimes) and phosphate (usually) and a high alkaline phosphatase (see Table 11.2 on blood testing for bone diseases). Definite diagnosis requires a bone

biopsy, which characteristically shows widened osteoid seams, revealing a high proportion of uncalcified bone matrix. Other tests include the measurement of serum vitamin D levels.

Management

Management of rickets consists of administration of vitamin D (often in high doses) and calcium to normalise bone formation. Care must be taken to monitor calcium and phosphate concentrations during treatment; there is both a risk of hypocalcaemia (rapid calcium absorption by bone) and a theoretical risk of hypercalcaemia, with attendant risk of abdominal pain or renal stones. Corrective osteotomies, particularly around the knee, may be required if deformities have become established.

Treatment of renal osteomalacia requires administration of hydroxylated vitamin D (dihydroxycalciferol) to bypass the mechanism of hydroxylation.

PAGET'S DISEASE (OSTEITIS DEFORMANS)

Scenario 3

The patient had developed bowing of her legs over the preceding 2 years. The orthopaedic surgeon described the fracture as a 'fatigue' fracture. He showed her the extensive areas of deformity on X-ray of the bones in her lower limb. The fracture was fixed with an intramedullary nail and was slow to heal. Treatment was later started with bisphosphonates, but despite this her tibial bowing deteriorated and she later had corrective osteotomies of her tibia.

Epidemiology

Paget's disease is a common disease of bone which usually presents in middle-aged or older patients. There is regional variation in the incidence of the disease; it is particularly common in the north of England.

Pathology

The pathology of Paget's disease involves accelerated bone turnover. Both osteoblastic and osteoclastic activity are markedly increased on bone biopsy. The accelerated turnover of bone results in rather disorganised architecture which ultimately leads to a significant change in mechanical properties.

Clinical features

Patients present with a variety of clinical features, such as aching pain in the bone. This pain may be severe, and if troublesome is one reason for active treatment. Alternatively, some patients present with deformity. This is frequently present in the skull, where expansion of membrane bones sometimes leads to marked enlargement of the size of the skull, frontal bossing and effects such as deafness due to compression of the auditory nerve in the petrous temporal bone. Patients with Paget's disease of the tibia usually present with a combination of bone pain and progressive deformity. The characteristic deformity is of a 'sabre' tibia, with varus and procurvatum of the tibia gradually increasing (Fig. 3.8, p. 21). Figure 11.5 demonstrates deformity in Paget's disease.

Fractures in Pagetic bones may occur with minimal or no trauma. In particular, the brittle nature of Pagetic bone, together with the deformities which develop, may result in so-called 'pseudo-fractures'. Essentially, these are fatigue fractures. The tibia is frequently involved, and healing may be difficult to achieve (Fig. 11.6). A further (although rarer) complication of Paget's disease is the development of a Pagetic osteosarcoma in an area of Pagetic bone. These generally occur in elderly patients who have had Paget's for many years. They are highly malignant and the outlook is poor. The diagnosis should be considered in any bone which has been affected by Paget's for some time and is rapidly changing.

Investigations

Diagnosis of Paget's disease is usually on the basis of identification of skeletal abnormality on X-ray,

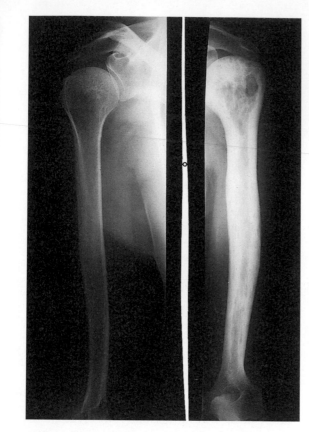

Figure 11.5 Normal appearances (left) and thickening of shaft of humerus (right) with increased sclerosis. Changes extend distally from the proximal joint surface.

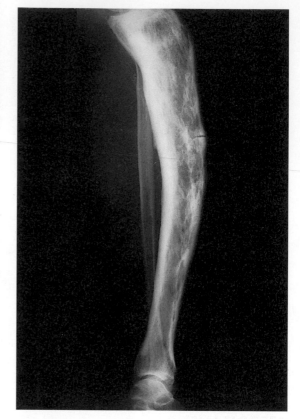

Figure 11.6 Fatigue fractures in Paget's disease. The fractures are on the concave surfaces of the femur.

sometimes followed by blood and urine testing. Biopsy, although diagnostic, is not usually required to confirm the diagnosis. X-ray features suggestive of Paget's disease include a single bone affected by an expansile, sclerotic process which is generalised throughout part of the bone. On occasion, the condition may be seen to progress along the length of a long bone, usually starting at the proximal end. Differential diagnosis on X-ray includes the presence of osteoblastic bony metastases, in particular those arising from prostatic and some breast tumours. Any bone (or several) may be affected by the condition. Characteristically affected are the skull, pelvis, femora and tibiae. Isotope bone scanning shows increased uptake at affected areas (Fig. 11.7).

Biochemical investigations are useful. The serum alkaline phosphatase is high, reflecting high osteoblastic activity, while serum calcium is normal. Incidental finding of a high alkaline phosphatase on blood testing may be the presenting feature of Paget's disease. The high levels of bone turnover result in accelerated rates of collagen formation and degradation; this may be detected by measuring urinary levels of hydroxyproline (an amino acid from collagen breakdown). Twenty-four hour urinary hydroxyproline levels are high in Paget's disease. Acid phosphatase and prostate-specific antigen levels are normal; this helps to differentiate Paget's disease from metastatic prostate cancer in men.

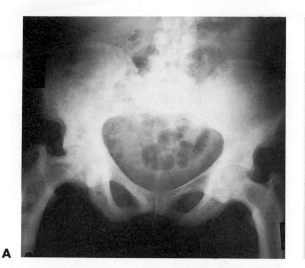
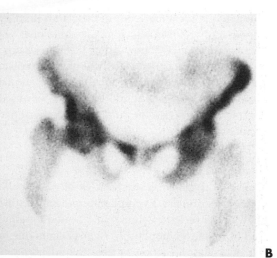

A   B

Figure 11.7 Plain X-ray appearances (A) and isotope bone scan (B) in a patient with Paget's disease involving the whole of the pelvis.

Management

Medical treatment of Paget's disease consists of the use of salmon calcitonin or bisphosphonates. Both of these inhibit osteoclast action and essentially markedly slow down the abnormal bone remodelling. Salmon calcitonin requires injections and may become ineffective after a period. Its use has now largely been superseded by bisphosphonates; these work by inhibiting osteoclast function and are usually given intravenously but may now be given orally. Their use in symptomatic Paget's disease is now widespread.

Deformities in Paget's disease are sometimes bad enough to require surgical correction. Because bone often heals relatively poorly when affected by this condition, fixation of the bone at the end of the operation must be secure and intramedullary devices are preferred. Occasionally, multiple corrective osteotomies are performed to achieve correction of a severely deformed bone.

HYPERPARATHYROIDISM AND HYPERCALCAEMIA

Pathology

Hypercalcaemia may result from hyperparathyroidism or bone malignancy (metastatic disease or multiple myeloma). There are also rarer causes, such as vitamin D intoxication, sarcoidosis and thyrotoxicosis.

Clinical features

Hypercalcaemia results in muscle weakness, lethargy, polyuria and dehydration, and mental changes including disorientation. Renal tract stones may occur. Primary hyperparathyroidism may present with these features of hypercalcaemia or with bone changes resulting from the excessive bone resorption caused by the excess parathyroid hormone. These are described as 'osteitis fibrosa cystica' (von Recklinghausen's disease of bone), as in end-stage disease there are multiple small cystic lesions in the bone. Primary hyperparathyroidism is sometimes detected due to a chance finding of hypercalcaemia on a plasma biochemical profile taken for other reasons.

Secondary hyperparathyroidism is associated with renal disease, malabsorption and osteomalacia; chronic hypocalcaemia leads to chronically raised levels of parathyroid hormone, which acts to maintain serum calcium levels (but will adversely affect skeletal integrity). The persistent overactivity of the parathyroid glands in such circumstances can lead to development of an autonomous adenoma in one of the glands (tertiary hyperparathyroidism). Such an adenoma does not respond to serum calcium, so that if serum calcium is corrected by other methods hyperparathyroidism continues, with continuing bone loss. The normal response of the parathyroid gland to increased serum calcium is for parathyroid hormone secretion to fall.

Investigations

Diagnosis is made on the basis of blood calcium testing. In primary hyperparathyroidism, testing shows high serum calcium and elevated parathyroid hormone. Hypophosphataemia occurs due to the phosphaturic action of parathyroid hormone leading to excessive loss of phosphate in the urine; the serum alkaline phosphatase is sometimes elevated in severe cases. Because primary hyperparathyroidism leads to bone loss and impaired renal function (due to renal stones or nephrocalcinosis), measurement of bone mineral density and renal function is required.

Management of hypercalcaemia

No treatment is necessary in patients with asymptomatic minimal elevation of calcium. However, severe hypercalcaemia is often a serious condition resulting in 'hypercalcaemic crisis' with gross dehydration resulting from polyuria. Prompt rehydration with intravenous fluids is a vital initial measure in managing these patients. Treatment to reduce the bone loss of calcium usually employs an intravenous bisphosphonate. This will reduce the blood calcium levels over 2 or 3 days, and reduce the risk of further dehydration. Glucocorticoids may be useful in hypercalcaemia.

Long-term treatment is directed towards preventing recurrence of hypercalcaemia. Appropriate treatment, including radiotherapy, should be given for skeletal metastatic disease. Primary and tertiary hyperparathyroidism are treated by parathyroidectomy. The four glands are usually explored and frozen sections taken to determine which gland is affected by an (autonomous) adenoma. In secondary hyperparathyroidism a subtotal parathyroidectomy is usually carried out (removal of three and one half glands). Risks of

surgery include hypocalcaemia and damage to the recurrent laryngeal nerve.

BONE TUMOURS

Primary bone tumours are relatively uncommon, but a variety of tumours frequently metastasise to bone and cause symptoms. Primary malignant musculoskeletal tumours are commonest in children and adolescents. The exact incidence of skeletal metastases and the fracture rate are unknown, but such lesions are a common presenting complaint in orthopaedic departments.

Metastatic bone disease
Scenario 4

The patient had had some aching in her leg for several weeks, and also had some back pain. She had undergone a mastectomy some 6 years before, but had not received any recent treatment for this.

After fracture fixation (from which a bone biopsy confirmed metastatic breast cancer), she had a bone scan which demonstrated several hot spots in her lumbar spine as well as that at the fracture. These were treated with a single dose of radiotherapy, which completely relieved her back pain.

Pathology

Tumours metastasising to bone include carcinoma of the breast, lung, kidney, thyroid, prostate and large bowel. Such tumours are commonest after the age of 40. Any bone may be affected by metastatic disease. Features include bone resorption, which is caused by the combined action of the tumour cells and (particularly) the bone's reaction to the tumour. This consists of an active inflammatory and macrophage response, which causes local bone damage. Reactive new bone formation is usually seen histologically in the area surrounding metastatic deposits.

Clinical features

The commonest clinical feature is pain. This may be unremitting, is frequently severe at night, and may occur in several sites if there is more than one site of metastases. Common sites of bony metastases include the thoracic and lumbar spine, the proximal femur and the proximal humerus. Pathological fractures are also a common presenting feature of metastases; such fractures often follow minimal violence. Patients may present due to hypercalcaemia.

All patients presenting with back pain should have the most likely primary sites (lung and breast) assessed. Similarly, patients with known metastatic deposits but unknown primary sites should be carefully examined for evidence of the source of metastases.

Investigations

Blood tests. Blood tests are important in screening for possible metastatic disease. Both ESR and the level of C-reactive protein (CRP) are useful but rather undiscriminating tests for inflammation and malignancy. ESR rises with age. Alkaline phosphatase is usually increased with metastatic bone disease, and hypercalcaemia (see above) may occur. Raised acid phosphatase or prostate-specific antigen (PSA) are almost pathognomonic of prostatic cancer. Investigation of multiple myeloma or similar tumours may be prompted by the finding of high total protein or globulin levels on routine biochemical testing (with a multichannel analyser). The appropriate investigation is then serum electrophoresis. Multiple myeloma demonstrates a single (monoclonal) band (a paraprotein). Bence–Jones' proteins are also detectable (these are monoclonal light chains excreted in the urine).

X-rays and scans. X-rays may remain normal for weeks or even months after the onset of severe bone pain. Therefore, a normal plain X-ray does not exclude bony metastases. When X-ray signs are present, most carcinomata will result in a lytic area with a variable amount of surrounding sclerosis. Multiple lesions are present in many patients. Periosteal elevation or reaction is uncommon (except with prostate cancer). Metastatic lesions represent a combination of bone destruction due to the effect of tumour cells, and an attempted repair reaction where bone is being laid down. In the majority of lesions, destruction predominates over formation, but some lesions may result in the formation of a large amount of disorganised new bone. These include prostate cancer and some types of breast metastases; these lesions result in sclerotic deposits when seen on X-ray. Conversely, multiple myeloma (a tumour of plasma cells) is associated with multiple lytic deposits but with essentially no osteoblastic response.

Radioisotope bone scanning (scintigraphy), commonly using technetium-99-labelled phosphonate compounds which are preferentially taken up in areas of active bone formation, is widely used for investigation of metastatic disease. This form of investigation is markedly more sensitive than plain X-rays and will generally be positive before any evidence of bone destruction can be seen. Most tumours are visualised as an area of markedly increased isotope uptake; frequently multiple deposits are visible (Fig. 4.7). Occasionally, lesions are visible as an area of markedly decreased uptake. This is particularly common in multiple myeloma. Bone scans are particularly helpful as they may reveal the presence of lesions at a presymptomatic stage. Thus, a lesion may be identified at an early stage and treatment offered before there is a substantial risk of fracture.

Recently, *magnetic resonance imaging* has been used to investigate metastatic deposits. This is a sensitive technique for this purpose, but is more expensive than bone scanning and can only practically be used to examine one or two sites per patient.

Management

Treatment of bone pain in these circumstances is palliative. Effective treatment often gives a gratifying improvement in the patient's well-being. Bone pain can be relieved by analgesics—NSAIDs (which can be particularly helpful) and radiation therapy. Additional treatment may be required if pain does not respond to these modalities, or if there is a substantial risk of fracture. Bones identified as being at risk of fracture should be treated prophylactically with internal fixation, as the results of treatment after fracture are poorer than with prophylactic intervention. There is a substantial risk of fracture if more than a third of the width of the bone has been destroyed by lesions. Fixation by an intramedullary rod is generally employed in long bones.

Disorders of bone

Surgery may also be required in spinal metastatic deposits. Indications include persisting pain and instability, or neurological compromise caused by extradural spinal cord compression. Modern techniques of spinal stabilisation, together with cord decompression if needed, are tolerated surprisingly well by most patients with metastases. Excellent palliation is often obtainable for spinal pain, but recovery of nerve function will only occur if decompression is undertaken promptly after onset of neurological symptoms.

Primary musculoskeletal tumours

Primary musculoskeletal tumours are uncommon. These almost all arise from cells of mesenchymal origin, and, accordingly, malignant tumours are known as sarcomas. A wide variety of both benign and malignant musculoskeletal tumours occur. It is impossible in this book to consider all varieties of such tumours, and as such, the principles of diagnosis and management of these conditions will be illustrated by considering four tumours.

Osteochondromas (Fig.11.8)
These tumours are relatively common, consisting of a pedunculated lesion arising from the cortex of a long bone adjacent to the epiphyseal plate. They may be solitary, but a hereditary condition exists of multiple exostoses. Osteochondromas characteristically have a cartilage cap during growth, which changes into bone at maturity.

Management of osteochondroma poses several issues. First, diagnosis of the lesion is not always obvious from clinical examination and X-rays, and if doubts persist as to the identity of the lesion, an excision biopsy is appropriate. Further, such lesions may undergo malignant transformation (usually starting at the tip) into chondrosarcomas. This is uncommon with solitary lesions, although the risks with multiple osteochondromata are higher.

Simple excision for osteochondroma provides definitive treatment.

Enchondromata
Enchondromata may be solitary or multiple (Ollier's disease). They are most frequent in the tubular bones of the hands and feet, but also occur

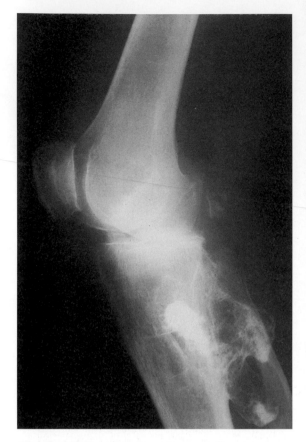

Figure 11.8   X-ray appearances of osteochondroma.

elsewhere. They occasionally present due to fracture through the lesion. Typical radiological features are as shown in Figure 11.9. Histologically, the lesions consist of areas of small chondrocytes. Malignant transformation occasionally occurs, but is extremely rare in lesions in the hands and feet.

Many of these lesions should be left untreated. Treatment of endochondromata, where required, consists of curettage of all cartilage tissue and bone grafting of the resulting defect.

Giant cell tumour of bone
Giant cell tumours of bone (Fig. 11.10) are of interest in that they are intermediate between benign and malignant primary bone tumours. These lesions consist of stromal cells together with numerous multinucleated giant cells. Giant cells are similar (or perhaps identical) to osteoclasts.

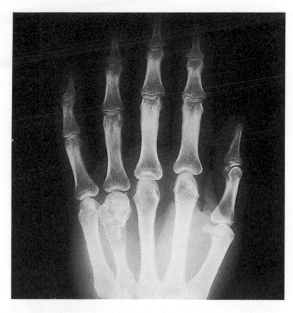

Figure 11.9 Radiological appearance of enchondroma in ring finger metocarpal.

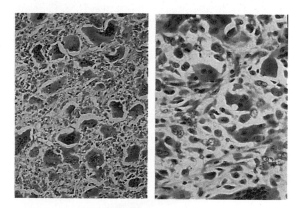

Figure 11.10 Low (left) and high power (right) views of histology appearances of a giant cell tumour showing multinucleated giant cells. Courtesy of Professor A J Freemont.

Giant cell tumours characteristically develop in the long bones after skeletal maturity. Most of them develop around the knee, but they also occur at the ends of other bones. They are rarely malignant de novo, but have a marked tendency to local recurrence after excision. Such local recurrence may be followed by malignant transformation with the risk of metastases. This transformation is particularly likely to be prompted by radiotherapy.

Giant cell tumours are usually lytic lesions, in a juxta-epiphyseal position. The cortex often appears to be destroyed by the tumour, and lesions often have poorly defined borders. There is sometimes a foamy appearance to the lesion on X-ray.

Treatment of the lesion should be informed by knowledge of histology and histological grading (which affects the risk of recurrence). Available methods of treatment include curettage and bone grafting or cryosurgery (destroying residual tumour cells with liquid nitrogen at the time of surgery).

Osteosarcoma

Pathology. Osteosarcoma is the commonest primary bone malignancy. It typically occurs during childhood and adolescence, but may rarely occur in older patients due to malignant transformation of Pagetic bone. The most common sites for the lesion are the bones around the knee (50%) and the proximal humerus (25%).

The pathognomonic feature of an osteosarcoma is the presence of osteoid matrix in a sarcomatous lesion. There are several variants of the tumour, and the starting point of the tumour is important for prognosis. In particular, periosteal osteosarcomas, arising on the outer cortical surface of a bone, have a better prognosis than most tumours which arise in the medulla of the bone. Histological diagnosis of osteosarcomas (and indeed many other bone tumours) may pose particular difficulties for pathologists. The services of a specialised bone and joint pathologist are usually required, and it is important that X-rays and scans are available to the pathologist to aid diagnosis (Fig. 11.11).

Clinical features. Patients may present with either pain or a palpable mass. Occasionally the pain results from a fracture through the tumour. The possibility of a bone tumour, particularly an osteosarcoma, must be considered in anyone who persistently complains of bony pain. This is particularly relevant at the knee, although it must

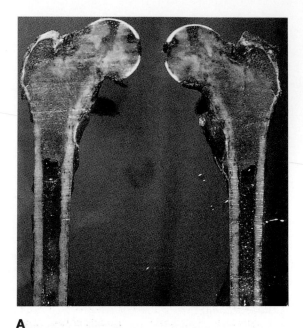

A

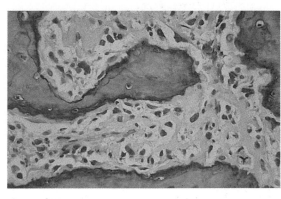

B

Figure 11.11   Macroscopic (A) and microscopic (B) appearances of an osteosarcoma. Note the abnormal bone formation. Courtesy of Professor A J Freemont.

be recalled that hip problems also cause pain in the thigh and knee in children; these will elude diagnosis unless the hips are properly examined. Sarcomata characteristically metastasise via a haematogenous route, leading to lung metastases. Initial screening of patients thought to have an osteosarcoma should include a chest X-ray.

Investigations. The features of osteosarcomata on plain X-ray are protean. Thus, there may be intramedullary osteosclerosis, radiolucency, cortical destruction or periosteal elevation, or any combination of these. They are seen most frequently at the juxta-epiphyseal area. As the tumour extends through the cortex, the periosteum may become elevated, stimulating reactive bone formation. This results in the so-called Codmann's triangle (Fig. 11.12).

MR scanning is important to determine the extent of tumour and of soft tissue involvement. Such investigations have become progressively more important as the prognosis for these tumours is critically dependent on correct treatment.

Definitive diagnosis of these lesions requires biopsy, but note that this should be carried out in specialised units where definitive treatment of such lesions is undertaken. Contamination of the tract of biopsy wounds is frequent during biopsy surgery, and this can lead to local (and fatal) recurrence in the area of the wound. Meticulous planning of biopsy wounds, followed on many occasions by subsequent excision of this wound at the time of definitive surgery, is required.

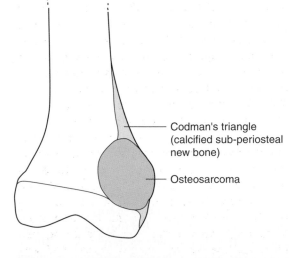

Codman's triangle (calcified sub-periosteal new bone)

Osteosarcoma

Figure 11.12   X-ray appearances Codmann's triangle.

Management. Treatment of osteosarcomata has been revolutionised over the past 25 years due to implementation of vigorous multi-drug chemotherapy regimes. The tumour previously had an extremely high mortality rate due to metastatic disease. An additional improvement has been the adoption of aggressive surgical measures to resect pulmonary metastases in some patients, prolonging survival. Current cure rates for osteosarcomata vary, but may reach up to 80%. Consequently, maintenance of good limb function has become increasingly important and limb amputation is now less widely used as the main surgical part of the treatment of the disease. In many patients, tumour resection after chemotherapy can be followed by limb reconstruction (e.g. with extended joint replacements).

OSTEOMYELITIS
Scenario 5

After her initial injury the patient's fracture was fixed with an intramedullary nail. Unfortunately the wound became infected, and despite antibiotics the infection proved very hard to eradicate. The wound discharged pus from a sinus intermittently for a period of 8 months. The patient was then seen by a specialist in bone and joint infection, who proposed that the (6 cm) area of femur which was demonstrated to be infected on a labelled white cell scan should be excised; this included the fracture. The patient agreed to this. It was explained to her that an external fixator frame would be on her leg for at least 6 months following surgery. This prediction turned out to be accurate, but she made good progress following her reconstruction using distraction osteogenesis, and the frame was removed 8 months after the surgery. She took a further 4 months to regain reasonable knee and ankle movement, but continued to have some aching pain, particularly in cold weather. Despite the protracted treatment, she felt that the undertaking had been worthwhile as she no longer had any discharge of pus from her leg, and she no longer had to wear a dressing on the area.

Pathology

Osteomyelitis is infection of bone or bone marrow. This is a serious condition which may be caused by a wide variety of organisms. It can arise as a result of direct contamination from outside the body (e.g. at a compound fracture, or after operation), or as a result of haematogenous spread. Infection due to haematogenous spread is particularly common in children and adolescents; this used to be by far the commonest cause of the disease.

The features of osteomyelitis reflect the relatively poor blood supply of many areas of bone. Further, inflammation in bone and associated swelling may result in dramatic increases in pressure and consequent ischaemia due to microvascular occlusion. Organisms which are frequently implicated in this condition include various micrococci (e.g. *Staphylococcus aureus*, *Staphylococcus epidermis*), *Pseudomonas* and tuberculosis, which presents particular features and problems (see below).

The pathological process of osteomyelitis consists of an infection with an associated inflammatory response, which is often brisk. This process frequently leads to areas of bone death; extensive areas of dead bone may occur. Dead bone arising due to osteomyelitis is known as a *sequestrum*. Subsequently, new bone may arise due to perforation of the cortex by pus, elevation of the periosteum and subperiosteal new bone formation. This may lead to an extensive area of new bone formation (an *involucrum*) in the case of untreated osteomyelitis. Such extensive osteomyelitis, with sequestra and an involucrum, is often associated with sinuses which discharge pus through the skin.

Clinical features

Osteomyelitis may occur at any site in the bone, but it starts most frequently in the juxta-epiphyseal area of long bones (adjacent to joint). Non-specific features of infection, including pyrexia and malaise, are often present. There is usually pain and marked bony tenderness at the site of infection, and there may be restriction of movement of adjacent joints, although this is rarely as marked as when septic arthritis is present. Confusingly, an effusion sometimes arises in the neighbouring joint despite the lack of septic arthritis (sympathetic effusion).

Investigations

Plain X-rays are of limited value in establishing the diagnosis of osteomyelitis early in the disease. The first sign of osteomyelitis is an area of vague rarefaction in the infected area, commonly adjacent to the epiphysis in a long bone. Subsequently, periosteal new bone formation occurs and this is visible as a thin line of subperiosteal new bone parallel with the cortex on X-ray. Areas of dead bone, which are commonly very sclerotic, may be seen. Large involucra are unusual in orthopaedic practice in developed countries. Blood tests are of value principally in excluding the presence of sepsis. Thus, patients with a normal white cell count, normal ESR and normal CRP are relatively (but not absolutely) unlikely to have musculoskeletal sepsis.

Bone and white cell scans. Because of the insensitivity of X-rays for early detection of osteomyelitis, alternative strategies must be employed. These consist of the blood tests mentioned above and radioisotope scanning. Technetium bone scans are of value as a relatively simple and rapid way of detecting early osteomyelitis. They are sensitive in the first few days of the condition, whereas X-ray changes are not usually seen until about 3 weeks following the onset of infection. The bone scan (using technetium-99 phosphonate compounds) demonstrates increased osteoblastic activity, which appears as a hot spot. Areas of dead bone are often difficult to see, but sometimes appear as a cold area on the scan.

Recently, alternative methods using white cells labelled with radioactive chromium have been developed. The white cells are obtained by spinning down a blood sample from the patient, and are then labelled with a radioactive marker. The cells are then reintroduced into the patient. The labelled circulating white cells will then be preferentially taken up in areas of active inflammation and infection. This technique is relatively specific for infection and is of value in discriminating between infective and non-infective causes of chronic bony conditions.

Management

Antibiotic treatment

The critical point in management of osteomyelitis is early diagnosis. The incidence of chronic osteomyelitis in children has fortunately markedly decreased in the last 50 years. A large part of this decrease is due to early active treatment of possible bone infections with antibiotics. The lugubrious sight of children with persistent bone pain, deformity and chronically discharging sinuses is now fortunately rare. Once diagnosis of osteomyelitis is strongly suspected, most clinicians would start antibiotic therapy, using intravenous administration of antibiotics against likely pathogens. In most forms of osteomyelitis, the commonest culprits are staphylococci, and the use of anti-staphylococcal drugs such as flucloxacillin is widespread. Strenuous efforts should be made to obtain appropriate tissue or pus samples for bacteriology, as antibiotic sensitivity amongst staphylococci (and all other organisms) can no longer be taken for granted. Methicillin (flucloxacillin)-resistant *Staphylococcus aureus*, in particular, is likely to be an increasing problem in the future in bone infections. The antibiotics administered should be adjusted once bacterial sensitivities are clear. Antibiotic treatment for bone infection should be protracted, usually including 2 weeks of intravenous antibiotic and 4 weeks of oral antibiotics.

Surgery

The role of surgery in early osteomyelitis is controversial. There is usually markedly raised pressure in the marrow cavity even in early disease, and previously surgeons sometimes drilled the bone to decompress the medulla. However, once established infection is present, surgery should certainly be undertaken if there is dead bone present. The dead bone is likely to act as a nidus of infection which may cause later recurrences or prevent the initial episode settling. Such dead bone will clearly not be penetrated by antibiotics.

Chronic osteomyelitis

Once osteomyelitis becomes chronic, management is extremely difficult. Recurrences or flares of acute sepsis are common. These may occur after many years of quiescence, so that a patient who has previously had osteomyelitis in the lower limb may suffer the first recurrence of infection 20 or 30 years after the first episode. In these circumstances, it is uncommon for antibiotic therapy alone to be curative. Most patients will require resection of an area of chronically infected bone, because it is impossible to fully clear the bone of the chronic infection, either by antibiotic treatment or by limited debridement. Several techniques are available for treatment of this condition, including excision of a segment of bone followed by reconstruction using callus distraction (distraction osteogenesis). These major operations are carried out using external fixation devices (Ch. 19). Other complications of chronic osteomyelitis include Marjolin's ulcers in chronically discharging sinuses (malignant transformation of the edges of an osteomyelitic sinus) and renal failure due to amyloidosis resulting from the presence of the chronic sepsis.

TUBERCULOSIS OF BONES AND JOINTS

Bone and joint tuberculosis is now relatively rare in Western countries. However, there is evidence that drug-resistant tuberculosis is increasing, and it is likely that an increase in bone and joint tuberculosis will be seen over the next decade.

Pathology

Any bone or joint may be affected by tuberculosis. Characteristically, the hip, knee and vertebrae are affected by this disease. The pathology involves infection with mycobacteria. Typically, *Mycobacterium tuberculosis* is involved, although other forms of mycobacteria do occur in bone and joint infections. *Mycobacterium tuberculosis* is acid- and alcohol-fast on Zeil–Nielsen staining. The material taken from the foci of infection is typically a very thick whitish form of pus, reflecting the caseation present in tuberculous lesions. Bone and joint tuberculosis is a reflection of secondary tuberculosis. It occasionally occurs in adolescence after primary infection, but more commonly presents in adults or elderly people. Bone and joint tuberculosis also occurs in patients with AIDS.

Clinical features

The clinical features are extremely varied, and tuberculosis should be borne in mind as a differential diagnosis of any atypical monoarthritis or bone or soft tissue tumour. Presentation of tuberculosis in peripheral joints generally involves chronic, rather indolent, swelling, pain, and frequently the development of a gradual deformity which usually includes some element of fixed flexion. Tuberculosis may affect the spine, causing an acute kyphosis (flexion deformity of the spine or gibbus) due to collapse of the vertebral body affected by the tuberculous process. The combination of collapse and the expanding volume of necrotic material due to infection often leads to paraplegia due to spinal cord compression.

Investigations

Diagnosis of skeletal tuberculosis can be difficult. There may be evidence of active or inactive tuberculosis on chest X-ray. X-ray appearances of bone tuberculosis include evidence of bone destruction and often areas of surrounding calcification. Skin sensitivity testing (Mantoux testing) is of value. Blood tests will indicate evidence of inflammation and sepsis with raised ESR and there is likely to be evidence of bone destruction occurring, with raised alkaline phosphatase. Definitive diagnosis requires biopsy for microbiological and histological evaluation.

Typical appearances of a tuberculous spine are shown in Figure 11.13.

Management

Management of tuberculosis of the skeleton is both medical and surgical. Adequate and vigorous treatment is required to control the tuberculous process, requiring the assistance of specialists in

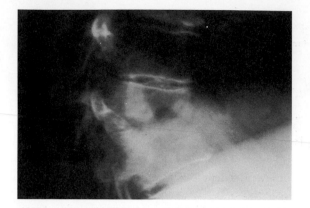

Figure 11.13 X-ray appearance of a tuberculous spine.

infectious diseases. Combination chemotherapy is employed for a period of several months. Drugs used include para-aminosalicylic acid, rifampicin and isoniazid.

Surgical management requires adequate debridement of the infected bone or joint to minimise the amount of infected material present. Treatment of spinal tuberculosis may be undertaken by prolonged bedrest and then plaster casting (to prevent development of spinal deformity), together with chemotherapy. Alternatively, surgical stabilisation of the spine may be undertaken to alleviate the risk of development of the spinal deformity and to allow patients early mobilisation.

12 | Medical conditions with musculoskeletal manifestations

Case history

A 40-year-old man presented with generalised aching and fatigue. He was a little stiff in the morning, but there had been no joint swelling. On examination he had some proximal muscle tenderness, but there was no very obvious weakness, no joint swelling and he had a full range of movement of all joints.

Initially, no cause could be found for his symptoms. However, these persisted, and he had increasing difficulty coping with his work. He was reassessed, and because symptoms were persisting but there were no specific findings on musculoskeletal examination, the doctor checked the full blood count, ESR and biochemical profile, including thyroid function tests. Results showed that he was significantly hypothyroid. Thyroid replacement was commenced and within 1 month his musculo-skeletal symptoms had resolved.

Key points

- **Diseases which are not primarily of the musculoskeletal system can be associated with musculoskeletal symptoms**

So far, this textbook has mainly dealt with conditions which primarily affect the locomotor system and connective tissues. However, in the same way that rheumatoid arthritis (for example) can be associated with multisystem involvement, so too can a variety of other medical conditions be associated with musculoskeletal complaints. Sometimes these can be the presenting feature of the disease.

This chapter describes some important conditions that can be associated with musculoskeletal features. Wherever possible, these have been grouped according to which organ, system or disease mechanism is primarily involved. Conditions included elsewhere, such as arthritis associated with inflammatory bowel disease, are not considered.

GENERAL MEDICINE

Case history

A 28-year-old woman developed a painful, swollen right ankle and painful, reddish-coloured lumps on the front of her lower legs. Other lumps developed subsequently and she felt feverish and unwell, and her right wrist became painful. She attended her GP, who asked what tablets she was taking and was interested in the fact that she had had a recent sore throat.

On examination her temperature was 37.7°C. Her tonsils were slightly enlarged but were not red, and there was no cervical lymphadeno-pathy. There were several tender, erythe-matous nodules of her lower legs. Her right ankle was tender, swollen and painful and her right wrist was tender.

She was referred to hospital where she was admitted to the rheumatology ward. Investiga-tions included a white blood count of $12.0 \times 10^9/$L and and ESR of 55 mm/h. Blood biochemistry was normal, as was a chest X-ray. When asked why a chest X-ray was necessary, the doctor explained that sometimes this condition (which was called erythema nodosum) was associated with chest problems. The doctor also explained

that, although it was unlikely that there was an infection in the ankle, it was best to make sure by aspirating the joint. Clear fluid was aspirated; microscopy showed no organisms and a white cell count of only 500/mm^3. Antibiotics were not prescribed.

The ankle swelling settled with ibuprofen and bedrest and gradually the lumps on her legs became a darker colour and less painful. After 3 days in hospital she was allowed home. It was explained to her that the erythema nodosum was most likely related to her recent throat infection. Six weeks later she was completely well.

Erythema nodosum

Erythema nodosum is an acute skin lesion caused by inflammation of subcutaneous fat, typically occurring in young adults. Tender nodules (Fig. 12.1) occur characteristically on the lower leg anteriorly. Erythema nodosum can occur in association with a number of conditions, including sarcoidosis, which is described below, and an underlying cause should always be sought (Box 12.1).

Many patients with erythema nodosum are febrile. The significance of this condition to the rheumatologist is that it can be associated with an acute arthropathy. The synovitis is self-limiting and usually settles with the skin lesions. Treatment is with rest and NSAIDs.

Sarcoidosis

Sarcoidosis is a systemic disease, the main histological feature of which is the presence of non-

---

Box 12.1   Conditions associated with erythema nodosum

- Infection
  - bacterial, e.g. streptococcal, tuberculosis
  - fungal

- Drugs, e.g. sulphonamides, oral contraceptives

- Sarcoidosis

- Lymphoma

- Behçet's syndrome

- Inflammatory bowel disease

---

caseating granulomata. Sarcoidosis can be associated with either acute or chronic polyarthritis and with bony changes. Other features of the disease can include pulmonary involvement (bilateral hilar lymphadenopathy [Fig. 12.2] or pulmonary infiltrates), skin changes (including erythema nodosum) and uveitis. Some patients are hypercalcaemic.

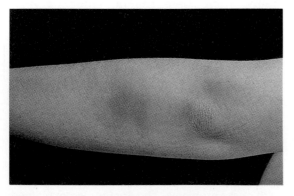

Figure 12.1   Erythema nodosum.

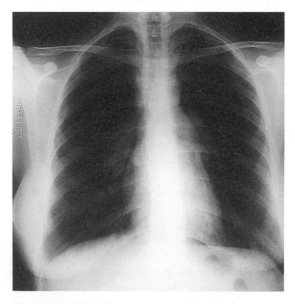

Figure 12.2   Chest X-ray showing hilar lymphadenopathy of sarcoidosis.

The commonest articular presentation of sarcoidosis is an acute arthritis, often associated with erythema nodosum and hilar lymphadenopathy. Usually, large joints such as the ankles and knees are affected. This form of the disease carries a good prognosis and is often self limiting.

Bone changes occur, especially in patients with chronic disease, characteristically affecting the digits; changes include bone rarefaction, punched-out lesions and bone destruction. Dactylitis may occur.

The diagnosis of sarcoidosis may be obvious from the clinical features and appearances on chest X-ray. Lymph node biopsy may be diagnostic. Serum levels of angiotensin-converting enzyme are raised in active sarcoidosis, but this test is not specific.

Acute arthritis usually responds to NSAIDs, whereas some patients with active, persistent disease are prescribed prednisolone.

PULMONARY
Bronchial carcinoma

This can be associated with hypertrophic osteoarthropathy, described later in the section on malignancy. Always take a smoking history.

GASTROINTESTINAL

There are many close associations between the gastrointestinal tract and the joints, e.g. spondyloarthropathy associated with inflammatory bowel disease and reactive arthritis (described in Ch. 8).

RENAL

Patients with chronic renal disease may develop 'renal bone disease' and are also at risk of gout (Ch. 7). In addition, patients undergoing dialysis may develop a number of musculoskeletal problems.

Renal bone disease
As described in Chapter 11, patients with chronic renal disease may develop hyperparathyroidism or osteomalacia. In this context, the terms 'renal bone disease' or 'renal osteodystrophy' are used.

Dialysis arthropathy
Patients on long-term haemodialysis have high circulating levels of β_2-microglobulin, already referred to in the section on amyloidosis (Ch. 8), and these contribute to a chronic arthopathy (sometimes destructive) which can develop in this patient group. β_2-Microglobulin amyloid may be found both within the joints and in periarticular tissue. Many patients on long-term peritoneal or haemodialysis develop carpal tunnel syndrome.

Patients on dialysis are also at risk of articular and periarticular problems related to deposition of calcium salts (usually apatite), which can trigger an acute inflammatory response.

NEUROLOGICAL
Neuropathic arthropathy

Patients with sensory neuropathy can develop an accelerated destructive joint disease. The so-called 'Charcot joint' was first described in association with tabes dorsalis, but is now most commonly found in diabetes, when the mid- and forefoot are usually affected. In syringomyelia, the large joints of the upper limb may be involved.

The joint becomes completely disorganised. Although usually there is little pain, the joint is swollen, often with an effusion, and unstable. X-rays show gross joint destruction, with bone resorption and new bone formation.

Treatment is palliative with the emphasis on joint protection. Joint replacement is seldom feasible.

HAEMATOLOGICAL
Haemophilia

The most common complication of haemophilia (deficiency of factor VIIIc or IXc) is intra-articular bleeding. The likelihood of intra-articular bleeding is related to the severity of the factor deficiency: less than 5% of normal is associated with a high risk of recurrent haemarthrosis. Presentation is with a monoarthritis (most commonly of knee, ankle or elbow), but if repeated haemarthroses occur, a more chronic arthropathy develops with joint destruction. Treatment of the acute episode is with rest, analgesics, factor replacement and physiotherapy.

Haemoglobinopathies

Patients with homozygous sickle cell disease are at risk of vaso-occlusive episodes due to sickling of the red blood cells. The major musculoskeletal manifestations occur as a result of occlusion of blood vessels in the bone marrow and are as follows:

- painful crises – these occur most frequently in the long bones but also in the spine and abdomen
- avascular necrosis (Ch. 10) – this most often affects the femoral head but can occur elsewhere, e.g. in the shoulder
- dactylitis – this can occur in young children.

Patients with other haemoglobinopathies, such as beta-thalassaemia, may develop similar problems.

Patients with haemoglobinopathies are at increased risk of osteomyelitis (*Salmonella* is the most common organism) and gout. Blood cultures should be taken in patients with fever, and synovial fluid sent for culture and microscopy if there is joint inflammation.

Leukaemia

Joint pains and arthritis can occur in patients with acute or chronic leukaemia, especially in children with acute lymphoblastic leukaemia. It is thought that articular manifestations are due to leukaemic infiltration of the synovium or periosteal elevation.

METABOLIC AND ENDOCRINE DISORDERS

Haemochromatosis

Idiopathic haemochromatosis is a genetic disease characterised by iron overload, typically presenting in middle-aged men. Although joint involvement is seldom severe, it may be a presenting feature and its recognition may allow early diagnosis of haemochromatosis and treatment by venesection at an early stage before irreversible organ damage (e.g. cirrhosis) occurs.

Typically the metacarpophalangeal (MCP) joints of the index and middle fingers are affected, although other joints can be involved. Calcium pyrophosphate dihydrate (CPPD) deposition occurs in a proportion of patients with haemochromatosis and therefore a diagnosis of haemochromatosis should always be considered in patients presenting with CPPD deposition disease.

Other features of disease include:

- skin pigmentation
- diabetes
- myocardial disease
- hypogonadism
- hypopituitarism.

The ferritin is high and liver function tests are often abnormal. Excessive iron on liver biopsy confirms the diagnosis. Treatment with venesection does not significantly affect the joint disease of which the treatment is symptomatic.

Hyperlipidaemias

Musculoskeletal problems that can be associated with hyperlipidaemias are

- Tendon xanthomas. These are a prominent feature of type IIa hyperlipoproteinaemia (familial hypercholesterolaemia) when they are usually symmetrical and occur especially over the finger extensors but also at other sites such as over the Achilles tendon. They also occur in type III hyperlipoproteinaemia (familial dysbetalipoproteinaemia).
- Arthritis. This can occur in familial hypercholesterolaemia or in type IV hyperlipoproteinaemia.
- Gout. There is an association between raised triglyceride levels and gout.

Diabetes mellitus

Diabetes can be associated with a number of rheumatological problems (Box 12.2), some of which are described elsewhere:

- increased risk of septic arthritis (Ch. 7) and osteomyelitis (Ch. 11)
- neuropathic (Charcot) joints (described above)
- diffuse idiopathic skeletal hyperostosis (DISH; Ch. 11)

- soft tissue problems, e.g. shoulder capsulitis, trigger finger, carpal tunnel syndrome
- 'diabetic foot' (this is a major clinical problem; see Ch. 16).

Patients with diabetes may also develop a condition of the hands termed 'diabetic cheiroarthropathy'. The clinical features are similar to sclerodermatous involvement of the hands, with tendon and joint contractures and skin thickening, leading to fixed flexion contractures of the fingers.

Thyroid disease

Musculoskeletal features may occur in association with both hypo- and hyperthyroidism. Proximal weakness can occur with either, and thyroid function tests should be checked in the patient with generalised aches and pains (as in the Case history). The muscle enzymes may be raised in hypothyroidism, and it can be associated with carpal tunnel syndrome. Hyperthyroidism is a risk factor for osteoporosis. Thyroid acropathy – soft tissue swelling of the fingers and toes, clubbing and periostitis, with pretibial myxoedema – can occur in patients with hyperthyroidism, often many years after diagnosis and treatment.

Parathyroid disease

Hyperparathyroidism is discussed under metabolic bone disease (Ch. 11). CPPD deposition disease can be associated with hyperparathyroidism – an episode of acute pseudogout may be the presenting feature of hyperparathyroidism.

Box 12.2   Musculoskeletal problems in patients with diabetes mellitus

- Diabetic cheiroarthropathy
- Increased risk of septic arthritis and osteomyelitis
- Neuropathic (Charcot) joint/ the 'diabetic foot'
- Diffuse idiopathic skeletal hyperostosis (DISH)
- Soft tissue problems, e.g. shoulder capsulitis, trigger finger

---

Acromegaly

Acromegaly, caused by excessive production of growth hormone, is associated with a variety of musculoskeletal complaints. Common symptoms include backache, arthralgia, muscle weakness and symptoms of carpal tunnel syndrome. Cartilage thickening occurs and there is a predisposition to early degenerative change.

MALIGNANCY

There are several associations between musculoskeletal disease and malignancy. Some of these have already been mentioned. For example, an underlying malignancy should always be considered in the adult patient presenting with dermatomyositis, and Sjögren's syndrome is associated with an increased risk of lymphoma.

However, in broader terms, malignancy should always be considered in the patient who presents with musculoskeletal symptoms, especially if other factors point to possible malignancy (e.g. weight loss and a raised ESR). Musculoskeletal symptoms may be the result of:

- skeletal metastases – metastatic bone disease is considered in Chapter 11
- paraneoplastic syndromes – these can include a polyarthritis, which may precede the clinical expression of the underlying neoplasm. A condition termed 'hypertrophic osteoarthropathy' is classically associated with bronchial carcinoma. Finger clubbing is usually obvious, with swelling and tenderness of wrists, fingers and ankles. X-rays show subperiosteal new bone formation in the distal parts of the radius and ulna, tibia and fibula.

CONCLUSION

A patient presenting with musculoskeletal symptoms may have any one of a variety of underlying medical conditions. This emphasises the importance of a detailed assessment of all patients. Look beyond the musculoskeletal system, especially if there is no obvious musculoskeletal cause to explain the clinical features.

13 | Inflammatory joint disease in childhood

Case history

A 4-year-old girl developed a slight limp, and her mother noticed that her left knee was swollen. One week previously, the girl had fallen in the playground, but as the knee was not painful her mother decided to leave it for a few days before going to the doctor. However, as the swelling did not settle she took her to see the GP who prescribed ibuprofen. Although the girl was well, the knee swelling persisted and she was referred to the paediatric rheumatology clinic.

At the hospital (4 weeks after the knee first became swollen) the doctor asked if she had had any rashes, fevers, or recent sore throat or other infections. On examination the knee was slightly warm and swollen with a small effusion, but only very minimally tender. There was a 20° flexion deformity. All the other joints were normal.

A blood sample was taken. The ESR was high at 30 mm/h, but the blood count was normal. Rheumatoid factor was negative but antinuclear factor was positive at a titre of 1/100. X-ray of the knee showed some soft tissue swelling but no bony abnormality. The doctor arranged for the knee to be aspirated under a general anaesthetic. Culture of the synovial fluid was negative but the synovial fluid white cell count was raised at 3000/mm³.

With physiotherapy and a small increase in the dose of ibuprofen, the knee swelling settled slowly. At a visit to the clinic 4 months after the onset of the problem, there was still mild synovial swelling but no tenderness, and the girl was not limited in her activities.

Her mother was surprised when the girl was referred to an ophthalmologist, who examined her eyes through a slit lamp and explained that she would require regular eye checks throughout childhood.

Key points

- Chronic inflammatory joint disease can occur in children (juvenile chronic [idiopathic] arthritis) and can be associated with major morbidity

- Juvenile chronic arthritis can cause blindness. Regular eye checks are mandatory for children at risk

- Although rheumatic fever is now rare, correct diagnosis is essential in order to prevent long-term cardiac sequelae

In the UK, the term 'juvenile chronic arthritis' (JCA) is given to that group of diseases characterised by arthritis beginning before the age of 16 years and lasting at least 3 months, in the absence of any other specific disease which may cause joint inflammation. However, the terminology of chronic arthritis is confusing and is currently under review. Discussion of this terminology is outwith the scope of this textbook, but it is likely that in future the term 'juvenile idiopathic arthritis' will be used internationally. At the risk of perpetuating a term soon to be outdated, we have chosen to stick with 'JCA' here. The term 'Still's disease' is now seldom used. While in this chapter we concentrate on juvenile chronic arthritis, with a brief description of rheumatic fever, it is important to remember that joint problems in children, as in adults, can occur as a result of many different disease processes (e.g. septic arthritis and connective tissue diseases) and injuries. Those musculoskeletal conditions in children which are dealt with primarily by orthopaedic surgeons, e.g. slipped femoral epiphysis and Perthes' disease, are described in Chapter 14.

JUVENILE CHRONIC ARTHRITIS

The classification of chronic arthritis in children is currently under review. However, it is accepted that there are certain broad subtypes of juvenile chronic arthritis, defined by the pattern of disease in the first 6 months:

- *Pauciarticular onset*, when arthritis occurs in four or fewer joints. Some children with pauciarticular disease go on to develop polyarticular disease. There is a high risk of chronic anterior uveitis in this subgroup, particularly in children with early-onset disease (6 years or younger) who are antinuclear antibody (ANA) positive.
- *Polyarticular onset*, when arthritis occurs in five or more joints. Some children (usually these are older girls) develop what is essentially rheumatoid arthritis (juvenile rheumatoid arthritis). Children with this subtype of polyarticular disease are usually rheumatoid factor-positive, unlike most other children with JCA in whom rheumatoid factor positivity is rare.
- *Systemic onset*, when systemic features such as a high spiking fever and rash are prominent and may precede the arthritis.

Psoriatic arthritis and ankylosing spondylitis can present in childhood, and in the UK have usually been considered under the umbrella term of juvenile chronic arthritis.

One cause for confusion in the terminology of JCA is that in the USA the term, 'juvenile rheumatoid arthritis' has been used to describe most children with juvenile chronic arthritis, as opposed to simply that subset who have the rheumatoid arthritis pattern of disease. Hence, the need for a revision in terminology referred to above.

Epidemiology

The true prevalence of JCA is not known, although it has been estimated that around 1 in 1000 children are affected.

Pathology

The aetiology of JCA is unknown. As with many rheumatic diseases, an infectious aetiology has been postulated, but there is no definite evidence of such. Certain HLA associations with different subtypes of JCA have been described. HLA-B27 is associated with the seronegative spondyloarthropathies in children as in adults. In JCA, synovial hypertrophy occurs, with a marked inflammatory infiltrate (mainly plasma cells and lymphocytes) and increased vascularity.

Clinical features

The first step is always to establish the diagnosis by a careful history and examination, with X-rays and other investigations as appropriate. Depending upon the age of the child, the history may be mostly taken from a parent. Musculoskeletal examination may be difficult, especially in the young child who is in pain. Unwillingness to move a limb is often an important clue as to where pain is originating.

Specific points to ask about or to look for in the child with JCA, or in the child in whom this diagnosis is suspected, are highlighted here.

History

Musculoskeletal. Key points to ask about are:

- *Are features of joint inflammation present?* As in adults, the main symptoms are pain, swelling and stiffness. The child may be most symptomatic first thing in the morning and have difficulty getting up and going to school. Some children with arthritis, particularly pauciarticular disease, complain of surprisingly little pain.
- *Which joints are involved, and how many?* The number of joints involved at the onset will distinguish between pauciarticular and polyarticular onset JCA. The neck and temporomandibular joints are often affected in children. Back pain may be a feature, especially in older boys who have a juvenile form of ankylosing spondylitis.

• *Were there any associated features at the onset of the arthritis?* Always ask about injury: a swollen knee may be the result of trauma. A recent sore throat or other infection means that viral arthritis, bacterial infection, rheumatic fever (described below) or another form of reactive arthritis are possibilities. Ask about rash and fever, which occur in systemic-onset JCA.

Remember that children (especially younger children) will not describe their symptoms in the same way as adults. A parent may describe how the child refuses to walk or crawl. The older child may no longer participate in games or may have difficulty dressing.

Systemic enquiry. In children as in adults, inflammatory arthritides are systemic diseases (especially systemic-onset JCA); therefore, take a full history. Ask about eye symptoms, although uveitis is often asymptomatic. Children with HLA-B27-related disease may develop an acute iritis which is symptomatic.

Family history. Ask about a history of HLA-B27-related disease, i.e. psoriasis, ankylosing spondylitis, inflammatory bowel disease.

Social history. It is important to establish the family background, and whether the child is happy in the home and school environments. Joint pains in children may be psychogenic, and the child with

JCA may have difficulty coping. In the child debilitated with this disease, a supportive family and school will have a major impact on the child's well-being.

Examination

A full examination is necessary. Pay special attention to the following.

General. A high spiking fever is characteristic of systemic-onset JCA (Fig. 13.1). The spikes usually occur in the evening, when the child is listless and unwell. Lymphadenopathy is common in systemic-onset disease. Children with JCA, especially those with systemic-onset disease, are often anaemic and are therefore pale.

Skin. The characteristic rash of systemic-onset JCA is salmon pink, macular and evanescent (Fig. 13.2). Typically, it is present when the child has a fever, and so may be gone in the morning during the doctor's ward round. Look for the rash of psoriasis.

Musculoskeletal. Look for signs of joint inflammation – swelling, tenderness, pain on motion (Fig. 13.3). Young children are often reluctant to allow the doctor to examine a painful joint. Remember to assess the neck, which is frequently involved in JCA (fusion of the apophyseal joints can occur in severely affected children). Particular points to look for in children are:

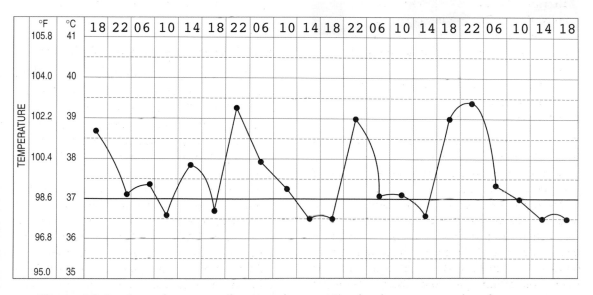

Figure 13.1   Fever chart in systemic-onset disease. Note the characteristic spiking fever.

Inflammatory joint disease in childhood

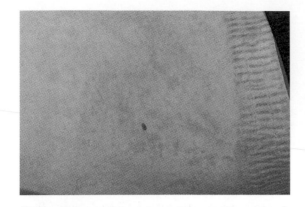

Figure 13.2   The erythematous macular rash of juvenile chronic arthritis.

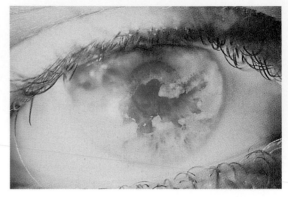

Figure 13.4   Uveitis. This is the left eye of a 7-year-old girl with JCA of pauciarticular onset. The figure shows severe band keratopathy secondary to uveitis. Courtesy of Mr N Jones.

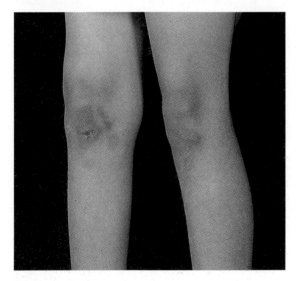

Figure 13.3   Knee swelling in a child with juvenile chronic arthritis.

- Contractures – these can develop very quickly in children with inflammatory joint disease, e.g. flexion contractures of the knees and elbows.
- Growth abnormalities – these can be divided into generalised and local, and can relate to both under- and overgrowth. *Generalised* growth is retarded in patients with systemic disease; while this occurs as a result of active inflammatory disease, steroid therapy may contribute. A number of *local* growth abnormalities can occur in JCA, common ones including:

— overgrowth at the knee: this is frequently seen in the child with arthritis of one knee, when accelerated growth and epiphyseal maturation can occur; the result is a leg length discrepancy, which leads to a scoliosis that must be corrected by using a shoe-raise
— micrognathia: mandibular hypoplasia is a result of temperomandibular joint involvement; it is important to refer these children for an orthodontic assessment.

Eye.   Those at highest risk of developing the chronic anterior uveitis which can lead to blindness (Fig. 13.4) are young girls who are ANA-positive. Irregularity of the iris is a late finding and most children are asymptomatic, therefore regular slit-lamp examination is required. A painful red eye may be due to the acute iritis which can occur in HLA-B27-associated disease.

Other.   Look for signs of pericarditis and hepatosplenomegaly in the child with systemic-onset disease.

Investigations

In a child presenting with inflammatory arthritis, the ANA and rheumatoid factor should be checked. ANA positivity confers an increased risk of uveitis. A positive rheumatoid factor is seldom found except in that subgroup of older children who develop rheumatoid arthritis, and is therefore associated with a high risk of progressive joint disease.

As in adults with inflammatory joint disease, a full blood count, biochemical profile and urinalysis should be carried out. Children with JCA may be anaemic, especially those with systemic-onset disease who often have high white cell and platelet counts. The ESR is high in active disease. Some children with systemic-onset disease have raised transaminases.

Always check the urine, and monitor this especially in children with systemic-onset disease. Proteinuria may reflect amyloidosis (Ch. 8), which occurs in a proportion of children with systemic-onset disease. Synovial fluid analysis will show inflammatory change, and is mandatory if there is any suspicion of sepsis.

Radiographs will initially be normal and may be difficult to interpret, e.g. sacroiliac joint X-rays in childhood and adolescence. A small proportion of children go on to develop erosive disease.

Differential diagnosis

The differential diagnosis of JCA is shown in Box 13.1. In children as in adults, always consider the possibility of joint sepsis. Reactive arthritis, e.g. following enteric infections, is a relatively common cause of joint swelling in children. Rheumatic fever, although now uncommon, is an important diagnosis to make because of the increased incidence of long-term cardiac sequelae if left untreated. It is discussed below. An important differential diagnosis in the child with painful joints is malignancy, and this possibility should always be considered.

Children with hypermobility may present with joint pains. Because hypermobility is common in children, key features of hypermobility syndrome are outlined in Box 13.2, although this is also an important differential diagnosis of joint pain in adults.

Box 13.1 Differential diagnosis of JCA

- Infectious/post-infectious
  — septic arthritis
  — osteomyelitis
  — viral arthritis
  — reactive arthritis/rheumatic fever

- Other inflammatory diseases
  — SLE
  — dermatomyositis
  — vasculitis

- Malignancy
  — acute lymphoblastic leukaemia
  — neuroblastoma
  — bone tumour

- 'Structural', e.g. slipped femoral epiphysis

- Hypermobility

- Psychogenic

Box 13.2 Hypermobility syndrome

Many children are hypermobile – they have an increased range of joint movement due to ligamentous laxity. Hypermobility decreases with age, especially during the childhood period. Tests used to identify this are most commonly the ability to:

- appose the thumb to the forearm
- dorsiflex the little finger (at the MCP joint) to 90°
- hyperextend the elbow by 10°
- hyperextend the knee by 10°
- place the palms of the hands flat on the floor with the knee extended.

It is now well recognised that children and adults who are hypermobile may experience musculoskeletal symptoms in the absence of any other rheumatic disease and this has been termed the 'hypermobility syndrome'. These symptoms include arthralgia, myalgia and back pain. Occasionally there may be a low-grade synovitis. Therefore, remember to examine for an increased as well as a reduced range of movement in children and adults presenting with joint pains. While the hypermobility syndrome is relatively common, a minority of patients who are hypermobile have an underlying hereditary disorder of connective tissue, e.g. Marfan or Ehlers–Danlos syndrome.

One reason why it is important to diagnose the hypermobility syndrome is that patients are often relieved to be given an explanation for their symptoms.

When no organic cause of joint pain can be found, a careful social history must be taken. Unhappiness at school or at home may be contributing to the child's problems.

Management

General measures

The principles of management of the child with JCA are similar to those of the adult with polyarthritis. A multidisciplinary approach is essential (Box 13.3). However, the child with JCA has particular needs. Optimising psychological and physical well-being means including the parents and school in the management of the arthritis. Referral to a child psychologist should be considered, as this may help the child and the family in coping with chronic pain and disability.

Many children benefit from hydrotherapy, in addition to other forms of physiotherapy (Figs 13.5 and 13.6) they gain confidence in moving their painful joints in the warm water. Night splints should be used in children with contractures for prevention and treatment.

A dietician is an important member of the multidisciplinary team, especially for children

with active disease who have lost weight and/or in whom growth is retarded. Ready access to the dentist is also important because of the tempero-mandibular problems which occur.

Drug treatment

With respect to drug treatment, the main drugs used are NSAIDs, corticosteroids and disease-modifying agents. Corticosteroids are indicated in children with systemic-onset disease who do not respond to NSAIDs. A particular concern with corticosteroid use in children is growth retardation. Wherever possible, an alternate day regime should be used to minimise the adverse effects of corticosteroids on the hypothalamic–pituitary–adrenal axis. Most of the disease-modifying drugs

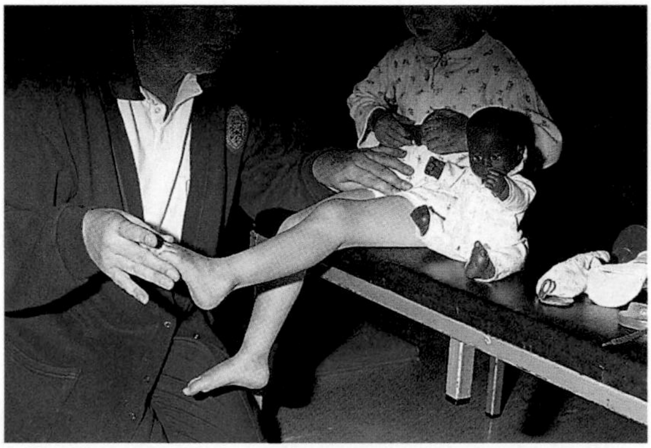

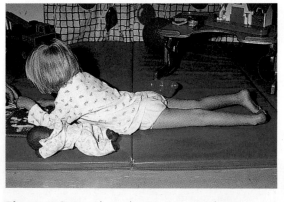

Figure 13.5 Physiotherapy – this child is being taught quadriceps exercises.

Figure 13.6 Physiotherapy – prone lying to correct flexion deformities at hips.

Box 13.3   The multidisciplinary team in juvenile chronic arthritis

- General practitioner
- Rheumatologist
- Ophthalmologist
- Orthopaedic surgeon
- Physiotherapist
- Occupational therapist
- Nurse
- Dietician
- Orthodontist/dentist
- Child psychologist
- Social worker
- Family
- School teacher

used in adult polyarthritis have not been shown to have significant benefit in JCA. However, methotrexate has been shown to be beneficial and is used in the management of children with active polyarticular disease, although it is of course important to consider the potential risks as well as benefits of treatment, and all children on methotrexate must have regular monitoring of their full blood count and biochemical profile.

Corticosteroid injections are helpful for single inflamed joints. In younger children these are given under general anaesthetic.

Surgery

Joint replacement poses particular problems in children because of the very small size of the bones and the long service which will be required, but it may be indicated for a painful destroyed joint. If joint replacement is required in childhood, this should be performed in a specialist centre.

Prognosis

This depends on the subtype of JCA. While it used to be thought that the majority of children have a good long-term outcome with respect to joint disease, it is now recognised that this opinion was overoptimistic and that a significant proportion of children still have active joint disease 10 years after its onset.

Long-term joint problems are unusual in patients with pauciarticular onset disease: the main morbidity in this group is from uveitis. Children with seropositive polyarticular disease usually go on to develop erosive disease and significant disability. While many children with systemic-onset disease go into remission, others develop destructive arthritis and a small but significant number die of amyloidosis or infection.

RHEUMATIC FEVER

Rheumatic fever is an acute inflammatory illness which usually follows 2–4 weeks after a pharyngeal infection with group A beta-haemolytic streptococci. Children are most commonly affected. This is a systemic illness affecting heart, brain and skin as well as joints.

Rheumatic fever is a diagnosis which should always be considered when a child presents with joint swelling, especially if migratory. Rheumatic fever can be considered as the 'prototype' of 'reactive arthritis': infection elsewhere triggers inflammation within joints. The major long-term morbidity of rheumatic fever results from chronic rheumatic heart disease which occurs in a proportion of patients. Systemic-onset juvenile arthritis is an important differential diagnosis.

Pathology

'Molecular mimicry' is thought to play an important role in the pathogenesis of rheumatic fever. The immune response triggered by the streptococcal throat infection cross-reacts with certain host tissues (e.g. sarcoplasmic membranes within the myocardial cells to produce a myocarditis). Most studies on the pathology of rheumatic fever relate to the heart. Inflammatory cell infiltrates are found in heart muscle and valves. The pathognomonic lesion of rheumatic fever is the Aschoff nodule, comprising cells derived from macrophages or monocytes. Later on in the disease course, valvular scarring results in chronic rheumatic heart disease.

Clinical features

Not all patients have a history of pharyngeal infection.

Constitutional. Fever is sustained. This is in contrast to the spiking fever of systemic-onset JCA.

Articular. The characteristic feature is a *migratory* 'flitting' arthritis. Typically, synovitis develops in one joint for 1–5 days and as it subsides another joint becomes affected. The arthritis is usually self-limiting, subsiding within 4–6 weeks.

Cutaneous. Erythema marginatum occurs in a minority of patients. Like the rash of systemic-onset JCA it is evanescent, but it is distinguished by the lesions having an irregular border, often with central clearing. Small subcutaneous nodules may be found in a similar distribution to rheumatoid nodules (e.g. extensor aspects of forearms).

Neurological (Sydenham's chorea) and cardiac. Details can be found in general medical texts. A key point is that cardiac involvement is the most worrying feature of rheumatic fever. If rheumatic fever is suspected, look for a tachycardia and listen carefully for murmurs or a pericardial rub.

Key investigations

The diagnosis of rheumatic fever cannot be made without supporting evidence of a preceding streptococcal throat infection. Sometimes streptococci can still be cultured from the throat and so a throat swab should be sent. Blood should be sent for assay of antistreptococcal antibodies, e.g. ASO titre.

Patients with rheumatic fever may be anaemic with a leucocytosis and a high ESR. If the diagnosis is suspected, always request an ECG, when prolongation of the P–R interval or more severe conduction abnormalities may strengthen a clinical suspicion of carditis. Look for cardiac enlargement on chest X-ray. Echocardiography may demonstrate pericardial, myocardial or valvular involvement.

Treatment

Elimination of haemolytic streptococci

Usually phenoxymethylpenicillin is given for 10 days.

Symptomatic measures for the acute attack

An NSAID is given to suppress the fever and inflammation. Most experience has been with aspirin. Bed rest is required for patients with active carditis. Corticosteroids are occasionally used in patients refractory to the above measures.

Prophylaxis against further attacks

This is essential, the rationale being that it is important to prevent further attacks which bring with them the risk of further cardiac damage. Usually, either oral phenoxymethylpenicillin or intramuscular benzathine penicillin are prescribed. Prophylaxis should be continued indefinitely in patients with established rheumatic heart disease.

14 | Paediatric orthopaedics

Case history

A 4-year-old girl with cerebral palsy was referred to the paediatric orthopaedic clinic with difficulty walking. She was articulate, personable and of normal intelligence. Her upper limbs were only slightly impaired, but she had severe impairment of both lower limbs and was experiencing increasing difficulty with walking. She walked with a scissor gait, most of the time on tip toes. Examination revealed that she had markedly increased tone in both lower limbs. Hip movements were restricted, and only 90° of flexion and 5° of abduction were possible.

Treatment was initially with physiotherapy and stretching exercises for 2 years, but after an initial improvement her walking again started to deteriorate. Surgery was proposed, and bilateral open adductor tenotomies were carried out, together with bilateral tendo Achilles lengthenings. This was at the age of 7 years. These procedures improved her gait considerably, permitting her to resume walking outside the home, although she still had to use crutches.

Children are *not* small adults, and the musculoskeletal conditions seen in children are frequently distinct from those seen in adults. However, delayed results of many of these conditions are important in adult orthopaedic practice, and it is therefore important that anybody seeing adult orthopaedic patients with musculoskeletal conditions has some knowledge of children's musculoskeletal disease. Juvenile chronic arthritis, discussed in the preceding chapter, presents particular issues and is an important differential diagnosis in the child presenting with joint problems.

Conditions affecting the musculoskeletal system in children may be congenital or acquired. Further they may be localised or generalised. It is important to realise that presentation with a fairly common and localised musculoskeletal difficulty (e.g. a limp) may be due to some important underlying condition such as muscular dystrophy. This is an example of how a generalised condition may present as a musculoskeletal problem.

As will be appreciated, a wide variety of generalised and localised conditions may affect the musculoskeletal system in children.

Key points

- Many musculoskeletal problems in children are caused by underlying generalised conditions; these should be sought during assessment

- Many children present with musculoskeletal problems which are in fact within the range of normal variation; such children (and their parents) are best managed by explanation and reassurance

- All treatment of children takes place against a background of development of the musculoskeletal system. Treatments should be appropriately timed to maximise the role of normal development in recovery of function

- Many childhood musculoskeletal conditions result in sequelae in adults, including accelerated degenerative changes

GENERALISED CONDITIONS

Cerebral palsy and Duchenne muscular dystrophy are discussed here, as both are relatively common neuromuscular conditions which may present to orthopaedic surgeons. Clearly, their orthopaedic management is only a small part of the total care required, which is delivered in conjunction with general practitioners, paediatricians, neurologists, nursing and physiotherapy staff and social support. There are many other paediatric neurological conditions which require attention in a similar fashion.

Cerebral palsy

Cerebral palsy affects many body systems, and a detailed discussion of the general management should be sought in a textbook on paediatrics. The musculoskeletal problems of cerebral palsy are an important contributor to the disability caused by this condition. The problems arising from cerebral palsy are due to muscle spasticity, muscle weakness and poor motor control. Secondary to these neuromuscular abnormalities, bony deformities may develop which sometimes require corrective surgery.

Clinical features

Cerebral palsy may affect all four limbs (quadriplegia), one or other side of the body (hemiplegia) or the upper or lower limbs (diplegia). The typical gait of a patient with cerebral palsy is the 'scissor' gait; the legs tend to cross due to tight adductor muscles. Patients often have poor knee excursion during walking, and also a shortened heel cord (gastrosoleus/tendo Achilles), as in the case described above. The persistent muscle imbalance around joints may lead to secondary bony or joint deformity. Common examples of this include acquired hip dislocation and scoliosis secondary to muscle imbalance.

Investigation and treatment

Initial treatment of the musculoskeletal problems associated with cerebral palsy includes physiotherapy, stretching and splints. Antispasmodics may be helpful.

The primary problems of cerebral palsy may be partly improved by adjusting the balance of muscle forces and moments around a joint. Antagonistic muscles are often of different strengths. Muscle balancing can be achieved by lengthening, dividing or transferring tendons. None of these will come close to restoring normal function, but some procedures may result in definite gains in limb function. Frequently, more than one procedure is required to improve the function of a limb.

Analysis of the specific muscle groups which require alteration can be dauntingly complex. This has resulted in the development of methods of analysing which muscle groups are inappropriately active at different phases of gait. Such analyses require sophisticated technology such as gait analysis laboratories and ambulatory electromyography (EMG) studies. Using such techniques, rate of walking, step length and cadence are accurately measured, and EMG studies demonstrate whether muscle activity is inappropriate to the task undertaken (e.g. persistent simultaneous high levels of activity in agonist and antagonists during walking). Such data permit rational planning of surgical intervention and may permit several procedures to be undertaken at once with reasonable certainty of the outcome. This contrasts with the previous scenario of having a protracted sequence of lesser procedures performed, due to the unpredictability of each of the operations.

Typical surgical procedures to improve the situation in the child with cerebral palsy include adductor tenotomies (tendon division) for the adductor muscles at the hip, and tendo Achilles lengthening for the calf problem, as performed in the case described. Surgical treatment of the secondary bony or joint deformities is also often worthwhile: it may reduce pain (e.g. due to hip dislocation) or restore the ability to sit, which may be impaired with severe neuromuscular scoliosis. Such active treatment includes open reduction and tenotomies for the hip, and surgical correction of scoliosis.

Muscular dystrophy

There are several types of muscular dystrophy, the commonest being Duchenne muscular dystrophy.

This is a serious condition which arises from an X-linked recessive gene, and accordingly almost exclusively affects boys. There has been much recent work on the genetic basis of Duchenne muscular dystrophy, much of it centring around the so-called 'Dystrophin' gene. This cytoskeletal protein is thought to decrease muscle cell fragility, although its function is not fully understood. Interestingly, another abnormality of the same gene causes Becker muscular dystrophy, a less severe condition. Accurate diagnosis of these diseases requires muscle biopsy.

Clinical features

Duchenne muscular dystrophy is a progressive disease which is ultimately fatal, usually in the teenage years. Children generally present initially with clumsiness or vague weakness. They may be noted to have enlarged leg muscles, particularly in the calves (pseudohypertrophy). The diagnosis is made more easily in the presence of a family history, but otherwise it is frequently delayed. The clinical course is of progressive weakness of walking and also of the upper limbs. Secondary joint contractures may occur, and scoliosis is a frequent and important complication of the condition.

When muscular function has deteriorated to the stage that the patient is no longer capable of maintaining an upright posture, rapid deterioration of any scoliosis may occur. This further compromises respiratory function. Children, in general, ultimately die from respiratory failure due to muscular weakness.

Treatment

There is no treatment which will affect disease progression. There is evidence that standing for several hours a day improves the prognosis for respiratory function and this is encouraged; therefore, input from a physiotherapist is beneficial. Use of devices such as a standing frame is required to maintain the standing posture in the presence of severe leg weakness. Operative intervention to treat the scoliosis by spinal instrumentation and arthrodesis may be required to help control the scoliosis, and may prolong life.

LOCALISED CONDITIONS

CONGENITAL JOINT DEFORMITIES

Most joints may be affected by congenital joint deformities. The two commonest, and arguably the most important, are the hip joint and the hindfoot and these will be discussed here.

Congenital dislocation of the hip (developmental dysplasia of the hip)

Congenital dislocation of the hip (developmental dysplasia of the hip, DDH) is a relatively common condition (between 1 and 15 per 1000 births). There is a strong familial tendency and it is commoner in females. It is also commoner in first-born children and in children who maintained a breech intrauterine position during late pregnancy. It is less common in black and Chinese babies.

Clinical features/diagnosis

Early diagnosis of congenital dislocation of the hip is vital. If the hip is not maintained in a normal reduced position before walking commences (usually by the age of 18 months), normal hip development will not occur even if surgery is subsequently undertaken. Thereafter, it is likely that such hips will be the site of early osteoarthritis and painful dysfunction during early adult life. Diagnosis is best established in the neonate by careful clinical examination. This includes the use of Ortolani's or Barlow's manoeuvres (Fig. 14.1). Both of these manoeuvres require experience to be carried out effectively.

If diagnosis is delayed, this may become more difficult, as the Ortolani and Barlow manoeuvres both require the hip to be reducible. Within a few months of birth the hip will become irreducible by closed means, making these tests of no value. There may be limb length discrepancy, and children may limp when they walk.

Investigations. X-rays are of limited value in diagnosis of congenital dislocation of the hip before the age of 6 months, as the normal capital femoral epiphysis may not form until this time. Radiographic appearances of congenital dislocation

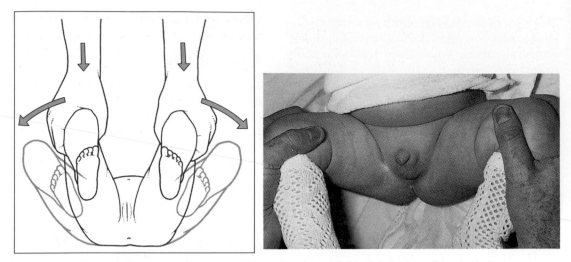

Figure 14.1   Ortolani's manoevre. Examiner's hands on child's knees, hips flexed, slight pressure along line of femur. Move hips into abduction. This results in a click as a dislocatable hip reduces in abduction.

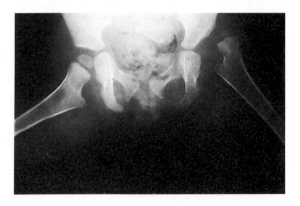

Figure 14.2   X-ray of congenital hip dislocation.

of the hip are shown in Figure 14.2. Recently, there has been increasing use of diagnostic ultrasound to achieve early diagnosis of congenital hip dislocation in doubtful cases. This has proved both accurate and sensitive, and there is now interest in the use of this modality as an additional screening technique in high-risk patients.

Treatment

Most congenitally dislocated hips are reducible without surgery, providing they are recognised at the neonatal stage and treatment is then started. The hips are generally stable in reduction whilst flexed and abducted and this position may be maintained using a variety of splints and harnesses, e.g. Van Rosen splint, Pavlik harness. For later diagnosis, open reduction of the hip may be required. A principal problem in late diagnosed congenital hip dislocation is poor acetabular development, and various osteotomies around the acetabulum have been described to partially correct this. These include the Salter and Chiari osteotomies.

Talipes (club foot)

There are two principal variants of talipes: congenital talipes equinovarus (CTEV) and congenital talipes calcaneovalgus (Figs 14.3 and 14.4). Talipes calcaneovalgus is usually a relatively unimportant condition which corrects with minimal treatment over the first few weeks or months postnatally.

Congenital talipes equinovarus may be a more serious problem. In this condition there is marked shortening of the heel cord (Achilles tendon), ankle flexion and hindfoot varus. This is frequently noted in the neonatal stage; it may be bilateral and there is frequently a family history.

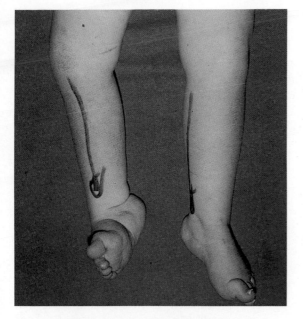

Figure 14.3 Congenital talipes equinovalgus.

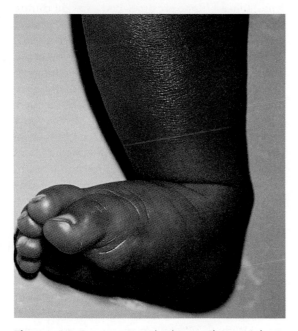

Figure 14.4 Congenital talipes calcaneovalgus.

Treatment

Relatively mild cases, which are passively correctable, may be treated by strapping techniques to good effect. However, this is insufficient in some children who will require surgical treatment. A trial of serial corrective casts may be used, but open corrective surgery may also be required. This involves lengthening the Achilles tendon, posterior release of the ankle joint and release of tight structures on the medial side of the foot. This allows adequate correction of both the ankle flexion and the hindfoot varus. As with congenital dislocation of the hip, it is important to achieve this correction at a relatively early stage as subsequent corrective surgery may be substantially less successful.

A SURVEY (BY REGION) OF ACQUIRED DEFORMITIES IN CHILDREN

Hip

Throughout childhood a variety of conditions, both inflammatory and non-inflammatory, can affect the hip. The age of the child may provide a clue to the nature of the hip problem. For example, hip pain in a 13-year-old boy would more likely be due to a slipped capital femoral epiphysis than Perthes' disease, which affects younger boys. Although septic arthritis is not included in this subsection, septic arthritis in children commonly affects the hip – always remember this possibility in the child who presents with hip pain. Also remember that hip pain in children is often referred to the thigh or knee.

Irritable hip

Irritable hip is a common condition in children up to the age of approximately 5 years. It frequently follows a minor viral illness and appears to be a transient synovitis of the affected hip. The child usually presents initially complaining of hip pain or a limp. The child is generally reasonably well and there are no signs of systemic sepsis. Examination of the hip reveals a decreased range of movement, but within this range there remains a limited pain-free arc. The principal differential diagnosis is septic arthritis of the hip, and all patients thought to have irritable hip should be carefully assessed in order to exclude this.

Imaging of irritable hip is possible using ultrasound, which will reveal the presence of an effusion. The condition will generally settle with rest and simple analgesic. It may occasionally be recurrent.

Perthes' disease

Perthes' disease is a hip condition which is commonest in boys aged between 4 and 11. The pathology is thought to be of recurrent episodes of avascular necrosis of the femoral head, a site which may be affected by vascular problems at any stage in life. The cause of these recurrent episodes is currently unknown.

The presenting complaint of the child is generally hip or knee pain and an associated limp. Examination of the limb may reveal a fixed flexion deformity and a decreased range of movement of the hip. X-rays may be normal on initial presentation, but may also reveal deformity. This reflects how many children may have long-standing disease which has been only minimally symptomatic. Indeed, patients may present in adult life with hips which appear very likely to have suffered from Perthes' disease in childhood, but with no history of symptoms at that time. X-rays reveal changes such as fragmentation of the capital femoral epiphysis, subluxation, lateral calcification and incongruity. A subchondral fracture line may be visible (Fig. 14.5).

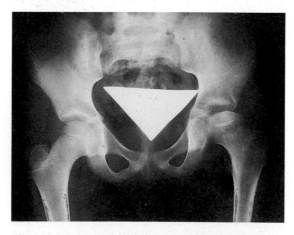

Figure 14.5 Perthes disease of the left hip. There is flattening and sclerosis of the upper femoral epiphysis; this may progress to complete collapse of the epiphysis.

Treatment of Perthes' disease is very controversial. There is currently little enthusiasm for the use of protracted bedrest or for the use of orthoses or splints, at least in the UK. Surgical management of the condition is directed to maximising 'containment' of the femoral head within the acetabulum, with the intention of using the acetabulum as a mould to maintain the shape of the head. This has been attended by greatly varying degrees of success. The outlook after Perthes' disease is relatively poor, and many of these patients will develop painful hips in early adult life. The prognosis is best in children in whom onset of the condition occurs at a young age.

Slipped capital femoral epiphysis

The capital femoral epiphysis generally fuses at the age of approximately 15 in boys and somewhat younger in girls. The geometric design of the hip results in substantial loads being carried across the femoral head (up to six times body weight during running). As a result of this, and the relative weakness of the cartilage at the epiphyseal line, slips of the capital femoral epiphysis may occur. These occasionally present as an acute epiphyseal slip after an injury, but more frequently they present after a protracted period of relatively minor symptoms. The condition most commonly occurs in boys between the ages of 9 and 14. These children are frequently hypogonadal and somewhat obese. There has been much interest in determining whether they suffer from endocrine abnormalities, but no specific pattern of such abnormality has been found to be associated with the condition.

The typical presentation of slipped capital femoral epiphysis is of either hip (groin/greater trochanter) pain, or, commonly, thigh or knee pain. The presence of thigh or knee pain in a child should prompt careful examination of the hip in all cases. With SCFE, this may reveal an external rotation deformity or a tendency for the hip to go into external rotation when it is flexed. There may be a small amount of shortening of the lower limb.

Anteroposterior X-rays of the hip may be normal. It is important to obtain a lateral X-ray of the hip in order to establish the diagnosis adequately (Fig. 14.6). It may be possible to detect

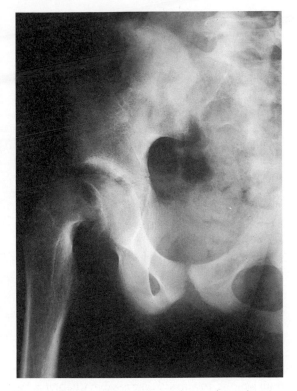

Figure 14.6 Slipped upper femoral epiphysis. This is best seen on lateral film; the abnormality may be invisible on AP X-ray.

whether the slip is old, revealed by the presence of reactive new bone formation.

Treatment of this condition is surgical, involving pinning of the slipped epiphysis in situ. Manipulation to reduce the slipped epiphysis is not a wise move, as it may precipitate avascular necrosis and consequent arthritis of the hip. The condition is very frequently bilateral (40%) and many surgeons would advocate bilateral fixation of the epiphyses in all cases.

Knee

Many parents bring their children to the doctor's surgery with genu varum (bow legs) or genu valgum (knock-knees). Similarly, many children present both to general practitioners and to orthopaedic surgeons with torsional problems (in-toeing or out-toeing) as discussed below. These problems are common in young children, and will usually to some degree lessen (although not

necessarily disappear) with growth. While it is rare for there to be an underlying disorder, remember the possibility of rickets in children with genu varum.

Occasionally, these problems are severe enough to warrant surgical attention, but far more frequently reassurance of the patient, and particularly of the parents, is all that is required. Good knowledge of where an acceptable range of normality ends and unacceptable deformity begins is required to decide whether reassurance is the most appropriate means of management. Conservative methods of management (footwear modification and the use of splints) are of little value in these deformities. If the deformities are severe, surgery may be considered. This usually requires bony correction with one or more osteotomies.

Torsional problems

Children may present (or be presented) with complaints of intoeing or out-toeing (Fig. 14.7). Intoeing is the more common. These problems often prove to be due to torsional abnormalities in the femur or tibia. Affected children may appear

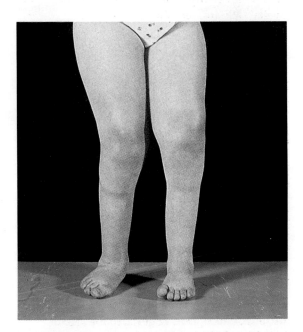

Figure 14.7 Out-toeing of the right foot. There is torsion of the right tibia.

clumsy or have a tendency to trip. There are two things to grasp about these common problems: they will frequently resolve (especially in children of less than 5 years), and careful examination and possibly specialised X-rays (often CT scans) are often required to determine the exact site of the deformity. The whole limb is often affected, and one common site of the deformity is the femoral neck (persistent femoral anteversion).

There is very little evidence that conservative measures have any effect at all. Surgery is occasionally used, but should usually be reserved until the patient is 12 or older.

Foot

Pes planovalgus (flat feet)

As with rotational deformities of the lower limb (e.g. intoeing) and minor angular deformities at the knee, flat feet are a common cause of presentation of children to general practitioners and orthopaedic surgeons (Fig. 14.8). The majority of these are within the normal range, will cause few or no problems and require no treatment.

However, there are some exceptions to this. First, a markedly abnormal foot in the neonate or infant may be due to a congenital vertical talus. Because of the largely cartilaginous nature of the hindfoot at this stage, X-ray assessment may be difficult and assessment by a paediatric orthopaedic surgeon is recommended. This abnormality results in the so-called 'rocker bottom foot'.

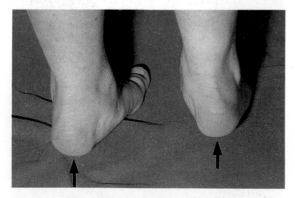

Figure 14.8 Pes planovalgus. The heel cord (Achilles tendon) is in valgus, and the medial plantar arch is not evident.

Secondly, pes planovalgus is usually pain-free, and painful flat foot occurring in early or mid-adolescence may require additional investigation. This may be caused by abnormal cartilage bars between the bones of the hindfoot. These bars (of which the calcaneonavicular bar is the most common) are generally formed of cartilage at birth. The cartilage is flexible, and accordingly they cause relatively few symptoms. During adolescence this cartilage can ossify, leading to increased rigidity of the hindfoot and a flat foot deformity. This deformity may be associated with spasm of the peroneal muscles and associated pain. It may be possible to recognise the bar on plain X-ray, but scanning techniques such as CT scans may be required. Excision of the bar may be successful in restoring normal hindfoot mobility.

Other foot deformities are discussed in Chapter 16.

Limb length inequality

Limb lengths are described by true and apparent limb lengths, as already discussed in Chapter 3. We mention limb length inequality again here because this should always be considered in children with musculoskeletal problems. True limb length inequality may result from a disorder of the bone or joint, or both. Thus, congenital dislocation of the hip may lead to a short leg; the most appropriate initial treatment for this would be directed to the hip. Some patients have limb length inequality due to inadequate growth of one or more bones in the limb. Inequality in the upper limb does not usually lead to any functional problems. Conversely, lower limb length inequality may lead to a markedly abnormal gait, stress on other joints and back pain due to the adoption of a curved posture of the back. Leg length discrepancy may occur in the femur or tibia, or both. Most patients are able to tolerate at least 1 cm of limb length discrepancy with minimal symptoms.

Correction of limb length abnormality may be attempted in several ways. First, the longer leg may be constrained from reaching its anticipated eventual length at maturity by ablation of the epiphysis at the growing end of the bone (epiphysiodesis). This must be carefully timed so that the short limb just catches up the length of the other side. Secondly, the short side may be lengthened. This may be done in a variety of ways; the most widely used method is currently 'distraction osteogenesis', where bone forming in a callus response after an osteotomy is distracted using an external fixation frame. Finally, the longer leg may be shortened. This may be technically the most straightforward, but may be unacceptable to the patient.

Spinal problems

We will consider three conditions affecting the spine in children. It is important to be aware of the existence of these conditions, but details of management are really a postgraduate subject.

Spina bifida

In spina bifida there is incomplete closure of the neural tube, usually at the lower levels. Varying degrees of neurological deficit occur, depending on the severity of the defect. Spina bifida occulta refers to a failure of closure of the bony elements of the spinal canal, and is usually asymptomatic. At the other end of the spectrum with an open neural tube defect, major neurological abnormalities can occur, with sensory loss, upper motor neurone

signs of spasticity and weakness, and a variable level of lower motor loss (flaccidity). Thus, children with associated neurological deficit vary from having a minimal amount of lower limb spasticity, but otherwise leading a normal life, to having very severe lower limb contractures, being effectively wheelchair bound and developing severe secondary deformities in the lower limbs and spine (where scoliosis is common). As well as physiotherapy and surgical treatment for spasticity and contractures of the lower limbs and associated joint problems, such patients often require substantial orthotic assistance (wheelchairs, splints, standing frames etc.) to achieve a reasonable degree of independence. Such patients often encounter increasing difficulties in middle age as their available muscles begin to weaken with age. This may result in progressive difficulties in walking at this stage.

Spondylolysis/spondylolisthesis

This condition most commonly occurs in the lower lumbar spine or the lumbosacral junction. Spondylolysis denotes that there is a defect (probably a fatigue fracture in most patients) in the pars interarticularis of a vertebra (part of the pedicle) (Figs 14.9 and 17.3). In effect, the bony

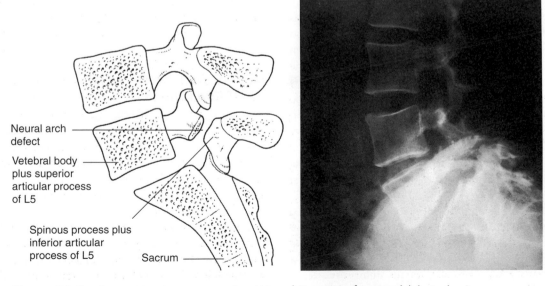

Neural arch defect

Vetebral body plus superior articular process of L5

Spinous process plus inferior articular process of L5

Sacrum

A

B

Figure 14.9 Diagrammatic representation (A) and X-ray (B) of a spondylolysis due to a pars intra-articularis defect resulting in a spondylolisthesis at the level of L5/S1.

Paediatric orthopaedics

continuity between the two parts of the vertebra is lost; this may result in painful instability, although many patients with this defect are asymptomatic. Secondary to this, the upper vertebra may slip forward on the one below (spondylolisthesis). Symptoms vary with the amount of forward slip; patients with severe slips are often symptomatic and may have sciatica as well as back pain. Spondylolisthesis may also develop in older people as part of degenerative spinal disease.

Scoliosis

Scoliosis denotes a lateral curvature of the spine (as opposed to a kyphosis which denotes a forward curvature in the sagittal plane). Scoliosis almost always includes an element of rotation as part of the deformity. The deformity is usually best seen by standing behind the patient; the spinal curve is visible and, on asking them to bend forward, the rotation of the ribs or lumbar regions is easy to see in profile.

This condition may be idiopathic, secondary to a neuromuscular condition, or secondary to a structural anomaly such as the presence of an additional hemivertebra (congenital scoliosis). Idiopathic scoliosis may occur in infants or adolescents. Infantile scoliosis often corrects spontaneously, but when it does not it is extremely difficult to control. Progressive adolescent scoliosis is more common. It is commoner in girls, and usually the curve is convex to the right. Children with onset at a young age fare worse, as the scoliosis will stop progressing in most patients when skeletal growth is complete, and the interval between onset of the deformity and cessation of growth is an important determinant of the eventual severity of the deformity. The deformity is worst when it affects the thoracic spine (lumbar curves are often hardly noticeable) (Fig. 14.10).

There is some debate about whether these patients require treatment to reduce the risk of back pain. Most evidence indicates that for the majority of adolescent patients this is principally a (sometimes severe) cosmetic deformity. Non-operative treatment with spinal braces is of debatable effectiveness. Surgical treatment, usually

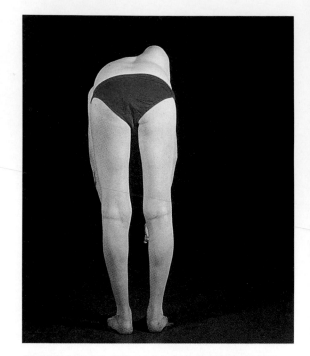

Figure 14.10   Thoracic scoliosis. The rib hump is best seen by asking the patient to bend forward.

including fusion of part of the spine and internal fixation, can dramatically improve the spinal shape, but occasionally results in spinal cord problems. The risk of this infrequent but severe hazard must be taken into account when making decisions about surgery.

SEPTIC ARTHRITIS AND OSTEOMYELITIS

Septic arthritis

Although septic arthritis has already been discussed in Chapter 7, we mention it again here because it is relatively common in children and is a differential diagnosis of most painful joint conditions in this age group. The effects of septic arthritis at any age may be devastating to the long-term function of the joint, and accordingly every care should be taken to exclude this in children with painful joints. Thus septic arthritis of the hip may lead to avascular necrosis of the capital femoral epiphysis, with subsequent failure of femoral growth and substantial limb length inequality. In addition, neither femoral head nor acetabulum will develop normally and early osteoarthritis is the rule.

Examination of a septic joint usually reveals that very little motion is possible either actively or passively. The joint is generally warm and tender to the touch. There are systemic signs of sepsis. X-rays may be normal.

It is essential to establish the diagnosis accurately. Aspiration of the joint is required, with appropriate culture for bacteriological diagnosis and establishment of bacterial sensitivity. Lavage of the joint to reduce the number of contaminating organisms is employed. Appropriate intravenous antibiotics are essential. In the hip joint, in addition to the active sepsis, very high intracapsular pressures may occur. This is partly responsible for the development of avascular necrosis and consequently there is a strong argument for surgical exploration (or arthroscopy) of any septic hip in order to decompress this pressure as well as obtain material for bacteriology.

Osteomyelitis

While less common than septic arthritis, osteomyelitis does occur in children and should always be considered in the child with fever, bone pain and tenderness. Osteomyelitis is discussed in Chapter 11.

BONE TUMOURS

Primary bone tumours are more common in children than in adults, although they are rare in all age groups. They may be benign or malignant, and are discussed further in Chapter 11. It is important to remember that the knee is the commonest site for osteosarcoma (the commonest primary malignant bone tumour) to occur. Children complaining of knee pain or swelling for longer than a few days should be X-rayed to try to exclude this possibility. Ewing's tumours, which affect the diaphysis of long bones and may mimic osteomyelitis on X-ray, occur in children. Also relevant in children is the fact that a neuroblastoma may metastasise to bone. Leukaemic infiltrates may also cause bone pain.

15 | Disorders of the upper limb

Case history

A 35-year-old right-handed typist presented with a history of pain and numbness of the radial side of the right hand and forearm. This came on mostly at work, but it also happened at night and sometimes woke her. She had never had these symptoms before and had not suffered any trauma to cause them. She attended the local orthopaedic department where she was told that she probably had carpal tunnel syndrome. Nerve conduction studies were arranged: surprisingly these proved to be normal. Subsequently, she developed some neck pain, and an X-ray of her neck showed spondylosis at C5/6, with marked narrowing of the disc space. Accordingly, it seemed likely that her arm and hand symptoms might be coming from her neck. She was advised to use only a low pillow at night, and with physiotherapy her symptoms improved to a stage where she was almost asymptomatic.

The introductory sections of this chapter highlight key points concerning upper limb function, the assessment of the upper limb, and conditions affecting the upper limb. The importance of always considering the cervical spine in the patient with upper limb complaints is stressed and common upper limb complaints (Box 15.1) are described. These have been grouped, very broadly, on a regional basis, i.e. shoulder, elbow, wrist and hand problems. However, between the elbow and wrist sections we have inserted a section describing upper limb problems arising from peripheral nerve dysfunction. This seemed the best position in the chapter for this as entrapment neuropathies commonly affect the distal upper limb.

Key points

- The upper limb is principally employed to position the hand in space. More proximal conditions of the upper limb often affect what patients can do with the hand
- Both sensory and motor function are vital to normal use of the hand and upper limb
- Nerve entrapment is more common in the upper than in the lower limb; the ulnar and median nerve are frequently compressed
- Disorders of the neck often cause upper limb symptoms
- A painful arc of shoulder abduction is a common problem
- The functional importance of the hand is reflected in the number of apparently minor conditions requiring surgery

The function of the upper limb

The function of the upper limb is strikingly different from that of the lower limb. The principal role of the upper limb in humans is to position the hand in space. This allows the hand to perform its many functions. These include power grip (holding a sledgehammer), fine grip (holding a pen), manipulation (threading a needle) or exploration (performing a rectal examination). All of these functions differ from the principal role of the lower limb, which is to permit stance and locomotion. The requirements from the physiology and anatomy of the upper and lower limbs are therefore different.

First, sensory nerve function is crucial to all upper limb functions in a variety of ways.

Box 15.1   Common upper limb complaints

Shoulder problems
- **Painful arc syndrome and rotator cuff tears**
- **Frozen shoulder**
- **Winging of the scapula**

Elbow problems
- **Tennis elbow (lateral epicondylitis)**
- **Golfer's elbow (medial epicondylitis)**
- **Olecranon bursitis**

Peripheral nerve problems affecting the distal upper limb
- **Cubital tunnel syndrome (ulnar nerve dysfunction at the elbow)**
- **Ulnar claw hand**
- **Median nerve compression (carpal tunnel syndrome)**

Wrist problems
- **Ganglia**
- **Tenosynovitis**
- **Carpal instability**

Hand problems
- **Dupuytren's disease**
- **Trigger finger**

Adequate positioning of the limb in space requires normal proprioceptive functions from both muscles and joints. Both fast and slow muscle fibres are required, but the levels of strength required in the muscles of the upper limb are much less than those in the lower limb. Also, the sensory functions of the hand are crucial to our ability to explore the world around us. The extensively developed tactile abilities of the hand are reflected in the large area of sensory cortex occupied by neurones subserving hand sensation; this area is completely disproportionate to the size of the hand, but emphasises the importance of this organ in human life.

Second, nerves are particularly vulnerable to local problems in the upper limb. Thus both median and ulnar nerves are frequently affected by local compression; this contrasts markedly with the situation in the lower limb.

As a minimum, adequate upper limb function requires the following.

The ability to position the hand in space. The ability to place the hand above shoulder level is not required for most activities of daily living, but is crucial to many occupations (e.g. decorators, electricians). A reasonable range of rotation of the shoulder is required, especially with the arm at the side. Flexion and extension of the elbow are important, particularly the ability to get the hand to the mouth. The final 30° of extension of the elbow is of relatively less importance. Elbow rotation is vital to permit the hand to subserve its normal range of functions: try accepting a handful of change in a shop with your forearm maintained in pronation! Finally, the wrist must be adequately stable and pain-free to permit free and powerful hand function. A normal range of flexion and extension movement of the wrist is arguably less important, but it does permit fine-tuning of the hand position.

The ability to use the hand freely and without pain. This requires normal finger and thumb movements, and normal stability of the joints of the hand. The extrinsic muscles (i.e. long flexor and extensor muscles and their respective tendons) must function normally, as must the intrinsic muscles of the hand.

Normal sensory function. This is required to provide control for grasping functions and to allow the hand to be used for exploration of the environment. An extreme example of this is the ability of blind persons to compensate for many of the handicaps they suffer by use of their tactile senses in the hand. However, we all constantly use the hand as a sensory instrument, and loss of this ability is frequently as serious as the motor disabilities which may occur after nerve injury.

The assessment of upper limb function

Adequate assessment of the upper limb (Ch. 3) must take all of the above elements into account. It is likewise vital to assess the functional requirements of the particular patient. Thus the upper limb requirements of a 20-year-old labourer differ substantially from those of an elderly lady living in a nursing home. Some requirements may, however, be unexpected: the elderly lady may well use her upper limbs for weight-bearing if she has to use a walking frame for mobility. Upper limb weight-bearing places particular demands on the shoulders and the wrists, as may be seen in sufferers from a variety of disabilities such as paraplegia.

Conditions affecting the upper limb

This chapter deals predominantly with problems local to the upper limb, e.g. 'frozen shoulder'. Nerve entrapment syndromes and enthesopathies, as described below, are common. However, the upper limb is freqently affected by generalised diseases, as are other areas of the body. Inflammatory arthritis, particularly rheumatoid arthritis, may severely affect the upper limb, notably the fingers (e.g. ulnar deviation of the MCP joints), wrists (tenosynovitis, destructive arthritis), elbow and shoulder (both may be affected by destructive rheumatoid arthritis). Osteoarthritis is less common in the large joints of the upper limb than in those of the lower limb. However, small joints (especially the interphalangeal joints of the fingers) are often first to be affected in primary generalised osteoarthritis. Gout frequently affects the upper limb (although the shoulder is spared): an acute monoarthritis of the wrist or elbow may be due to gout, and in patients with long-standing disease, tophaceous deposits may develop at the elbow. Therefore, always consider the possibility that a patient presenting with an upper limb problem may have a more generalised disease.

Interrelationship between problems of the upper limb and cervical spine

In almost all conditions of the upper limb, cervical spinal disorders are part of the differential diagnosis. Proximal parts of the upper limb may be affected by cervical root compression and/or referred pain from spondylosis (Ch. 17), while the hand is also affected by root disorders. In particular, the possibility of nerve root compression should be remembered when assessing patients suspected of having median nerve compression (as in the Case history). Therefore, the cervical spine should always be assessed in patients presenting with upper limb complaints.

SHOULDER PROBLEMS

The shoulder is a complex joint which normally integrates movements at four different sites:

- the glenohumeral joint
- the acromioclavicular joint.
- the subacromial 'joint'
- the scapulothoracic articulation.

The first two are synovial joints and as such are subject to the range of problems occurring at synovial joints. Disorders of the subacromial 'joint' are common at all stages of life, from late adolescence. The scapulothoracic articulation rarely gives problems other than winging of the scapula (described below). The sternoclavicular joint is also usually considered as part of the shoulder girdle. For example, if a patient raises their arm above the head then movement occurs at the sternoclavicular joint as well as at the other articulations already mentioned.

Painful arc syndrome and rotator cuff tears

Painful arc syndrome is a common condition; pain is felt arising from the shoulder but only in a restricted arc of movement (Fig. 15.1). Rotator cuff tears are less common, and clinically are frequently confused with a simple painful arc. Although relatively easy to test for, they are frequently missed.

Painful arc syndrome. Several pathologies can cause a painful arc syndrome. The commonest are supraspinatus tendinitis and subacromial bursitis (which can be associated with impingement). In the latter, the subacromial bursa is inflamed. This lies between the acromion process and the rotator cuff muscles (specifically the supraspinatus) (Fig. 15.2) and is thus subject to movement whenever the glenohumeral joint moves; hence, if inflamed, such movements may cause pain. Subacromial bursitis may occur due to a generalised

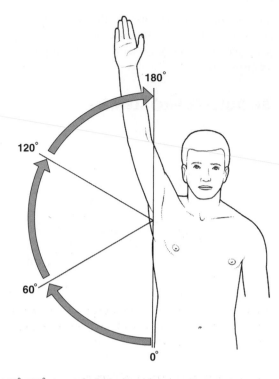

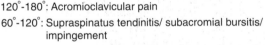

120°-180°: Acromioclavicular pain
60°-120°: Supraspinatus tendinitis/ subacromial bursitis/
          impingement

Figure 15.1   Causes of a painful shoulder arc.

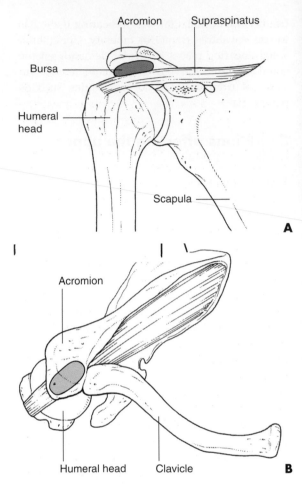

Figure 15.2   The subacromial bursa. **A.**
Anteroposterior view—subacromial bursa lies
between supraspinatus and the acromion. **B.** View
from above – the acromioclavicular joint (and any
osteophytes) directly overlies the bursa and the
humeral head.

inflammatory arthropathy, due to local 'impingement' (when development of a beak-like
osteophyte on the tip of the acromion, which
occurs with ageing, increases local pressure on the
supraspinatus and the intervening bursa) or due to
trauma (which is usually indirect, e.g. a fall onto
the hand causes a twisting movement of the
shoulder).

Rotator cuff tears.   These may arise as a result of
trauma or degeneration due to age. Degenerative
tears are extremely common at postmortem; some
of these tears appear to be asymptomatic. Both
causes may contribute; thus tears are common after
shoulder dislocations in the elderly, presumably
because the cuff is already weak. The
supraspinatus is the most commonly affected
muscle, a tear in this leading to weakness of
initiation of abduction. The size of the tear may
vary from tiny (and functionally irrelevant) to

complete, where the 'bald' humeral head
articulates directly with the acromion.

Clinical features

History.   The defining feature of a painful arc
syndrome is the presence of an arc of abduction of
the shoulder which is painful. If the pain is caused
by supraspinatus tendinitis or subacromial
bursitis, the arc is usually between 60° and 120° of
abduction; if it is caused by acromioclavicular
arthritis, the arc is usually from 120° to 180° of

abduction. The position of the pain varies. Pain from supraspinatus tendinitis/subacromial bursitis is frequently felt vaguely over the deltoid, while pain arising from the acromioclavicular joint is generally accurately located to that joint (Fig. 3.32, p. 43). The pain may be worse with movement in one direction, especially bringing the arm back to the side.

Very similar pain to subacromial bursitis may be felt with rotator cuff tears; in addition, the patient may complain of clicks from the shoulder on movement, or of weakness. In particular, working with hands above shoulder height frequently becomes impossible in the presence of a significant rotator cuff tear.

Examination. When examining the patient, first inspect the shoulder contour and rhythm. The contour will be normal in most cases, and if it is not this may be due to a bony abnormality (e.g. a missed posterior dislocation) or a soft tissue problem (e.g. muscle wasting due to axillary nerve injury). The rhythm describes the way in which the entire shoulder – glenohumeral, acromioclavicular and scapulothoracic 'joints' – moves together. This is frequently disordered with any shoulder pathology. The painful arc is also sought at this stage, noting the position of the arc and any clicks which are felt on movement. After inspecting the active ranges of movement, the passive ranges should be ascertained. The strength of the rotator cuff muscles is next tested, usually examining resisted external rotation of the forearm with the arms at the side (Fig. 15.3).

Investigation. Plain X-rays may be uninformative, although with acromioclavicular impingement an osteophyte may be visible on the tip of the acromion (Fig. 15.4). There may be calcification within the supraspinatus tendon or subacromial bursa. A severe rotator cuff tear may lead to direct contact between humeral head and acromion. This is revealed by reduction in the space between the humeral head and the acromion on the anteroposterior X-ray, and sclerosis of the opposing bone ends. Adequate imaging of rotator cuff tears may be obtained by magnetic resonance imaging. Remember that, as with all other soft tissue and 'degenerative' lesions, the full blood count, ESR and biochemical profile should be

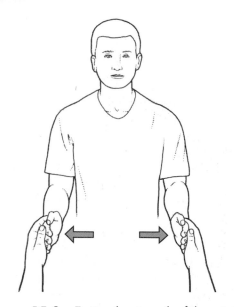

Figure 15.3 Testing the strength of the rotator cuff muscles: the examiner's hands resist external rotation of the shoulders.

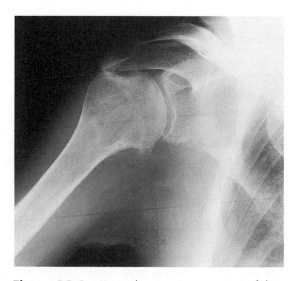

Figure 15.4 X-ray showing impingement of the humerous (greater tuberosity) on the acromion. There is sclerosis of the acromial lip and a small osteophyte.

normal. If not, ask why and look for an underlying condition which could explain the abnormality.

Pinpointing pain from the several different possible sources is notoriously difficult. In the patient presenting with shoulder pain and a painful arc, a useful way of clarifying this is to perform serial local anaesthetic injections of the possible sources of pain. A small amount of local anaesthetic is injected in sequence into the subacromial bursa, the acromioclavicular joint and the glenohumeral joint. A period of 10–15 minutes is allowed between injections, and the effect of each injection on the pain noted. If one of the injections dramatically reduces the pain on movement, it may not be necessary to perform the other injections.

Management

Most shoulders with painful arc syndrome are initially managed by local anaesthetic and steroid injection into the subacromial bursa (supraspinatus tendinitis/subacromial bursitis/impingement) or acromioclavicular joint (acromioclavicular joint arthritis). The injection may need to be repeated (once) after an interval of several weeks. Physiotherapy may be helpful for painful arc syndrome and for rotator cuff tears. Surgical treatment, if required, consists of decompression of the subacromial bursa and rotator cuff, by excision of the osteophyte and coracoacromial ligament, and/or excision of the lateral 1.5 cm of the clavicle with adjoining osteophytes. For rotator cuff tears these procedures may be combined with a cuff repair, although some very large cuff repairs, especially in older patients, may be irreparable and are better left alone.

'Frozen' shoulder

Frozen shoulder, often termed (adhesive) capsulitis, is a common condition of uncertain aetiology. The condition is most common in middle-aged females. Essentially, an acute fibrosis occurs within the gleno-humeral joint, leading to severe stiffness which takes a considerable time to resolve. Patients may have associated conditions, e.g. immobilisation associated with an elbow or wrist fracture, or the process may occur spontaneously.

The condition starts with aching of gradual onset and may become very painful. At the same time, range of joint motion is lost over a short period, usually of a few weeks. The pain frequently settles with time, but untreated frozen shoulders may take much longer (many months) to regain normal movement. Examination reveals the lack of joint motion, while investigations are normal. Treatment usually consists of persistent physiotherapy, often combined with intra-articular steroids. However, it may be impossible for the patient to improve the range of motion, and a manipulation under anaesthetic is sometimes required to break down strong intra-articular adhesions. If this is undertaken, it is essential that it is followed by early postoperative physiotherapy, starting on the day of operation or the following day.

Winging of the scapula

The scapula is held onto the chest wall by the serratus anterior muscle. This has an unusual nerve supply, in that it is supplied by the long thoracic nerve which is superficial to the muscle and hence vulnerable to damage. Occasionally, the serratus anterior may become acutely paralysed; this causes 'winging' of the scapula. The condition may be caused by trauma, but more commonly it occurs for no obvious reason. It is best seen by asking the patient to push against a wall: this will reveal an obvious asymmetry between the two scapulae, with the affected one standing proud of the chest wall. No satisfactory treatment is available, although many patients are only mildly symptomatic.

ELBOW PROBLEMS

The commonest soft tissue lesions around the elbow are enthesopathies and olecranon bursitis.

Enthesopathies – tennis elbow (lateral epicondylitis) and golfer's elbow (medial epicondylitis)

Entheses are the anatomical structures where muscles arise from bone. They are specialised to transfer the muscular force to the structure of the bone. Most entheses can cause pain occasionally, but the entheses around the elbow are particularly prone to become painful. Such enthesopathy is often due to inflammation, but the pathological basis is not well understood, and most cases arise in patients without systemic inflammatory disease or obvious overuse injury.

Clinical features

Patients complain of pain at the lateral epicondyle (tennis elbow) or medial epicondyle (golfer's elbow). The pain is usually poorly localised to the bone and radiates distally from the elbow. The symptoms are usually worse with use of the forearm, particularly with lifting of heavy weights or repetitive tasks such as using computer keyboards. Examination reveals that there is tenderness along the bony origin of the muscle. The pain of tennis elbow is exacerbated on resisted wrist extension, whereas the pain of golfer's elbow is exacerbated by resisted wrist flexion (Fig. 15.5). Investigations are usually normal, although the elbow is usually X-rayed in persistent cases. Blood tests to investigate inflammatory arthropathy (especially the seronegative spondyloarthropathies, in which enthesopathies are common) should be considered.

Management

Treatment for enthesopathies usually includes NSAIDs and physiotherapy in the first instance.

A Patient extends wrist [against resistance]

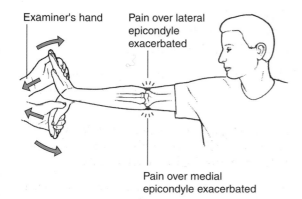

B Patient flexes wrist [against resistance]

Figure 15.5 Exacerbation of pain with resisted wrist extension in tennis elbow (A), and with resisted wrist flexion in golfer's elbow (B).

Sometimes an elbow splint may be of benefit. If there is no improvement, injection of local anaesthetic and a long-acting steroid preparation may provide prolonged relief. This treatment may need repeating. If these treatments are unsuccessful, surgical release of the common extensor origin should be considered, although the procedure rarely yields instant relief and a significant number of patients fail to improve despite it.

Olecranon bursitis

This can occur either as an isolated soft tissue lesion or in association with generalised conditions, such as rheumatoid arthritis or gout. Pain and swelling (often tender) occur over the olecranon. The pain is exacerbated by pressure over the elbow, e.g. by leaning on it. If infection is suspected, the bursa must be aspirated and antibiotics commenced.

PERIPHERAL NERVE PROBLEMS AFFECTING THE DISTAL UPPER LIMB

Nerve entrapment is common in the upper limb, and the median and ulnar nerves are those most commonly affected. The consequences of median and ulnar nerve dysfunction are described here. Nerves can be compressed for a variety of reasons. For example, median nerve compression can result from injury to the wrist or from pressure from hypertrophied synovium in rheumatoid arthritis.

Cubital tunnel syndrome/ulnar nerve dysfunction at the elbow

The ulnar nerve passes behind the medial epicondyle (through the cubital tunnel), against which it may be stretched each time the elbow is flexed. The nerve also passes between the two heads of the flexor carpi ulnaris, limiting its ability to move with elbow flexion. Most cases of cubital tunnel syndrome are idiopathic, but several predisposing causes are recognised. These include a cubitus valgus deformity, often due to a malunited childhood supracondylar fracture of the elbow, and instability of the ulnar nerve, such that it tends to dislocate anteriorly around the epicondyle on elbow flexion.

Clinical features

The clinical features of cubital tunnel syndrome consist of pain at the medial side of the elbow, with radiation to the medial forearm and usually to the ulnar nerve distribution in the hand (ulnar $1\frac{1}{2}$ fingers). The pain is usually worse with the elbow flexed; it may be related to activity. Examination may reveal tenderness of the ulnar nerve behind the medial epicondyle, and occasionally obvious instability where the nerve can be dislocated anteriorly. Local pressure over the nerve may provoke the symptoms of which the patient complains. There may also be evidence of motor dysfunction of the ulnar nerve (weakness in the hand due to intrinsic weakness) and possibly an ulnar claw hand (described below).

Recently, increasing numbers of keyboard operators have complained of pain in the upper limb related to their work. The pain is often diffuse and may not resolve with rest. The clinical management of these patients has not been helped by the acrimonious medicolegal disputes about the relationship of such symptoms to the patient's work.

Ulnar claw hand

Clinical features

This condition is caused by ulnar nerve dysfunction, which may occur at the elbow or wrist, or due to injury in the forearm. The features of the deformity are hyperextension of the MCP joints of the little and ring fingers, with flexion of the proximal and distal IP joints. The deformities arise due to lack of activity in the intrinsic muscles of the hand, which are (almost all) supplied by the ulnar nerve. This leads to an inability to extend the PIP and DIP joints, as the intrinsics are the main extensors of these joints. There is a compensatory hyperextension of the MCP joints. The middle and index fingers are usually little affected as the median nerve supplies the lumbricals to these fingers. The deformity is usually passively correctable for a period after the nerve initially fails

to work, but subsequently the deformities may become fixed (not passively correctable). If recovery of nerve function is anticipated, it is important that physiotherapy and splintage are used to prevent these deformities from becoming fixed, as subsequent recovery of muscles is most unlikely to give enough muscle power to overcome any fixed joint deformity.

Investigation.   Nerve conduction studies are the most important investigation for this condition. Sensory and motor testing will reveal with reasonable reliability whether the diagnosis is correct. It is important to exclude nerve entrapment at a root or plexus level as a cause of the symptoms. Nerve conduction studies will show conduction slowing across the elbow in the ulnar nerve in most cases, usually combined with a reduction in motor response.

Management

Surgery is the only useful treatment option in most cases of this condition. However, treatment is not always needed if sensory symptoms are tolerable and there is no evidence of weakness or muscle wasting. If surgery is contemplated, nerve conduction studies should be used to confirm the diagnosis. At operation, the nerve may be decompressed by dissecting it free from compressing bands or fascial tissue and separating the heads of flexor carpi ulnaris.

Median nerve compression/carpal tunnel syndrome

The median nerve passes under the transverse carpal ligament at the wrist; the space between this ligament and the carpal bones is known as the carpal tunnel. If the tunnel becomes narrowed for any reason, or the contents of the tunnel become enlarged, compression of the nerve may result. The condition is extremely common, especially in middle-aged and elderly women. Although usually idiopathic, it may be associated with a large number of underlying conditions, including diabetes mellitus, hypothyroidism, trauma (especially wrist fractures) and rheumatoid arthritis. The condition may first present during pregnancy.

Clinical features

Carpal tunnel syndrome usually consists of pain and/or paraesthesiae felt in all or some of the median nerve distribution in the hand. This is over the radial $3\frac{1}{2}$ digits on the palmar and dorsal surface, except for the dorsal surface of the thumb. The symptoms are often worse at night and classically wake the patient from sleep. Sometimes the symptoms are not confined to the hand, occasionally spreading as far proximally as the shoulder. The symptoms may vary with menstrual period and be worse with use of the hand.

On examination, there is often little to find. However, examination may reveal sensory changes in a median nerve distribution (Fig. 3.47), although these are often episodic and may not be present at the time. Wasting of the thenar muscles may be seen in later cases (Fig. 15.6). There are several provocation tests as already mentioned in Chapter 3: the symptoms may be provoked by maintained wrist flexion (Phalen's test) or by tapping over the median nerve proximal to the transverse carpal ligament (Tinel's test).

Investigations. Adequate diagnosis of carpal tunnel syndrome requires nerve conduction studies. The median and ulnar nerve conduction velocities across the wrist are examined, including both sensory and motor modalities. Other investigations, e.g. thyroid function tests, may be indicated to exclude the possibility of associated medical conditions.

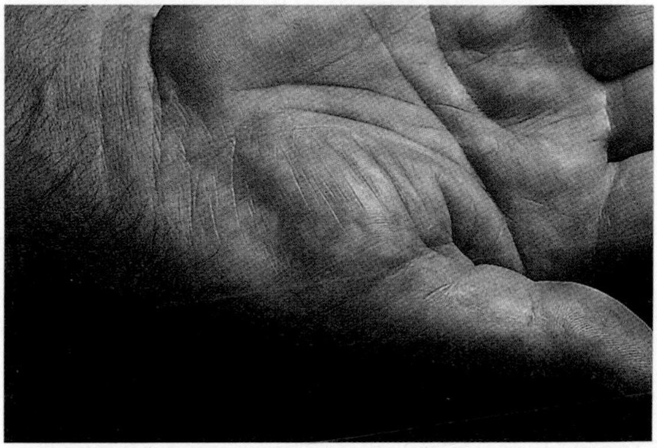

Management

Treatment of carpal tunnel syndrome is usually surgical; the results are relatively reliable, with relief of symptoms often being rapid and complete. The procedure – division of the transverse carpal ligament to decompress the carpal tunnel – is fairly simple and may usually be performed under local anaesthetic. Sometimes other measures may be tried first, including wrist splintage (especially if symptoms are only felt at night) and steroid injection into the carpal tunnel. Occasionally the nerve is so badly damaged by the time of surgical decompression that its function does not subsequently improve.

WRIST PROBLEMS

The wrist is commonly involved in different forms of inflammatory arthritis, e.g. rheumatoid arthritis and calcium pyrophosphate dihydrate deposition disease. However, pain and swelling around the wrist occur in certain specific conditions discussed here.

Ganglia

Ganglia are small cysts filled with viscous fluid. They arise due to outpouchings from synovium, either from joints or from synovial tendon sheaths (Fig. 15.7). They are common around the wrist, where they arise on the palmar surface (often close

Figure 15.6   Thenar muscle wasting in carpal tunnel syndrome.

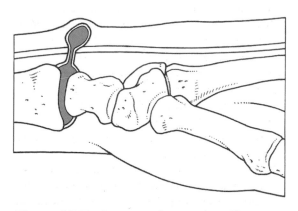

Figure 15.7   Diagram of a ganglion. This can arise as a pouch from any synovial sheath or joint. This one arises from the wrist joint, and would be palpable adjacent to the extensor tendons.

Disorders of the upper limb

to the radial artery) or on the dorsum. They may be uncomfortable or painful; examination reveals a swelling of variable size which may be fluctuant and transilluminates.

Treatment is not always required, although the traditional treatment of smiting the lesion a blow with the family Bible to rupture it at least has the merit of being non-invasive (there is little else to recommend this line of treatment). Other possible treatments are aspiration with a wide bore needle, yielding a 'glairy' viscous fluid which is often difficult to draw into the syringe, steroid injection or excision. All of these treatments lead to a substantial rate of recurrence.

Tenosynovitis

Many of the tendons around the wrist are surrounded by synovial sheaths. These synovial sheaths may become inflamed in the same way as synovium elsewhere, leading to tenosynovitis. Common causes of this condition include overuse (being common in oarsmen and keyboard workers amongst others) and inflammatory arthritis, notably rheumatoid arthritis.

Clinical features

Rheumatoid arthritis commonly affects the tendon sheaths on the dorsum of the wrist, leading to substantial swelling of the sheaths around the extensor retinaculum. This may be associated with tendon ruptures, due to impaired tendon nutrition or the development of sharp spikes of bone in damaged joints (e.g. the distal radioulnar joint). Extensor tendon rupture leads to an inability to extend the MCP joints of the fingers.

A common site for tenosynovitis in the absence of inflammatory arthritis is the radial side of the extensor surface of the wrist, involving abductor pollicis longus and extensor pollicis brevis (Fig. 15.8). This is known as de Quervain's tenosynovitis, and is commonly associated with overuse. Pain is felt around the radial styloid, with radiation proximally and distally. There is local tenderness around the appropriate tendon sheath, often with swelling. Forced ulnar deviation (or resisted radial deviation) of the wrist may cause severe pain.

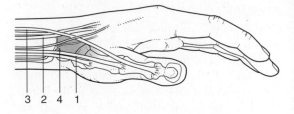

[1] anterior: extensor pollicis brevis/ abductor pollicis longus
[2] posterior: extensor carpi radialis longus/ brevis
[3] more posterior: extensor pollicis longus
[4] in the floor of the 'snuff box' : superficial radial nerve, radial artery, scaphoid

Figure 15.8   The relationship of the extensor tendons to the distal radius and the anatomical snuffbox.

Management

Treatment of tenosynovitis is initially with NSAIDs or rest with wrist splintage. Injection of local anaesthetic and long-acting steroids into the tendon sheath or inflamed synovium is also widely used. Surgical treatment may be required; this consists of 'decompression' of the tendon sheath (essentially dividing the roof of the sheath). Bowstringing of the tendons does not appear to be a particular problem after this procedure, although prevention of this is one of the anatomical functions of tendon sheaths and associated retinacula.

Carpal instability

The wrist is a complex joint, and not yet fully understood. The carpus consists of eight linked bones, with complicated relative motions during wrist movement. Recently there has been increased recognition of several problems arising from failure of the wrist bones to maintain this coordinated function; these are one cause of chronic wrist pain. A detailed analysis of this problem is beyond the scope of this book, but an example of the problem is the damage which can occur after rupture of the ligament that joins the scaphoid and lunate. This leads to a gap developing between the two bones, and lack of coupled relative motion. The wrist may be weak and painful at this stage, or it may be relatively asymptomatic. Over time, various secondary deformities develop in the relative position of the carpal bones, and severe radiocarpal arthritis develops. This situation is known as scapholunate advanced collapse (SLAC wrist); at this stage only palliative (fusion) treatment is possible. A very similar set of deformities may develop after un-united fractures of the scaphoid. It is therefore important to recognise damage to intercarpal wrist ligaments early, as this may give the best chance of a satisfactory long-term outcome.

HAND PROBLEMS

The importance of the hand as a motor and sensory organ has been emphasised above. However, there are relatively few conditions which are peculiar to the hand; most conditions affecting it are generalised (e.g. rheumatoid arthritis) or caused by a condition at some distance from the hand itself (e.g. cubital tunnel syndrome). Thus an adequate history and examination of the neck and remainder of the upper limb are vital in correctly assessing hand disorders. Perhaps the commonest condition which principally affects the hand is carpal tunnel syndrome; another common condition is Dupuytren's disease. Trigger finger is also discussed here.

Reflex sympathetic dystrophy affects primarily the extremities – hand and wrist, foot and ankle or knee – and can be a cause of severe pain and impaired hand function. It is discussed in Chapter 6.

Dupuytren's disease

Dupuytren's disease is a common fibrotic disorder, principally affecting the palm of the hand. The condition is commoner in patients with liver disease (including alcoholics), diabetes, and those taking anticonvulsant medication. However, the strongest predisposing factor to Dupuytren's disease is the presence of a family history: in many families, most of the male members are affected. The overall prevalence rate of the disease is much higher in men, in whom the incidence rate rises at a younger age than in women (between 35 and 50 years). However, after the age of around 55 years the incidence rate is similar in men and women. As

the condition is often present for many years before it causes sufficient deformity to require operation, the rate of female patients requiring operative treatment is much lower than that in males.

The condition consists of fibrosis in, or just anterior to, the palmar fascia, which is deep to the subcutaneous fat of the palm. Initially, cells (myofibroblasts or fibroblasts) proliferate to form a nodule which is palpable in the palm of the hand or finger. This is attached to fibrous bands which radiate longitudinally in the palm and fingers, and contraction of the nodule as it evolves causes gradual retraction of the affected finger(s).

Clinical features

The ulnar side of the hand, especially the little and ring fingers, is most commonly affected. However, any area of the palm of the hand may become involved, as may the sole of the foot (Lederhose's disease). Peyronie's disease of the penis is also an associated condition. Patients usually present complaining of an inability to fully extend the finger(s), or occasionally with discomfort caused by a palmar nodule. The functional limitations caused by the condition are often surprisingly modest, reflecting the relative importance of the radial side of the hand for most tasks. Nevertheless, loss of effective function on the ulnar side of the hand may be a significant functional problem for some patients. Many patients also report a tendency to catch fingers with fixed flexion deformities, and also find the appearance of the deformed finger objectionable.

On examination, the only finding may be a palmar nodule in either the palm or finger, or both. This represents the earliest stage of the disease. More commonly, however, there is a flexion contracture (fixed flexion deformity) of one or more fingers. Detection of this may be by use of the 'table-top test' (Fig. 15.9). Commonly, the MCP or PIP joints are involved (Fig. 15.10). The patient is normally able to flex the fingers fully. Ultimately, very severe deformity may develop, with the finger curled right down into the distal palmar crease. At this stage, adequate correction of the deformity may be extremely difficult, and amputation may have to be considered. Relatively early surgical treatment is therefore often indicated for hands

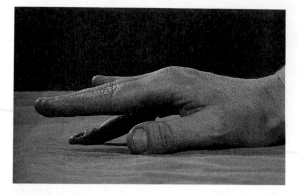

Figure 15.9   Table-top test. This patient with a contracture of the MCP joint cannot bring the palm of her hand down onto the examination table.

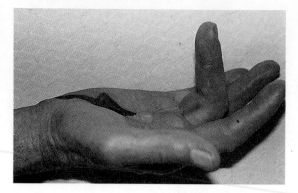

Figure 15.10   Dupuytren's contracture affecting the proximal interphalangeal joint.

which fail the table-top test. This is particularly true for contractures of the PIP joint, which have a higher tendency to recur after surgery.

Management

The only effective treatment for Dupuytren's disease is surgery. A wide variety of operations have been described, ranging from simple division of fascial bands (fasciotomy) to complete excision of the palmar fascia and partial skin grafting of the palm. The most commonly performed procedure is partial fasciectomy, where the obviously diseased palmar tissue is excised from the ray where contracture is present. The diseased tissue is usually closely applied to the digital nerves, and patients should be warned pre-operatively about the risk of damage to these nerves, and also about the risk of incomplete correction of deformity. The main postoperative risks are (early) stiffness of the hand and (later) recurrence of deformity, which may be due to new diseased fibrous tissue or to joint damage caused before the operation.

Trigger finger

Trigger fingers are common problems: any finger (or thumb) may be affected. The condition is particularly common in patients with rheumatoid arthritis, and occurs in other conditions including diabetes. 'Triggering' consists of a snapping or

flicking sensation on active flexion or extension of the digit. It is usually caused by a nodule developing on one of the flexor tendons (occurring as a result of degenerative changes in the tendon) and/or fibrosis and constriction of the finger flexor tendon sheath. The nodule tends to catch as it enters or leaves the flexor tunnel on the finger, during extension or flexion of the finger, respectively. Occasionally the nodule gets stuck within the flexor sheath; this leads to a fixed flexion deformity which may damage the affected joints.

Some trigger fingers cause little trouble and will resolve spontaneously. Treatment is usually surgical, or by injection of steroid into the tendon sheath. Surgery is a relatively minor procedure which may be performed under local anaesthetic in most cases. Treatment becomes urgent if the triggering nodule becomes stuck, causing a fixed flexion deformity.

CONCLUSION

Upper limb problems are common and the functional effects of these disorders are being increasingly appreciated. It is vital to appreciate the complex interplay of sensory and motor elements in upper limb function in order to evaluate problems fully. There are few areas where some knowledge of the subtleties of anatomy pays greater dividends than in understanding upper limb disorders.

16 | Disorders of the foot

Case history

A 58-year-old woman, who had always suffered with her feet, presented to the orthopaedic clinic having spent many hours and many pounds at chiropodists over the years. Her complaints were of the appearance of her feet, with large unsightly bunions, and of pain over her bunions and under her forefoot. She also had pain in her second toes which were now crossing over the first toes and hence being rubbed against her shoes and causing pressure and soreness. Inspection and standing X-rays confirmed hallux valgus and a varus first metatarsal. Initially, she was given advice about footwear and was told that foot surgery was often rather painful, and so should be avoided if her main worry was really the appearance of the feet.

By the time of her second appointment, the woman had decided that she would like surgery due to the persisting pain in her feet. She underwent a bilateral basal osteotomy of the first metatarsal to correct the hallux valgus, and an extensor tenotomy of the second toe to allow the toe to come down to the floor. After her surgery she was comfortable although slightly restricted in plasters for 6 weeks. After this she had more severe pain for the next 2 months, but thereafter her feet improved. Eventually she was pleased with the appearance and had less pain than before over the bunion area, but still had to go to the chiropodist because of callosities on the sole of her foot and over the fifth metatarsal head.

The foot frequently starts as an anatomical mystery to medical students early in their careers, is ignored later on in their course and is subsequently

Key points

- Foot disease is very common; most cases are managed in the community

- 'Foot' disorders may be secondary to anatomical problems elsewhere in the lower limb, to neurological conditions or to systemic disease

- Forefoot problems, especially of the great toe and first metatarsal, are very common. Most patients can be managed conservatively, but surgery can be very effective in more severely affected feet

- Hindfoot problems can be often managed with orthotics

- Foot surgery is often surprisingly painful for the first few months, and it is important to be realistic about the goals and outcomes of surgery when discussing it with patients

regarded with bewilderment by many doctors. This should not be so: the amount of discomfort and morbidity caused by foot disease makes study of this area worthwhile. Here we cover only the commonest foot disorders (Box 16.1), with cross-references to other conditions covered elsewhere in the book. As chiropodists (or podiatrists) and orthotists play a major role in the management of foot problems, we include a section at the end of the chapter outlining some of their specific roles.

The lower limb has several functions, including stance, balance and walking. Normal foot function is a prerequisite for all of these. Patients frequently present with complaints of deformity, pain and difficulty with footwear. 'Foot' deformity is a frequent reason for presentation to orthopaedic

---

Box 16.1   Common foot problems

Forefoot problems
- **Forefoot deformities**
  - **hallux valgus**
  - **hallux rigidus**
  - **minor toe deformities**
- **Morton's interdigital neuroma**
- **Stress fractures**
- **Systemic conditions with major forefoot involvement**
  - **rheumatoid arthritis**
  - **diabetes**
  - **gout**
  - **osteoarthritis**

Mid- and hindfoot problems
- **Pes cavus**
- **Plantar fasciitis**
- **Achilles tendinitis**

---

clinics, but it is important to realise that some patients may have an evident foot deformity due to an abnormality (or variant of normality) elsewhere in the limb. Common causes for concern in children and adolescents include forefoot deformities (especially hallux valgus) and torsional deformities (e.g. intoeing). Some deformities which occur during childhood and adolescence will correct spontaneously (Ch. 14), including most cases of intoeing, genu varum (bandy knees) or genu valgum (knock-knees). Many of these deformities are sufficiently mild that any possible treatment will be worse than the disease, leaving only a small number which are best treated actively, usually by surgery. Other common childhood foot disorders, e.g. flat feet, talipes or club foot, are covered in Chapter 14. Therefore, this chapter concentrates on foot problems in the adult.

The foot can be divided into the forefoot, the midfoot and the hindfoot. Broadly speaking, foot problems can be considered under two headings: forefoot problems, and mid- and hindfoot problems (see Box 16.1).

FOREFOOT PROBLEMS

Forefoot deformities, primarily hallux valgus and hallux rigidus, are common complaints in adults and are among the commonest presentations to a variety of medical and paramedical services, including podiatry/chiropody and surgical fitters for construction of appropriate wide toe box shoes. These deformities are an excellent example of the failure to examine results of treatment in a critical and structured way: there are over 50 different described operations for hallux valgus, many of which are still in common usage. However, it is still not clear which is the most appropriate operation in any particular situation. Pain under the forefoot is termed metatarsalgia and is a common symptom of forefoot disease.

Because forefoot problems frequently occur in patients with rheumatoid arthritis, diabetes, gout and osteoarthritis can be a major source of pain and disability, these associated problems are included in this chapter, with cross-references to previous chapters.

Forefoot deformities

Hallux valgus

Hallux valgus (Fig. 16.1) generally consists of two deformities. First, there is a valgus deformity of the first MTP joint. This causes the medial side of the neck of the first metatarsal to be thrust medially, causing an exostosis (a bunion) to develop. Second, the first metatarsal lies in an abnormally varus position, with a larger than usual angle between

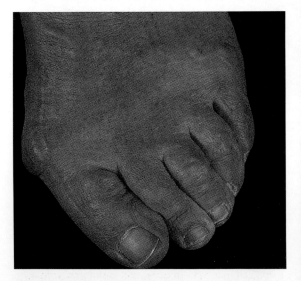

Figure 16.1 Hallux valgus.

first and second metatarsals; this deformity is the primary problem in many feet with hallux valgus. Ultimately, further problems develop, including malrotation of the hallux and subluxation of both flexor and extensor tendons. Bunions are a common deformity, especially in women. They may occur in adolescence, in which case they often progress rapidly, or at any time subsequently during adult life. Patients complain of pain over the bunion, especially when wearing shoes, and pain from the first MTP joint, which may develop osteoarthritis over time.

Most patients with hallux valgus require little treatment. Adoption of more comfortable footwear should be a first step in management. If this is unsuccessful, surgery may be considered, particularly in younger patients in whom the condition is likely to deteriorate. One common procedure, Mitchell's osteotomy, is shown in Figure 16.2. Other procedures include osteotomies close to the base of the first metatarsal to reduce the angle between first and second metatarsals. All patients having such forefoot surgery should be warned that, although the operative intervention is not major, recovery of normal foot function may be prolonged (several months).

Hallux rigidus

Osteoarthritis of the first MTP joint is termed

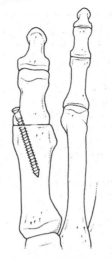

Figure 16.3   First metatarsophalangeal joint fusion. The cartilage has been removed from the joint surface, and the resulting bare bone surfaces compressed together with a screw.

hallux rigidus. This may develop at any age of life, but is (curiously) rather commoner in young men. Initially, conservative treatment such as analgesics should be employed. A variety of operative procedures can be employed if these measures fail. The commonest is fusion (arthrodesis) of the first MTP joint (Fig. 16.3). This works best if the adjacent first toe interphalangeal (IP) joint has normal mobility. An alternative is Keller's procedure, involving excision of the proximal third of the proximal phalanx of the great toe. This is an example of an *excision arthroplasty*. This procedure is often effective, but does carry the risk of substantially defunctioning the toe.

Minor toe deformities

These include hammer and claw toes (Ch. 3): the former (Fig. 16.4) has a flexion deformity at the proximal IP joint; and the latter has a deformity at both proximal and distal IP joints. Some of these deformities may cause sufficient discomfort to merit surgical correction e.g. by proximal IP joint arthrodesis.

Morton's interdigital neuroma

Neuromas (Morton's neuroma) may develop between the metatarsal heads in the forefoot. In

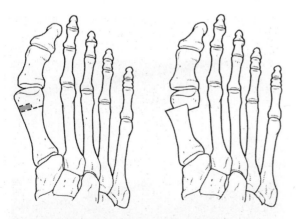

Figure 16.2   Mitchell's osteotomy for hallux valgus. A step cut is made in the first metatarsal neck, and the metatarsal is transposed laterally. This reduces the effective inter-metatarsal angle, reducing the degree of hallux valgus.

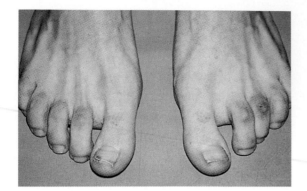

Figure 16.4   Hammer toes.

this location, particularly between second and third metatarsal heads, transverse pressure between the adjacent bones and minor degrees of synovitis of the intermetatarsal bursa may cause nerve compression and damage. This leads to severe pain in the forefoot which radiates down the adjacent borders of the affected digital cleft. The pain is usually worse (and very severe) on walking, and may be mimicked by transverse forefoot compression. Examination of the foot usually reveals some sensory changes in the affected cleft. Treatment may include moulded insoles which relieve weight on one of the metatarsal heads, or surgical excision of the neuroma and affected nerve (relieving the pain, but also reducing sensation in the adjacent toes).

Stress fractures

Stress fractures most commonly occur due to unaccustomed vigorous exercise. They are relatively common in army recruits. The fractures are similar to fatigue fractures seen in other materials, arising due to repeated stresses below that required to cause an acute fracture. The usual complaint is of persisting aching in a long bone, made worse by weight-bearing. In the foot, the second metatarsal is the bone most commonly affected; the tibial shaft is another common site. Usually pain predates any X-ray changes by weeks or months. However, the diagnosis may be confirmed by isotope bone scan which is generally strongly positive. An area of dense sclerosis, which usually (but not always) contains a fracture line, is seen on X-rays later in the disease. Treatment is usually conservative, providing support for the fractured bone during healing, which is often extremely slow.

Systemic conditions with major forefoot involvement

The rheumatoid forefoot

Patients with rheumatoid arthritis (Ch. 8) often have severe forefoot deformities (Fig. 16.5). Many of these arise because synovitis of the MTP joints leads to subluxation or dislocation of these joints, with the metatarsal heads being forced downwards into the sole of the forefoot. These problems occur due to the

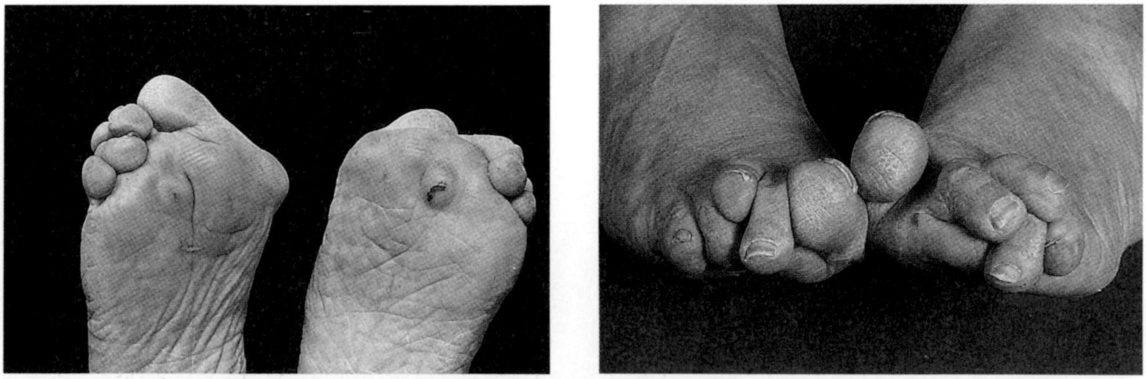

Figure 16.5   Two views of the forefoot of a patient with rheumatoid arthritis, showing callosities beneath the subluxed MTP joints, and hallux valgus.

capsular damage caused by the synovitis. The subluxed joints are painful in their own right, and also the metatarsal heads become prominent in the sole of the foot, giving a sensation of 'walking on pebbles'. Severe hallux valgus is also common with this condition. While initial treatment includes control of the rheumatoid process with drug treatment, local measures are usually required, including the provision of broad toe box shoes with padded insoles. Surgical measures include the forefoot arthroplasty, with excision of the prominent lesser (second, third, fourth and fifth) metatarsal heads. This is usually combined with fusion of the first MTP joint or Keller's procedure (excision of base of proximal phalanx of great toe). The forefoot arthroplasty procedure is *only* employed in the presence of inflammatory arthropathy.

Diabetes

Diabetes causes forefoot problems as a result of microvascular and associated neuropathic changes. Wounds heal poorly, so minor injuries may lead to persisting local sepsis, and then to osteomyelitis which may not be treatable without amputation. In neuropathic feet (whether due to diabetes or other causes), recurrent injuries may occur without the patient being aware of the problem. Therefore, education in foot care and appropriate footwear are essential for such patients, as prevention of injury is both easier and more effective than treatment. If ulcers do occur, treatment is usually prolonged. Assessment and treatment of proximal vascularity (where vessels may be occluded due to atheroma) are important, but most ulcers are associated with (currently untreatable) microvascular disease. Conservative treatment sometimes usefully includes the wearing of a 'contact cast'. This is an unpadded plaster of Paris cast which is used as a dressing. It is changed very regularly (initially every day or two) and used until healing occurs.

Gout

Although any one of a number of joints may be affected by gout, characteristically the great toe MTP joint is involved. In an acute attack, this joint is painful, swollen, erythematous and exquisitely tender. Treatment is discussed in Chapter 7.

Osteoarthritis

Hallux rigidus has been described above, when the great toe MTP joint may be the only joint obviously affected by osteoarthritis. However, in primary generalised osteoarthritis, this joint is one of many commonly involved (Ch. 10).

MIDFOOT AND HINDFOOT PROBLEMS

While forefoot problems are particularly common, mid- and hindfoot problems also occur.

Pes cavus

Pes cavus describes a high arched foot (Fig. 16.6). It may be associated with claw toes. Patients with pes cavus often present with forefoot pain, especially under the metatarsal heads. This pain occurs because, due to the arched foot, the total load-bearing area is markedly diminished, leading to high local pressures. While pes cavus may occur for no detectable reason, it is a frequent consequence of many types of neurological disorder, arising due to muscle imbalance. Patients presenting with this condition should therefore be examined carefully for abnormal neurological signs, and investigated or referred as appropriate. Associated conditions include spina bifida and hereditary motor sensory neuropathies.

Sometimes the degree of pain due to pes cavus may be severe. Under these circumstances, conservative treatment with shoe modification/orthotics may not suffice and surgery, such as

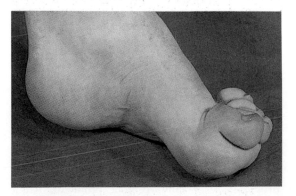

Figure 16.6 Pes cavus.

a closing wedge osteotomy of the midtarsal area, should be considered. A wedge of bone is excised from the midtarsal area (cuneiforms and cuboid and midtarsal joint) allowing the angulation between forefoot and hindfoot to be reduced. This is fairly major surgery; more minor surgery may be successful in mobile pes cavus in younger patients.

Plantar fasciitis

Plantar fasciitis is a common cause of heel pain, usually affecting the sole of the foot at the heel. It is thought to be an enthesopathy (see tennis elbow, Ch. 15) at the attachment of the plantar fascia onto the calcaneum. It is commonest in middle-aged and older patients. In young patients it may be associated with HLA-B27-associated arthropathy (e.g. ankylosing spondylitis, Ch. 8). X-rays may show a spur on the calcaneum at the site of attachment of the plantar fascia, but the relevance of this to both diagnosis and treatment is hotly disputed. The pain is usually much worse on walking. Management includes advice about padded footwear and insoles, physiotherapy and steroid injections into the area. Surgery is indicated occasionally, but is not always effective.

Achilles tendinitis

Achilles tendinitis results in pain, tenderness and swelling over the tendon near the site of its insertion. It can arise as a result of overuse (e.g. in runners or dancers) or in association with generalised inflammatory conditions. Pain is exacerbated by passive dorsiflexion at the ankle or by standing on tip-toe (which is not possible if the tendon has ruptured). Bursitis can also occur in the region of the Achilles tendon. Treatment is with rest, NSAIDs, ultrasound treatment and shoe modification, if appropriate. Rupture of the Achilles tendon is discussed in Chapter 23.

OTHER PROFESSIONALS INVOLVED IN THE MANAGEMENT OF PATIENTS WITH FOOT PROBLEMS

Chiropodists (or podiatrists) provide an important service in the treatment of foot problems, especially forefoot problems. Their input varies from management of skin lesions,

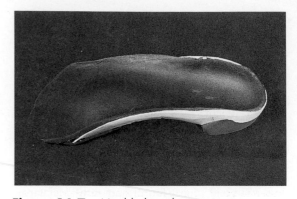

Figure 16.7   Moulded insole.

such as corns and calluses, to surgical treatment of some forefoot problems. Podiatrists are an important source of advice to many patients at risk of developing severe foot disorders, especially

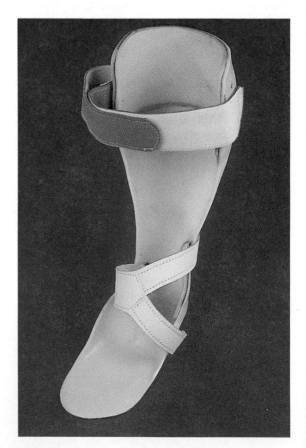

Figure 16.8   Ankle–foot orthosis.

diabetics and those with rheumatoid feet. Advice includes instruction on how to cut toenails (mistakes can lead to disastrous local sepsis, particularly in diabetics), footwear (Fig. 16.7) and management of local infective conditions (e.g. plantar warts/verrucae).

Orthotists and 'surgical appliance' officers commonly contribute to treatment of lower limb problems. An orthosis is an additional piece of equipment (e.g. an ankle–foot orthosis, Fig. 16.8) worn external to the body to support, correct or protect a body part. In contrast, a prosthesis is a replacement for a body part, e.g. a hip replacement or an artificial leg. Orthoses are commonly used in correction of deformity, e.g. painful grossly planovalgus (flat) feet. There is a wide range of orthoses, ranging from relatively lightweight in-shoe devices such as moulded insoles, to complex calipers of metals and leather. Newer materials such as epoxy composites and plastics are making modern orthoses dramatically lighter and more user-friendly, and the field of orthotics is evolving rapidly.

It is impossible to return some patients to a functional level of walking mobility. Such patients may require a wheelchair to give them reasonable independence. Others need even more complex rehabilitative machines, e.g. swivel walkers and standing frames for children and adolescents with cerebral palsy or Duchenne muscular dystrophy.

17 | Disorders of the spine

Case history

A 51-year-old taxi driver attended his GP complaining of low back pain. The pain had been present intermittently for over 2 years, but he had always tried to ignore it. However, now the pain had become constant and was interfering with his work. He was having great difficulty lifting suitcases into the boot of his taxi, and even bending down to pick up lighter objects was difficult. Sitting for more than 20 minutes, standing or walking all made the pain worse. A worrying feature to him was that, whereas the pain had originally been confined to the lower back, now he also felt pain down his left leg into his foot, and he was experiencing some pins and needles in his left leg. He was otherwise well. He smoked 30 cigarettes per day.

His GP asked if he had been having any difficulty recently passing water or with his bowels, or if he was stiff in the morning. He did feel stiff in the morning, but this was only for about 15 minutes and the worst time was later on in the day after he had been working for a few hours.

On examination the taxi driver was found to be overweight, and his lumbar spine movements were slightly reduced: back extension was limited and painful and his Schober's test was 4.5 cm. Straight leg raising was limited at 50° on the left and 70° on the right. Lower limb reflexes were present, but he had some diminution of light touch and pinprick sensation in an L5 distribution, with slight weakness of ankle dorsiflexion.

His GP prescribed an analgesic, arranged a lumber spine X-ray – which showed 'degenerative' disease of the lumbar spine with loss of disc height at L4/5 and L5/S1 and anterior and posterior osteophytes – and referred him to the rheumatology clinic when a blood sample was checked and a magnetic resonance (MR) scan arranged. The MR scan showed lumbar spondylosis with osteophytosis at several levels and apophyseal (facet) joint hypertrophy. At the L5/S1 level there was a small left-sided disc herniation and this, together with the foraminal stenosis caused by the facet joint hypertrophy, was compromising the L5 nerve root.

The taxi driver was referred for consideration of surgery to decompress the L5 nerve root. He asked the surgeon if the surgery would relieve the pain in his back, because this was far more of a problem to him than the pins and needles in his left leg. When he heard that there was no guarantee of this, he decided not to have an operation, and was referred to a physiotherapist who taught him a series of exercises to strengthen the muscles which supported the back; he was also taught different ways to protect his back, e.g. how to lift properly. He wished he had been taught these exercises years before. He found that over the following months his pain became less of a problem to him, or perhaps he had just become accustomed to it. Losing weight probably helped too. He managed to continue taxi driving: he just had to be careful.

This chapter deals predominantly with the approach to the patient presenting with either low back pain or neck pain. Both these complaints are extremely common and many patients have both.

Key points

- Neck pain and low back pain are common symptoms. If severe or chronic, they are a major source of morbidity, disability and time off work (this is especially true for low back pain). Conversely, many patients experience minor symptoms which are self-limiting

- The aetiology is often 'mechanical', overuse or trauma often being contributory factors. Spondylosis ('degenerative' disease of the spine) occurs most frequently in the cervical and lower lumbar regions. Abnormalities of the intervertebral disc and osteoarthritis of the apophyseal joints both contribute and usually occur together. The patient's occupation may be a contributory factor

- Neck pain and back pain are symptoms, not diagnoses. Always ask yourself what the underlying pathology is, although it may not be possible to pinpoint this. History and examination may suggest that further investigation, with imaging techniques, is required. Always look for neurological involvement. Pain in the neck or back may be referred from elsewhere (e.g. retroperitoneum).

- An important aim of treatment is to prevent pain from becoming chronic, when it is more difficult to treat

- Treatment of patients with chronic low back pain is multidisciplinary

- Only a minority of patients require surgical intervention

The patients seen in hospital with low back pain and neck pain are 'the tip of the iceberg'; these patients usually have severe or chronic pain. But many patients with low back pain or neck pain are successfully treated in the community and are never referred to hospital. Many patients do not even attend their GP's surgery, especially if the pain settles quickly.

Thus it is important to have an understanding of how to deal with the patient who presents with low back pain or neck pain. Remember that the spine is an extremely complex structure,

incorporating the vertebral column (Fig. 17.1), the spinal cord and its exiting nerve roots, the supporting muscles and ligaments and blood vessels. A wide variety of pathologies can affect the spine: some are localised to one particular level (e.g. a discitis, or a disc prolapse), whereas others may affect the spine at several levels (e.g. spondylosis or osteoporosis). Box 17.1 lists important causes of spinal pain. Often it is not possible to give the patient a precise diagnosis for the cause or origin of the pain, in which case it may be appropriate to label it as 'mechanical low back pain' or 'neck sprain'. While this is not entirely

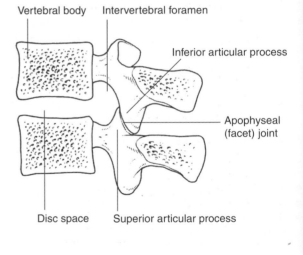

A Lateral

Vertebral body   Intervertebral foramen

Inferior articular process

Apophyseal (facet) joint

Disc space   Superior articular process

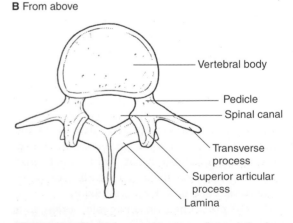

B From above

Vertebral body

Pedicle

Spinal canal

Transverse process

Superior articular process

Lamina

Figure 17.1   Schematic sections through lumbar spine to show bony architecture.

Box 17.1   Causes of spinal pain

'Mechanical'
- **Trauma (includes 'whiplash injury')**
- **'Degenerative' disease**
  - **spondylosis (with loss of disc space and osteoarthritis of the apophyseal joints)**
  - **disc herniation**
  - **spondylolisthesis (this may not be degenerative)**
  - **spinal stenosis (to which a variety of pathologies may contribute)**
- **Post-surgical back pain**
- **'Mechanical' pain not due to any of the above (sometimes termed 'muscle strain' or 'ligamentous strain')**

Inflammatory (non-infectious)
- **Spondyloarthropathy, e.g. ankylosing spondylitis**

Malignant
- **Metastatic disease**
- **Multiple myeloma**
- **Primary tumour of bone, spinal cord or nerve root**

Infection (including tuberculosis)
- **Osteomyelitis**
- **Paravertebral abscess**
- **Discitis**

Bone disorders, **including:**
- **Osteoporotic vertebral collapse**
- **Paget's disease**

Pain arising from outwith the spine

present with pain in their thoracic spine, e.g. as a result of osteoporotic vertebral collapse, but this is less common than neck pain or low back pain.

As already stated, neck pain and low back pain are common in adults (as opposed to the situation in children, in whom back pain should always be taken seriously), occurring in both males and females. However, low back pain is more common, and when chronic poses a huge burden of morbidity on the population. It is a major socioeconomic problem (Fig. 17.2). The reason for the huge rise in days off work with low back pain in developed countries is not known, but social and psychological factors may play a role.

AETIOLOGY AND PATHOLOGY

In dealing with causation of a symptom, we are essentially concerned with differential diagnosis. Each of the causes of spinal pain listed in Box 17.1 has its own aetiology and pathogenesis, many of which are dealt with elsewhere in this textbook. Some of the points below are worth emphasising.

Spinal pain

In most patients with neck pain or low back pain, this pain is 'mechanical'. This means that it is due either to overuse of a normal anatomic structure ('strain') or to deformity or trauma of an anatomic structure. Clearly this is a fairly comprehensive

satisfactory, the important point is not to miss serious underlying pathology, and to institute treatment at an early stage before the pain becomes chronic.

Disorders of the spine may present with symptoms other than pain. Patients may present with deformity, e.g. scoliosis, or with paraesthesiae from compression of a nerve root. However, most spinal problems cause pain, which may be of either acute or insidious onset, depending on the nature of the problem. There are many similarities between the approaches to neck and lower back pain, and so these symptoms are dealt with together, while highlighting points specifically relevant to one or the other. Patients may also

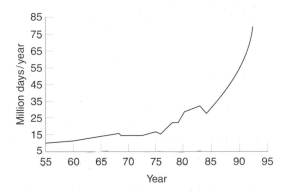

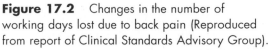

Figure 17.2   Changes in the number of working days lost due to back pain (Reproduced from report of Clinical Standards Advisory Group).

definition and 'mechanical pain' usually includes pain which is due to cervical or lumbosacral spondylosis, when loss of disc space and osteophyte formation alter the mechanics of the spine. 'Degenerative' disease of the spine includes osteophyte formation on either side of the intervertebral disc (*spondylosis*) and osteoarthritis of the (synovial) apophyseal (or 'facet') joints. However, the terminology is confusing, and often 'spondylosis' is taken to mean abnormalities of the disc *and* of the apophyseal joints; these usually occur together.

'Mechanical pain' is usually worse on movement, or after standing or sitting for any length of time, and this is another way in which it is sometimes defined. It could be argued, therefore, that several other of the conditions listed in Box 17.1 give rise to mechanical pain (e.g. osteoporotic collapse), but generally speaking if there is a pathology present other than 'degeneration'/overuse/trauma then most clinicians would not use the term 'mechanical'.

Spondylolisthesis

This refers to forward displacement of a vertebra relative to the one below. As already discussed in Chapter 14, it can be due to a congenital or traumatic break in the pars interarticularis (neural arch) (Fig. 17.3), or to degenerative disease. Spondylolisthesis may be asymptomatic, or it may be associated with back pain, radicular pain or symptoms of spinal stenosis (see below), depending upon the mechanical consequences of the displacement. The term 'spondylolysis' refers to the break in the neural arch which allows spondylolisthesis to occur (although spondylolysis is not necessarily associated with spondylolisthesis).

Spinal stenosis

This refers to narrowing of the spinal canal (generally taken to mean of the lumbar spinal canal). There are several possible causes which may act singly or together:

- congenital narrowing – when the canal has a so called 'trefoil' shape
- an acquired lesion – degenerative change with disc bulge/prolapse or spondylolisthesis
- a combination of both.

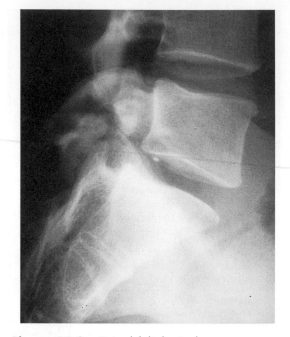

Figure 17.3   Spondylolisthesis due to a pars interarticularis defect of L5.

Symptoms of spinal stenosis are described later (Scenario 5).

Other causes of spinal pain

The pathologies of the other causes of spinal pain listed in Box 17.1 are covered in other chapters and will not be discussed further here.

Occupational factors

Back pain and, to a lesser extent, neck pain are often work-related and may therefore result in litigation against employers. The situation is often very complex. While heavy work may cause mechanical pain, it may also exacerbate an unrelated back condition. Employers now have an obligation to ensure that the work environment minimises the possibility of back problems, and employees should be taught methods of back protection.

Other factors

Age

The patient's age will suggest which diagnoses are likely or unlikely. For example, acute pain in a 70-

year-old woman is more likely to be osteoporotic vertebral collapse than a herniated inter-vertebral disc, whereas the opposite would be the case in a young adult.

Radicular pain

Nerve root compression causes radicular pain (Ch. 6), which is felt in the distribution of the affected nerve. The cause is usually a disc herniation (Fig. 17.4) or impingement of the intervertebral canal by osteophytes resulting in intervertebral foraminal stenosis (or a combination of both pathologies, as in the case history described). Lower lumbar radicular pain is termed *sciatica* and is frequently described as a shooting pain.

CLINICAL FEATURES

History

Although the history will concentrate on the neck or low back pain and any associated features, because spinal pain can be part of a generalised disease process it is also important to take a full history, as this may give clues to the diagnosis.

Pain

Key points to ask about are as follows:

- *Where is the pain, and does it radiate?* 'Mechanical' pain from the cervical spine is most often felt in the lower neck. Cervical spine problems may cause headache, or pain may be referred to the shoulder. Rarely, cervical spondylosis may be the cause of chest pain.

  Pain from the lower lumbar spine is often referred to the buttocks or thighs, but pain which radiates below the knee is usually neurogenic and is described as sciatica. The pain of nerve root compression is often exacerbated by changes in cerebrospinal fluid pressure; therefore, ask the patient: 'Is the pain worse if you cough?' ('impulse pain').

- *How long has the pain been present, and did anything special seem to bring it on?* Mechanical pain is often precipitated by an injury or by an abnormal movement, e.g. by lifting a heavy weight. Usually it settles gradually; many cases of low back pain resolve within a week, and in the order of 90% settle within 8 weeks. While this still means that a substantial number of

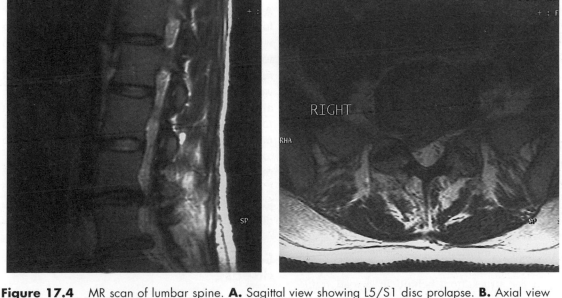

Figure 17.4 MR scan of lumbar spine. **A.** Sagittal view showing L5/S1 disc prolapse. **B.** Axial view showing central disc prolapse extending towards the right, with foraminal narrowing and crowding of the nerve roots. Courtesy of Dr C Hutchinson.

patients go on to develop chronic mechanical pain, nonetheless if pain is persistent always consider an underlying pathology, such as an inflammatory arthritis or malignancy. An acute onset to pain may indicate a prolapsed intervertebral disc (if there is nerve root entrapment this will be associated with radicular pain – Scenario 1) or vertebral crush fracture (often against the background of a more chronic pain – Scenario 2). In contrast, mechanical pain due to spondylosis is often insidious, as is pain caused by malignancy or spondyloarthropathy.

Scenario 1 – acute lumbar disc prolapse

A 28-year-old man experienced sudden onset of severe pain radiating down his right leg after pulling a shrub out of his garden. On examination he stood with a scoliosis, he was tender over the lower lumbar spine, lumbar spine movements were reduced (especially flexion and lateral bending to the right) and straight leg raising provoked pain at 30° on the right. On the affected side he had diminution of light touch and pinprick sensation in an L5/S1 distribution, weakness of ankle dorsi- and plantarflexion, and an absent ankle jerk. An MRI scan showed a large L5/S1 prolapse causing nerve root compression.

Scenario 2 – osteoporotic vertebral collapse

A 68-year-old woman experienced sudden onset of back pain. She had been on treatment with prednisolone for several years for asthma. On examination she was very tender around the T10 level. Lateral thoracic spine X-ray showed collapse of T10 and wedging of several other vertebrae. Full blood count, ESR and bone biochemistry were all normal.

Soft tissue injuries of the cervical spine ('whiplash' injuries) are becoming increasingly common. The typical scenario is of an occupant of a car struck from behind in a road traffic accident. The pain (usually felt in the neck, sometimes in the head or shoulder) typically comes on at a short interval (a few hours to days) after the injury. X-rays are almost always normal. The symptoms may persist for months or (occasionally) years, but usually settle eventually.

- *Does anything seem to make the pain better or worse? Is the patient stiff in the morning? Is sleep disturbed?* Particular movements tend to aggravate mechanical pain, depending on the nature of the underlying problem. Patients with mechanical low back pain find that standing or sitting for long periods of time and walking exacerbate the pain. This is in contrast to the young patient who is developing a spondyloarthropathy such as ankylosing spondylitis (Ch. 8), when activity eases the pain (Scenario 3). Patients with inflammatory disease are often very stiff in the morning. *Beware of the patient with intractable night pain, or elderly patients with a recent onset of sciatica;* this symptom should make you ask yourself whether the patient has an underlying malignancy (Scenario 4). Many patients who have chronic neck or back pain are depressed and so this may also be a reason for disturbed sleep.

Scenario 3 – ankylosing spondylitis

A 24-year-old man found that in the morning his lower back felt stiff. This gradually became worse, to the extent that he had significant pain for about an hour in the morning, with a nagging pain at other times. He found that walking or swimming relieved the pain. He attended his doctor who suggested that he rest for a few days. This made the pain and stiffness much worse. He went back to his doctor who examined him and found that all lumbar spine movements were reduced (Schober's test was 2 cm) and he was tender over the sacroiliac joints. X-rays showed mild sacroiliitis and a diagnosis of ankylosing spondylitis was made.

Scenario 4 – metastatic bone disease

A 55-year-old woman developed neck pain. X-rays showed some spondylotic change and she was told to take paracetamol and issued with a soft cervical collar. However, the pain became worse, to the extent that it was disturbing her sleep at night. She saw another doctor, who noted that she had undergone a mastectomy for breast carcinoma 8 years previously. Her ESR was 50 mm/h. An isotope bone scan showed multiple 'hot spots', including in the neck, consistent with metastatic bone disease.

If a patient describes pain in the legs when walking which is relieved by rest (usually in association with low back pain but not always), consider the diagnosis of lumbar spinal stenosis (*Scenario 5*). The main differential diagnosis is intermittent (i.e. vascular) claudication.

Scenario 5 – spinal stenosis

A 60-year-old man with a 5-year history of low back pain developed a heavy feeling in his legs when walking, relieved by sitting down or leaning forwards. His GP initially suspected peripheral vascular disease (he smoked heavily), but peripheral pulses were easily palpable. The diagnosis of spinal stenosis was considered next. Spinal movements were only slightly restricted and straight leg raising was full. MRI scan showed a narrow canal at the L3 and L4 levels, and the canal dimensions were further reduced by posterior disc bulges at the L3/4 and L4/5 levels.

- *Are there any associated symptoms?* Ask about paraesthesia and weakness, which may indicate neurological involvement. In a patient with neck pain, ask about dizziness or blackouts. Remember that the vertebral arteries ascend though foramina in the transverse processes of the cervical vertebrae and that patients with cervical spondylosis and bony overgrowth may develop features of vertebrobasilar insufficiency; osteophytes may distort the vertebral arteries and thereby impair blood supply.

In the patient with low back pain, especially if there has been a recent onset/exacerbation, ask about disturbance of sphincter control or bladder sensation, as *this may indicate a cauda equina syndrome which is a surgical emergency* (the spinal canal must be decompressed). Cauda equina syndrome is usually the result of a large central disc herniation compressing the cauda equina; rarely this may be the result of abscess of tumour (Scenario 6).

Scenario 6 – cauda equina syndrome

The patient in Scenario 1 was listed for decompression of his disc prolapse. However, before surgery could be performed he experienced an exacerbation of his back pain and he developed urinary retention. On examination, neurological testing again suggested L5/S1 compression, but now straight leg raising was significantly reduced bilaterally and there was saddle (i.e. perineal) anaesthesia. An urgent MRI scan was performed and this showed that the L5/S1 prolapse had increased and was now compressing the cauda equina. He was taken to theatre that night for urgent decompression and removal of prolapsed disc material.

General and systemic enquiry

Features of malignancy or infection. Always ask about a patient's general health. Have they lost weight or felt feverish or been having night sweats? Answers in the affirmative may indicate an underlying malignancy (spinal metastases are common, primary spinal tumours are rare) or infection. While tuberculosis of the spine is rare, cases do occur, especially in 'at risk' groups. Infections giving rise to neck pain or back pain include paraspinal abscesses or, rarely, septic discitis.

Risk factors for osteoporosis. This is more relevant to lower back or thoracic pain than to neck pain. Risk factors for osteoporosis are detailed in Chapter 11, and include an early menopause, corticosteroid therapy, inflammatory joint disease and a sedentary life style.

Features suggestive of an inflammatory joint disease. Ask about features of HLA-B27-related disease (Ch. 8), e.g. psoriasis, especially in the younger patient with neck or back pain and early morning stiffness.

Past medical history and other medical conditions

These can be highly relevant. A past history of breast carcinoma, for example, immediately raises the possibility of spinal metastases (Scenario 4). Ask also about other medical conditions. There is an association between diabetes and a condition called diffuse idiopathic skeletal hyperostosis ('DISH'), which is characterised by florid new bone formation, especially at entheses, and which is often associated with back pain. Remember that metabolic bone disease (Ch. 11) may result in back pain, so a history of, for example, malabsorption or renal disease may be important. A variety of general medical conditions such as asthma are treated with prednisolone, putting the patient at risk of osteoporosis (Scenario 2).

Family history

A family history of a HLA-B27-related disease is particularly relevant if the clinical features are suggestive of a spondyloarthropathy.

Social history

Always ask about occupation, as this may be an important contributory factor; and even if neck or back pain is causally unrelated to work, then a patient's occupation may be an aggravating factor and it may be necessary to advise them to seek lighter duties. As already stated, low back pain may prevent an individual from working and may therefore have a devastating effect, including on the family. It may be possible to offer some simple advice for the workplace which may alleviate the problem, e.g. providing a higher desk for a patient with neck pain. Sporting activities may also be relevant – e.g. rugby players are prone to neck injuries.

Examination

General

Look for any clues which point to underlying systemic disease: fever, signs of anaemia, lymphadenopathy. It is important to assess the patient fully, not only as this may provide clues to the diagnosis, but also because findings may influence treatment decisions. For example, if a patient has ischaemic heart disease and is breathless with a degree of cardiac failure, it would be inappropriate to suggest a programme of isometric exercises for chronic back pain.

Always remember: pain in the neck or lower back may be referred from elsewhere (Box 17.2). Be especially alert to this possibility if the patient has a good range of pain-free neck/back movements.

Note the patient's weight. Patients who are overweight are at increased risk of mechanical low back pain, due to increased spinal loading.

Box 17.2   Non-spinal causes of spinal pain

Neck pain
- Disorders of the shoulder
- Visceral pain, from:
  — heart (ischaemic heart disease)
  — oesophagus (oesophageal spasm)
  — pleura (pleural inflammation)
  — vasculature (dissecting aneurysm)
- Diaphragmatic pain (subphrenic abscess, gall bladder disease)
- Systemic infection (meningitis)

Low back pain
- Disorders of the hip
- Visceral pain, from:
  — gastrointestinal tract (pancreatitis, colonic carcinoma)
  — genitourinary (renal calculus, endometriosis, ovarian carcinoma)
  — vasculature (abdominal aneurysm)

Musculoskeletal

Only certain key diagnostic points will be highlighted here, as examination of the spine has already been described in Chapter 3. Remember to assess posture (this means that the patient with low back pain must be examined standing as well as supine and prone), to identify areas of tenderness, and to check the range of movement, noting which movements cause pain. *In patients with spinal problems, you must assess the patient neurologically* (see below), as spinal cord or nerve roots may be compromised.

Neck pain. Patients with a local mechanical neck problem often have an asymmetrical lesion and this means that movement may be limited and/or painful asymmetrically. This is in contrast to the patient with an inflammatory or malignant problem when all three planes of movement (flexion/extension, rotation and lateral flexion) are restricted and painful.

Back pain. Look at the patient standing. There may be an obvious deformity, e.g. in the young patient with a scoliosis or in the postmenopausal female with a thoracic kyphosis secondary to osteoporotic collapse. Check for a leg length discrepancy (Ch. 3).

Remember that the sacroiliac joints form part of the axial skeleton and that pain arising from the sacroiliac joints is felt in the lower back. Therefore, when assessing for areas of tenderness, check for sacroiliac tenderness as well as tenderness over the lumbar spine. Sacroiliac tenderness may occur not only in patients with spondyloarthropathies, but also with sacroiliac strain. Pain arising from the sacroiliac joints may radiate down the thigh posteriorly, but not below the knee. Patients with ankylosing spondylitis or other spondylo-arthopathies characteristically have reduction of lumbar spine movements in all planes (flexion/extension and lateral bending). If this diagnosis is suspected, the chest expansion should be checked, as this is often reduced.

The straight leg raising and femoral stretch tests described in Chapter 3 (p. 64) should always be performed in the patient presenting with lumbar spine problems. Pain on stretching the sciatic nerve (L4/5, S1) or femoral nerve (L2–4) indicates nerve root irritation.

Neurological

Signs associated with cervical spine pathology. Look for signs of nerve root compression. Cervical spondylosis most commonly affects the lower cervical spine, and so C6, C7 and C8 are the nerve roots most commonly involved. For example, in a patient with cervical spondylosis with left-sided C6 compression, classically the left biceps jerk will be reduced or absent, there will be weakness of the biceps and diminution of light touch, and pinprick sensation of the thumb and index finger and lateral border of the forearm. In practice, it is often not possible to localise the lesion precisely on clinical grounds as there is some overlap in the clinical findings between different nerve roots.

Involvement of the higher cervical roots is rarer but may occur with trauma or inflammatory disease.

Remember that cervical spine disease can also cause pyramidal tract signs due to spinal cord compression. *If* a patient presents with pyramidal tract signs, remember that the pathology may be in the neck and not in the brain, especially if there are accompanying neck problems and/or upper limb radicular symptoms or signs.

Cord compression can be due to a combination of disc degeneration with protrusion, osteophyte formation and thickening of the ligamentum flavum (Fig. 17.5). Usually, spinal cord compression resulting from cervical spine disease occurs in

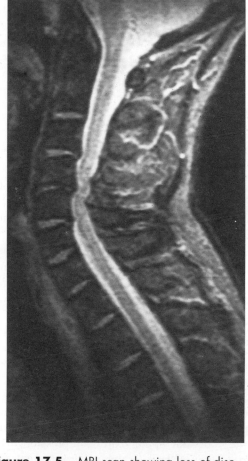

Figure 17.5 MRI scan showing loss of disc height and thecal space narrowing at C4/5 with associated cord compression. Courtesy of Dr C Hutchinson.

association with neck pain, but occasionally a patient will present with long tract signs in the absence of significant neck pain. In a patient with severe cervical spondylosis, there may be a combination of upper limb nerve root signs (with weakness, absent reflexes and sensory loss) and long tract signs (lower limb spasticity and extensor plantar responses). The exact combination of symptoms and signs will depend on the level of the lesion, and on whether the degenerative cervical spine disease has resulted in foraminal stenosis (causing nerve root compression) in addition to spinal canal stenosis (causing cord compression). Remember that rheumatoid arthritis (Ch. 8) may be associated with cervical spine instability and cord compression.

Signs associated with lumbar spine pathology. The patient presenting with lumbar spine problems should have a neurological assessment of the lower limbs. The commonest reasons for root entrapment are either a prolapsed intervertebral disc or osteophytic narrowing of the exit foramina. If there is any suspicion of a cauda equina syndrome (Scenario 6) check for saddle (perineal) anaesthesia and for changes in anal tone.

Investigations

The same principles of investigation apply to both neck and back pain. If a patient presents with a short history of neck or low back pain which is not severe and is generally well, and the history is suggestive of a mechanical problem, then no investigation is necessary. However, if pain persists, or if there is evidence of neurological involvement or systemic disease, then further investigation is indicated. You should be aware that in the past 10 years, the increased availability of computed tomography (CT) scanning and magnetic resonance imaging (MRI) has revolutionised the investigation of spinal problems. These techniques are non-invasive (although intrathecal contrast may be used with CT) and they have superseded myelography in the investigation of nerve root and spinal cord compression. The introduction of these techniques has dramatically improved the ability to choose suitable candidates for spinal surgery.

Blood tests

The full blood count, ESR and plasma biochemistry should all be normal in the patient with mechanical neck or low back pain, including pain due to spondylosis. In a patient with persistent pain or any suggestion of systemic disease, these should be checked and any abnormality explained. For example, a patient with anaemia, a raised ESR and a raised alkaline phosphatase may have spinal metastases and needs further investigation. Other blood tests are indicated according to the clinical situation. For example, the immunoglobulins should be checked in the patient presenting with osteoporotic vertebral collapse (Ch. 11).

Plain radiographs

These are not indicated in patients with a short history of neck or low back pain, unless there is a history of trauma or systemic ill-health. However, they are generally requested in older patients, those with persisting pain, and those with evidence of neurological involvement or in whom inflammatory or neoplastic disease is suspected. In some patients with metastatic spinal disease, bone destruction may be obvious. In others, only early signs may be apparent – in particular, look for evidence of damage to the vertebral pedicles on AP (anteroposterior) X-rays.

In patients with cervical or lumbosacral spondylosis, as in osteoarthritis (Ch. 10), there is a poor correlation between radiographic spondylotic change and symptoms. Many patients with spondylotic change on X-ray are asymptomatic; this leads on to the important clinical point that spondylotic change on X-ray (Fig. 17.6) may not be responsible for a patient's symptoms. This also applies to other X-ray abnormalities, e.g. spina bifida and spondylolysis, which may be clinically asymptomatic. Conversely, patients with normal X-rays may have severe pain.

In patients in whom spinal instability is suspected, both flexion and extension views should be requested.

Computed tomography

CT scanning gives excellent anatomical definition of bony lesions, demonstrating for example spinal

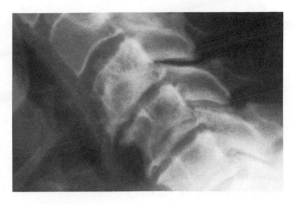

Figure 17.6 X-ray of cervical spondylosis, showing anterior osteophytes and loss of disc space.

stenosis and cortical bone destruction by tumour. However, intradural lesions are not demonstrated unless intrathecal contrast is used. The technique of CT myelography is used where MRI is not possible or unavailable.

Magnetic resonance imaging

MRI has several advantages over CT scanning in the assessment of the cervical and lumbosacral spines, but is currently less widely available. No ionising radiation is involved, and intradural soft tissue lesions can be visualised without the need for intrathecal contrast (Fig. 17.7). It is the investigation of choice for evaluating mechanical disorders of the spine and spinal/paraspinal infections. It is the technique of choice for visualisation of the rheumatoid neck. A disadvantage is that claustrophobic patients may not tolerate the procedure. Also, if there is any 'metalwork' in the spine, this will make the technique unsafe if the material is ferromagnetic, and even if the metal is not ferromagnetic then the surrounding image will be of poor quality.

One problem common to all investigations, but a particular problem with CT scanning and MRI is that many of the abnormalities detected are asymptomatic and clinically irrelevant. Therefore, it is always necessary to assess the results of imaging in conjunction with the clinical features.

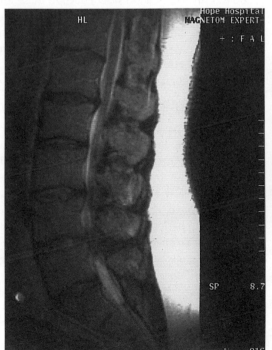

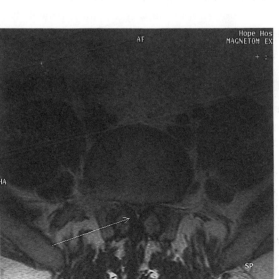

A
B

Figure 17.7 MRI of the lumbar spine. **A.** Sagittal view showing narrowing of the thecal canal from L2 downwards (most marked at L4/5). **B.** Axial view at the L4/5 level showing typical 'trefoil' appearance (arrow) and marked thickening of the ligamentum flavum. Courtesy of Dr C Hutchinson.

Isotope scans

Isotope scanning is a sensitive but non-specific technique for identifying pathology. It is useful when a generalised pathology is suspected, as the whole skeleton is visualised. Multiple bony metastases may be shown before they are visible on X-rays (Scenario 4), or a characteristic pattern of increased uptake in a patient with polyarticular disease.

MANAGEMENT

Most patients with neck and lower back pain are managed conservatively (non-surgically). Treatment will depend on the diagnosis, but for patients with mechanical pain (the vast majority) the mainstays of treatment are reassurance and patient education, analgesia and physiotherapy. However, a minority of patients will require surgery, depending upon the nature of the underlying problem, and patients with specific underlying conditions will require treatment of these.

A proportion of patients with low back pain go on to develop intractable back pain and are severely disabled. A proportion of these have had 'failed' lumbar spine surgery. For these patients it is particularly important to adopt a multidisciplinary approach to management.

General

Patient education, occupational therapy and physiotherapy

The patient with mechanical neck or back pain can usually be reassured that this is not a progressive condition, and that the pain is likely to settle or at least become less severe. The occupational therapist and physiotherapist both play an important educative role, advising on issues such as seating and desk/table height, and sleeping with a low pillow/firm mattress as appropriate. Wearing a cervical collar (soft or firm, not rigid) may help the patient with neck pain by 'resting' the neck, although this should not be worn continuously as it may well lead to spinal muscle weakness.

The physiotherapist will teach the patient with low back pain back protection measures, e.g. the correct way in which to lift, and a range of exercises to strengthen the supporting musculature of the back. Some countries operate 'back schools' which offer groups of individuals advice on how best to protect their backs and to cope with existing back problems. There are a variety of other treatment modalities used by physiotherapists, e.g. heat or cold packs. A proportion of patients with back pain benefit from use of a TNS machine (transcutaneous nerve stimulator). The rationale behind the TNS machine is that stimulation of low-threshhold fibres 'blocks out' nociceptive impulses.

For a patient with severe acute back pain, 'controlled physical activity' is now preferred to prolonged bedrest. If a patient does rest in bed, then the duration of this rest should be limited to 2–3 days.

Manipulation techniques

A wide variety of manipulation techniques are advocated for neck and back pain, although there is some controversy as to how effective these are, as there have been few clinical trials addressing their efficacy. Nonetheless, many patients attend osteopaths and chiropracters and find their interventions helpful.

Drug treatment

Neck and back pain are usually non-inflammatory and so a simple analgesic should be tried in the first instance. If this is not helpful, then an NSAID may be added in. Tricyclic antidepressants, commenced in low dosage, e.g. amitriptyline 10–25 mg, may relieve chronic pain and improve a patient's sleep pattern, but it may be several weeks before they take effect.

Injection therapy

A proportion of clinicians give epidural corticosteroids to patients with nerve root compression. However, the value of this form of therapy has been much debated.

Surgery

There are three main indications for surgery in the

patient with neck or lumbar spine pain/pathology (note that here we are not dealing with patients with infection or tumour, or other spinal pathology requiring specific treatment):

- Nerve root compression (decompression may be indicated).
- Spinal cord compression (decompression may be indicated).
- Instability (fusion may be indicated). The precise indications for surgery for instability are unsettled, but note that most spinal surgeons now include some form of formalised (often questionnaire-based) physical and psychological assessment of the patient prior to surgery. On the basis of such assessments, surgery may not be offered even in the presence of pain.

The commonest indication for spinal surgery is nerve root compression, either due to disc protrusion or due to foraminal stenosis resulting from osteophytes on the intervertebral apophyseal joints. For surgery to be indicated, the radicular pain (i.e. upper or lower limb pain) should usually be worse than the back or neck pain. It is important to realise that the natural history of disc-related radicular pain in many (though not all) patients is for it to settle gradually over a period of about 2 years; surgery may therefore be seen as a method of speeding this resolution or of treating radicular pain when it is of such severity that waiting for this period would be unacceptable. In appropriate patients the results are dramatic, with an immediate reduction in pain, permitting an early return to normal function. The general and specific risks of surgery need to be set against these benefits. The specific risks include epidural scarring and fibrosis, and postoperative spinal instability. Both of these may wreck the result of an otherwise successful procedure; they have become less likely with a widespread acceptance of less extensive surgical approaches to the spine. Improved imaging has also improved the chances of success in disc surgery, as greater diagnostic accuracy means few spinal 'explorations' are now undertaken.

Surgical treatment of spinal stenosis or intervertebral foraminal stenosis is often successful. The surgery, in expert hands, is possible even in older patients providing they are otherwise reasonably fit. As with any surgery in this age group, the risks and benefits need to be carefully weighed, as there may be little point in surgical treatment of spinal stenotic symptoms in a patient whose walking ability is also severely limited by ischaemic heart disease. In appropriate patients – severe symptoms and clear evidence of foraminal or spinal canal stenosis at only one or two levels on MRI or CT – results may be extremely satisfactory.

Always remember that *acute onset of spinal cord compression or a cauda equina syndrome is a surgical emergency*.

Most patients with metastatic spinal disease can be managed by conservative methods, especially radiotherapy. Some patients, however, may benefit from surgery, including those with disabling pain due to spinal instability arising from the malignancy and those with spinal cord compression (which must be dealt with urgently).

The patient with intractable back pain

Patients with intractable back pain are often extremely difficult to manage. They have unremitting pain, difficulty walking/performing activities of daily living, and are often very angry, as the problem may have resulted from an injury at work or may have been exacerbated by previous 'failed' surgery. There may be litigation pending. Once the nature of the pathology has been established (as accurately as possible), and no further specific medical or surgical intervention is indicated, these patients should be referred for a pain management/multidisciplinary approach to their problem (Ch. 6). Many have psychological difficulty in accepting and managing their pain and it may be possible to help them with improved strategies of pain management.

18 | Management of the multiply injured patient

Case history

A 35-year-old driver was injured in a car crash in which someone else was killed. He was brought into the A&E department, fully conscious and complaining of leg and abdominal pain and headache. He had previously been fit. He was not knocked out in the accident. On examination, he smelled of alcohol. Primary survey showed:

- airway – clear, talking.
- breathing – respiratory rate 36/min; breath sounds both lungs; trachea central
- circulation – pulse 126/min; blood pressure 120/95; cool and clammy peripherally
- orientated, pupils equal and reacting to light. Glasgow Coma Score = 15.

His clothes were removed to allow a more detailed examination, which demonstrated a laceration and bruising over the right temporal region. Cranial nerves were normal. In his abdomen there was bruising, and he was diffusely tender in all quadrants. No bowel sounds were heard. In his right leg there was external rotation with an obvious deformity above the knee. There were no wounds, but the thigh was swollen and tender. X-rays showed a femoral fracture.

The patient was resuscitated and peritoneal lavage revealed frank blood. He was taken to the operating theatre whilst resuscitation was continuing, and a laparotomy and splenectomy were performed. The fractured femur was fixed with an intramedullary nail.

Six hours postoperatively, the on-call house officer was called because the nurses had noticed a deterioration in the patient's level of consciousness. Having returned from theatre alert and orientated, he was now only making incomprehensible sounds and his Glasgow Coma Score had fallen to 7. On examination his pulse rate was 48/min, respiratory rate 8/min and blood pressure 180/110. He could not move his left arm or leg and had a dilated right pupil which did not react to light. Following an emergency CT scan, surgery was performed to remove an extradural haematoma.

The patient made an excellent recovery following his surgery, and was discharged from hospital 2 weeks after admission. He was able to return to his work as a labourer after 4 months, when X-rays showed that the femoral fracture had united.

Key points

- Patients with multiple injuries should be treated in a systematic fashion, as many deaths after trauma are due to simple problems with airway, breathing and circulation. A primary survey of these three areas should be undertaken, correcting or treating problems as they are found.

- Treatment and assessment must proceed in parallel.

- Initial resuscitation measures should be given to all patients at the time of primary survey. These include oxygen therapy and intravenous fluid (crystalloid).

- A secondary survey is then carried out to detect injuries in other body systems.

- Protection of the cervical spine is vital after trauma, especially in patients with impaired consciousness.

- Successful resuscitation depends on expert team members and one team leader who coordinates their efforts.

Many multiply injured patients have fractures and soft tissue injuries which are treated by orthopaedic surgeons. Accordingly, even junior orthopaedic medical staff may be part of the team caring for such patients, and it is important to know the steps to be taken in their management. The management of such critically ill patients has recently been formalised into systems which offer a standardised approach to patient care, such as that taught on 'advanced trauma life support' courses. The principles which underlie this system are that many patients die from unrecognised problems with ventilation (airway and breathing) and circulation, and that these problems may be corrected at an early stage using simple methods if they are recognised during the *primary survey*. More complex problems are then discovered and treated using a systematic survey of all the body system (*secondary survey*).

Multiple injuries are a common cause of death in children and young adults. In Europe they mainly result from road traffic accidents and falls. In the USA, shooting injuries are more frequent, both hand guns and high-velocity weapons being involved. Injuries are an important cause of death and persistent disability in all countries, and consume an inordinate proportion of the medical resources of developing countries. It must be realised that if treatment of multiple injuries is to be worthwhile and reasonably economical, early effective resuscitation is vital. Further, most of the accidents leading to multiple injuries are theoretically avoidable, and effective road safety legislation (for instance) is vitally important to the management of public health.

PATHOLOGY

Multiple injuries have many varied and often complex metabolic effects. The total metabolic demands of the body after injury may be very large, due to hormonal changes, the requirements of repair and the burden of infection. This results in a large increase in metabolic rate, increasing oxygen demand and utilisation of metabolic substrates. The practical implications of this are that all patients with multiple injuries will benefit from supplementary oxygen administration even if they have no obvious cardiorespiratory injury. Further, early and adequate nutritional supplementation is vital. The depressing sight of patients becoming progressively more malnourished after injuries, with little attention being paid to correction of the situation, is still common in many hospitals.

Inadequate circulating volume is a frequent complication of multiple injuries. This may occur due to external or internal bleeding. Alternatively, fluid may be lost (in large amounts) from damaged skin areas (especially burns). Fluid is also frequently lost by changes in capillary permeability, releasing circulating fluid into the extracellular space, with multiple injury patients frequently exhibiting marked peripheral oedema. The loss of circulating volume and the massive afferent barrage of painful stimuli may lead to inadequate tissue perfusion (**shock**). Initially, moderate degrees of shock are reversible, with circulation tending to be maintained in areas with very poor tolerance of reduced perfusion (e.g. brain) and restricted in less sensitive areas (e.g. gut, skeletal muscle). Subsequently, the changes become irreversible, so early restoration of adequate tissue perfusion and oxygenation is vital. This has led to the concept of the 'golden hour', with the initial hour of resuscitation being of paramount importance in eventual outcome.

An example of the damage which may occur after ineffective resuscitation (persistent hypotension and poor oxygenation) is the multiple organ dysfunction syndrome (MODS). This occurs partly as a result of generalised toxaemia or sepsis due to poor perfusion of the gut wall, which leads to increased wall permeability and transmigration of enteric organisms to cause infection. MODS leads to progressive multiple organ failure, with pulmonary, renal and hepatic function being severely affected. It is a common cause of death in multiple injury patients after the initial 2–3 days following trauma.

Multiple injuries may affect any body system, and hence be followed by multiple local or system specific sequelae. The following are all common in such patients:

- neurological injuries
  - intracranial injuries, e.g. extradural and subdural haemorrhages, diffuse brain injury

— spinal cord injuries, which may be caused by obvious fractures or vascular/soft tissue damage
• cardiopulmonary injuries
— penetrating injuries to the heart, which may cause cardiac tamponade
— aortic injuries, commonly caused by closed deceleration injuries
— haemothorax and pneumothorax
— adult respiratory distress syndrome (ARDS; this follows local lung damage and is part of MODS)
• intra-abdominal injuries
— splenic injuries and mesenteric vascular tears, which are common causes of intra-abdominal bleeding
— hepatic injuries
— diaphragmatic ruptures
• musculoskeletal damage.

MANAGEMENT OF MULTIPLE INJURIES

Primary survey

Remember that assessment and urgent treatment must proceed in parallel. Patients should first be assessed for airway, breathing and circulation.

Airway

Ask the patient: 'Are you all right?' Patients who can readily answer this question are conscious – and have a patent airway! Those who cannot answer, or who have evident breathing difficulty, may have an obstructed airway. Throughout the management of all multiply injured patients, care must be given to the cervical spine to prevent damaging the cervical spinal cord due to the presence of unstable fractures. Patients should be treated in a hard collar, with sandbags at each side of the head to prevent lateral movement.

Examine the mouth for obstructions, and ensure that the jaw is not falling back to obstruct the airway (jaw thrust manoeuvre). Use an oropharyngeal airway. If still obstructed, perform endotracheal intubation; if this fails pass a needle through the cricothyroid membrane.

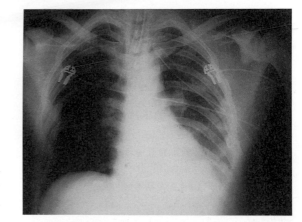

Figure 18.1 X-ray of right pneumothorax. Note loss of lung markings on the right side.

Breathing

Look for evidence of cyanosis. Observe the chest for evidence of breathing rate and rhythm. Check the position of the trachea, and percuss and auscultate the chest to ensure equal resonance and air entry all over chest. If any of these are asymmetrical, consider the possibility of tension pneumothorax, haemothorax or ruptured diaphragm, and treat appropriately. If the patient is not breathing, or if air entry is poor in all areas, assisted ventilation should be given – initially by mask and bag, and then by endotracheal tube, with a bag or ventilator. *All* multiple injuries patients should receive 40% inhaled oxygen by mask initially due to the increased metabolic demands after injury.

Circulation

Patients should be assessed initially by measurement of the pulse and blood pressure, and should be inspected for evidence of wounds and bleeding. Major sites of occult blood loss include the abdomen and chest. Cardiac auscultation may reveal muffled sounds, suggesting cardiac tamponade. Hypovolaemia is a major cause of death in patients after trauma. Adequate venous access (two large-bore intravenous cannulae) and an initial bolus of 2 L of crystalloid fluid are used in all adult patients. Blood is taken for cross-matching in all multiply injured patients.

Radiography

All patients with multiple injuries should have the following minimum set of X-rays:

- cervical spine – to look for fractures or dislocation which may threaten the spinal cord (the lateral view must show down to the C7–T1 junction)
- chest – to look for haemopneumothorax and signs of lung or cardiac damage
- pelvis – to look for pelvic fractures, which may be the cause of massive unexplained blood loss.

Other

The primary survey should be repeated at intervals to ensure that the patient is not 'going off'. Obtaining history from witnesses from the scene of accident (e.g. ambulance staff or police officers) is important. This is to establish the likely energy and mechanisms of injury: a patient is statistically more likely to have severe injuries after an accident in which another person has been killed.

Secondary survey

The primary survey is designed to address possible immediately life-threatening injuries. The secondary survey is designed to find injuries which may cause problems in the next hours or days, and must be comprehensive. Detailed consideration of the treatment of these problems is beyond the scope of this book.

Cardiovascular and respiratory systems

A complete examination of the chest, heart and peripheral pulses is required.

Abdomen

A careful examination of the abdomen, looking for tenderness, distension and bruising, is required. An abdominal paracentesis (diagnostic peritoneal lavage) may be required to establish the diagnosis of intra-abdominal bleeding.

Examination of the urethral meatus in men may show bleeding; this suggests a urethral injury associated with pelvic fracture. A rectal examination is required in men to ensure that the prostate is normally positioned. Tears of the membranous urethra are associated with a high riding prostate. A vaginal examination in women may reval a pelvic fracture.

Central nervous system

Head injuries are a common cause of death and morbidity in trauma patients. A useful method of recording the level of consciousness is the Glasgow Coma Scale (GCS, see Box 18.1). Adequate neurological examination includes observation of the size and reactivity of the pupils, and assessment of power, tone and reflexes in the limbs. In most patients with a deteriorating level of consciousness after injury there is an extracranial cause, such as hypovolaemia, hypotension or hypoxaemia due to airway problems. Deteriorating level of of consciousness must prompt a

---

Box 18.1   Glasgow Coma Scale

Sum of three scores: E-score (eye-opening); M-score (best motor response in any limb); V-score (verbal response)

	Points
E-score	
Normal (spontaneous and blinking)	4
To speech	3
To pain	2
None	1
M-score	
Obeys commands to move	6
Moves purposefully to pain	5
Withdraws from pain	4
Flexion (decorticate)	3
Extension (decerebrate)	2
No movement	1
V-score	
Orientated	5
Confused conversation	4
Random words	3
Incomprehensible sounds	2
None	1

Minimum possible score = 3
Severe head injury ≤8
Moderate head injury = 9–12
Minor head injury = 13–15

further review of airway, breathing and circulation as well as assessment of any head injury.

Musculoskeletal system

Fractures, especially open fractures, may be visually impressive, but they are most unlikely to cause early demise. Management of these injuries is thus usually secondary to that of more life-threatening problems. Exceptions to this include:

- cervical spine injuries, which have such potential for causing devastating spinal cord injuries that they must be addressed at an early stage in all patients
- pelvic fractures, which may cause very severe, occult, extraperitoneal bleeding.

TRAINING IN MANAGEMENT OF MULTIPLY INJURED PATIENTS

All medical students should familiarise themselves with basic methods of resuscitation, including cardiopulmonary resuscitation. Many of the principles of such treatment are common to management (especially primary survey and associated treatment) of patients with multiple injuries. Those who intend to develop an interest in trauma management should obtain, at an early date, advanced trauma life support training.

Management of the multiply injured patient

19 | Principles of fracture management

Case history

A 50-year-old right-handed HGV driver fell on to his outstretched right hand while ice-skating with his daughter. He presented to the A&E department complaining of severe pain in his wrist, which showed obvious deformity (Fig. 19.1). Sensation and circulation in the hand were normal. X-rays of the wrist (Fig. 19.2) showed a dorsally displaced distal radial fracture which did not involve the joint surface. The fracture was treated by manipulation under anaesthetic and application of a plaster back slab and the patient was scheduled to go home on the morning following this operation.

Prior to his discharge, he was reviewed on a ward round by the consultant orthopaedic surgeon who felt that the check X-rays taken in theatre were acceptable. However, the patient said that overnight he had developed a feeling of numbness and some pain in the thumb, index and middle fingers. This had not been present prior to his manipulation and did not improve with release of the back slab or with elevation of the arm. The orthopaedic team explained that it was necessary to release the compressed median nerve in his wrist. They also said that it might be advisable to fix the fracture more securely, as delivering adequate care to the wound on the wrist would require occasional removal of the plaster. The patient returned to the operating theatre and underwent a carpal tunnel release and fixation of the fracture with Kirschner stainless steel wires (Fig. 19.3). After his return to the ward he reported that the symptoms of pain and numbness in his hand had improved dramatically. He was discharged the following day.

He was seen in clinic a week after surgery and a check X-ray showed that the position of the fracture had been adequately maintained. Sutures were removed a fortnight after surgery and he wore a cast for a period of 4 weeks. The wires were removed in the day case surgical unit at 6 weeks, under local anaesthetic. The patient's wrist was noted to be rather stiff at this stage, although he had good finger movement. He only had 20° each of dorsiflexion and palmar flexion, and pronation and supination were similarly limited to 30° in each direction. He was therefore referred for physiotherapy, which he received twice weekly for 6 weeks. After this, his wrist movements were much improved, with almost normal movements in all directions by 3 months after the injury. He noted that his grip strength was the slowest problem to resolve, and this only really returned to normal 6 months after the injury, although he was able to go back to work at 3 months after the accident.

Key points

- The mode of bone healing depends on the type of fixation employed.

- Fractures are prone to a number of serious complications.

- Rehabilitation of soft tissues (joints, muscles) is crucial.

- The choice of operative or conservative treatment is a balance of risks and benefits.

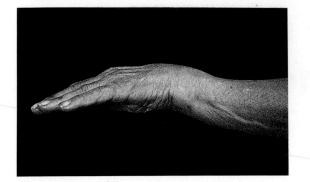

Figure 19.1 'Dinner fork' deformity of wrist after Colles fracture.

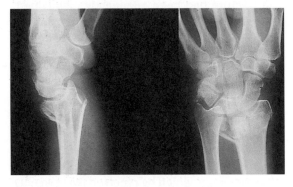

Figure 19.2 Distal radial (Colles) fracture.

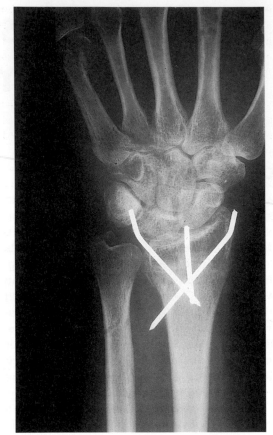

Figure 19.3 Colles fracture reduced and fixed with wires.

PATHOLOGY

A fracture is an abnormal break in the substance of a bone due to an applied load greater than the bone can bear. Such forces are usually substantial as bone is intrinsically a strong material; fractures which occur due to the structure of the bone being abnormally weak are traditionally termed *pathological fractures*. Pathological fractures caused by local processes (particularly primary and secondary tumours) are discussed in Chapter 11. Although fractures in osteoporotic bone are, strictly speaking, pathological fractures, their management is bound up with other issues of looking after elderly patients and will be dealt with in Chapter 21.

Mechanics of bone failure

Bone and cartilage are physical materials whose properties and behaviour may be described in similar ways to those of other materials, e.g. steel or plastics. Consideration of such properties is useful in understanding how fractures arise. Loading of bone or cartilage will cause stress (force per unit area) and, in consequence, strain (change of dimension per unit dimension). The loading may be in tension or compression, may be a bending load or a torsional load; each produces characteristic patterns of fracture. Although some fractures are caused by direct loading, others are caused by indirect injury, with additional force gained by the lever-arm of the limb. For example, a soccer player who receives a direct kick to his shin may sustain a transverse tibial fracture at the level of the blow; another who has a twisting injury while his boot is firmly anchored in the turf may acquire a spiral fracture half way up the shaft of his tibia. Depending on the nature of the abnormal loading, a long bone may fail in its mid-shaft (diaphyseal fracture), at the joint surface (intraarticular) or at the junction between these two zones where the bone is mainly cancellous (metaphyseal). The total amount of energy absorbed by the bone at the moment of its failure is the main factor determining the degree of *comminution*, i.e. the number of fracture fragments formed. A *simple* fracture consists of just two parts; butterfly fragments and a frankly comminuted pattern result from greater energy input. Figure 19.4 summarises these variations in fracture pattern.

Force may be transmitted along the line of a limb and result in a surprising variety of fractures. Thus, a fall on to the outstretched hand can result in a scaphoid fracture, distal radial fracture, fracture of the radius and ulna, a fracture of the radial head, a humeral fracture, or a shoulder dislocation. Similarly, a fall onto the heel from a height can cause fractures in the os calcis, talus, tibia, femur or lumbar spine.

Fracture repair

Fractures are repaired by a highly organised process which, in most cases, results in full functional restitution of the bone; this is termed *union* of the fracture. The phases of fracture repair

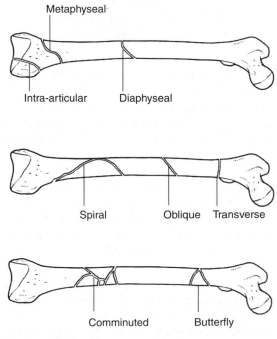

Metaphyseal

Intra-articular   Diaphyseal

Spiral   Oblique   Transverse

Comminuted   Butterfly

Figure 19.4 Variations in fracture pattern.

seen in the shafts of bones (the callus response) are shown in Box 19.1. These stages are the same as those seen in soft tissue wound repair, except that the matrix elaborated by the proliferating cells is bone: first woven bone and then eventually the mature form of lamellar bone. The woven bone matrix becomes calcified and sufficiently strong to afford mechanical stability to the fracture.

Mechanical stability is much enhanced if the fracture callus is located circumferential to the outside of the bone, the so-called *periosteal* callus. The initial physical property of the bone to return to a functional level is stiffness; the stiffness of the structure increases with the fourth power of the radius of the material laid down around the fracture. Thus an increase in radius of one-quarter the original radius will more than double the stiffness.

If the external callus described above fails to form, perhaps because of severe periosteal damage in a high-energy fracture, the fracture will be unable to heal promptly. A state of *delayed union* is said to have occurred. Provided the fracture is adequately splinted, however, it can still heal by the formation of *intramedullary*, or *endosteal* callus; this is a slow process. However, endosteal callus formation can also be a rapid event in an undisplaced fracture, in which case little periosteal callus will be seen.

The callus response described above is prevented if all fracture site movement is abolished. Under these circumstances, fracture union may be achieved by the normal process of normal bone remodelling – directly across the fracture gap; this is known as 'primary cortical healing'. It is frequently seen in fractures which are rigidly fixed with stainless steel plates attached to the bone (Fig. 19.7). The disadvantages of this type of bone healing are the risk of introducing infection at the time of plating, and its slowness, with the bone frequently taking over a year to return to a functional level of strength. Therefore, the use of rigid stainless steel plate fixation for fractures is now less widespread than it was 20 years ago.

When fractures occur in cancellous bone, the method of healing is different again. There is usually a weak external callus response, but healing proceeds by 'creeping substitution'. Here the fractured cancellous bone ends join directly by

Box 19.1   Fracture healing

Fracture healing is a process with many similarities to wound healing. It is important to realise that most fractures in the middle of long bones (the diaphysis) heal by external callus. This means that the fracture is effectively bypassed by new bone. Only after this has occurred does the original cortical bone heal. The four stages of fracture healing by callus formation are:

- haematoma
- inflammation and granulation tissue
- formation of woven bone matrix
- remodelling to lamellar bone.

The first step in fracture healing is for collars of new bone to form under the periosteum (Fig. 19.5). The fracture gap between these collars of bone is filled with haematoma, which is replaced with granulation tissue. The granulation tissue differentiates into cartilage, which undergoes endochondral ossification. This results in the fracture having a complete bony bridge (Fig. 19.6). At this stage, the fracture is usually functionally healed. The new bone in the fracture then undergoes gradual remodelling. The eventual outcome is a fracture which is fully healed, and in young patients remodelling may result in a bone which is indistinguishable from normal. Fracture in cancellous bone usually heals with only minimal external callus. This involves formation of intra-medullary new bone, and is termed "creeping substitution".

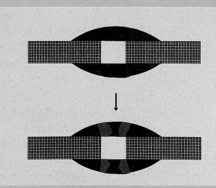

Figure 19.5   The subperiosteal collars of bone have formed. The fracture gap contains first haematoma, and then granulation tissue. The granulation tissue then differentiates into cartilage.

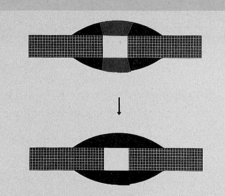

Figure 19.6   The cartilage completes the bridging of the fracture gap, and undergoes a process of endochondral ossification. When the cartilage is completely ossified, the fracture is bridged externally by woven bone, even though the cortex and medullary canal are not yet healed.

establishing a bridge of woven bone. Such healing may be seen in fractures such as intertrochanteric femoral fractures, and in fractures of the condylar ends of long bones, including intra-articular fractures.

The three principal modes of fracture healing are summarised in Box 19.2. If all these possible modes of healing fail to occur, a state of established *non-union* may be reached. Such a fracture will not heal without surgical intervention; this problem is discussed below.

Soft tissue injury

Soft tissue injury is an inevitable accompaniment of fractures. It sometimes receives less attention than it

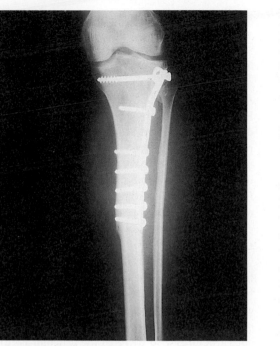

Figure 19.7   Plated upper tibial fracture.

Box 19.2   Three modes of fracture healing

- External callus
- Intramedullary (endosteal) callus
- Primary cortical healing

---

should as it is not readily visualised by imaging techniques such as X-ray. However, the soft tissue injury may frequently be the cause of greater long-term morbidity than any accompanying bone or joint injury. Soft tissue injuries heal with the classical injury repair response, but instead of restoring the original histological structure (as occurs with bone) repair is effected by fibrosis. Such fibrosis may result in contracture and stiffness, producing severe limitation of movement of adjacent joints – hence the importance of early joint movement as part of management.

Problems with fractures

The foregoing description is adequate for a large proportion of fractures, where the natural healing process leads to speedy restitution of bone structure by first-class new bone tissue. However, many fractures are much more problematic, for a variety of reasons, some of which lead to devastating late effects. All fractures must therefore be assessed for their risk of these potential complications.

Wounds and infection

Some fractures are open (compound). All fractured limbs must be carefully inspected for wounds which might connect with the fracture site, as the dire consequences of osteomyelitis mean that such wounds must be rigorously debrided and cleaned, and adequate antibiotic treatment given. All fractures result in necrosis of parts of the bone ends adjacent to the fracture, and these non-vascularised areas are very liable to bacterial colonisation. Open wounds have important consequences for the types of fixation which may be used for the fracture affected. In general, internal fixation is avoided after open fractures, as introduction of (avascular) fixation devices into the fracture area may result in persistent colonisation of the implants. In addition, the dissection necessary to insert implants (particularly plates) may increase the risk of necrosis or infection of marginally viable tissue, as well as introducing additional contaminating organisms.

When fractures become infected they are very unlikely to heal. The most commonly incriminated organisms are staphylococci (both *S. aureus* and coagulase-negative staphylococci). Dramatic measures may become necessary, including excision of relatively large segments of infected bone. Prevention of this serious complication is a prime objective of treatment.

Vascular injuries and compartment syndromes

Fractures and dislocations are often associated with vascular injuries, the cardinal sign of which is disappearance of pulses in the limb below the injury. However, pulses may be present initially and then disappear, e.g. with intimal flap tears of the arterial wall. The only adequate guard against ischaemia due to arterial injuries is repeated examination of temperature, sensation and pulses of limbs.

Compartment syndrome is one of the most important complications of fractures. It is commonest after tibial fractures, but may occur after any fracture. Muscles in the limbs are invested in a fascial sheath, which only provides limited volume for expansion of the muscle. When this volume change is exceeded (with swelling due to oedema or haematoma), the pressure in the sheath rises rapidly and soon exceeds capillary pressure. Tissue function, including gas exchange and nutrition, is then disrupted due to lack of capillary flow. **This condition may occur before there is any change in distal pulses**, because capillary pressure is so much lower than arterial pressure. The result of compartment syndrome may include muscle death and permanent deformity with contracture (Volkmann's ischaemic contracture). The key clinical feature which should alert suspicion is the pain – greater than would be expected from the fracture, especially if this has been adequately immobilised. This occurs because muscle ischaemia is exceptionally painful. Paraesthesiae can also develop due to ischaemia affecting the nerve in the compartment. Compartment syndrome may be present very soon after fracture, but more commonly develops in the days afterwards as swelling increases.

Physeal injuries

In children, fracture healing is generally both fast and reliable. However, fractures around (and especially across) the growth plate may pose problems. The physes are the site of most skeletal growth; premature fusion may lead to limb length abnormalities and abnormal development of adjacent joints. In particular, fracture often leads to a localised fusion of part of the physis; the remainder continues to grow, potentially leading to remarkable joint deformity. The best way to prevent such problems is to insist on accurate reduction of injuries crossing a growth plate to an anatomical position; fixation of the fracture is often necessary to maintain this position until union.

Fractures around epiphyses are classified according to a system devised by Salter and Harris. In general, epiphyseal fractures which do not traverse the growth plate rarely cause problems with growth. Those where the fracture line does cross the growth plate may cause partial fusions, and accurate reduction of these fractures is vital.

Intra-articular fractures

Fractures may involve the ends of a long bone and extend into the adjacent joint. Such fractures require special consideration, for two main reasons. Firstly, the articular bony architecture is one of the main stabilising factors of joints, so fracture may result in instability, with subluxation or dislocation. *Fracture-dislocations* are common, especially in the ankle and in many of the joints in the upper limb.

The second important factor in intra-articular fractures relates to the articular cartilage itself. The bone adjacent to joints is generally composed of cancellous bone, and healing (by creeping substitution) will usually be reliable. However, such fractures also traverse the articular cartilage which has a limited ability to repair itself. In addition, steps in the articular surface (which may occur if perfect reduction of the fracture is not achieved) cause local overloading of areas of cartilage. The direct cartilage damage and the overloading may be more than the cartilage can tolerate, leading to progressive cartilage break-down and *secondary osteoarthritis* in the joint.

Thus, management of intra-articular fractures is largely dedicated to obtaining and maintaining an anatomical position of the fracture fragments to restore joint stability and prevent osteoarthritis. Open reduction and internal fixation of articular fractures are often necessary to achieve and maintain this reduction (see Fig. 19.8). Such fixation also permits early joint movement, the importance of which, for maintaining cartilage nutrition and preventing stiffness, is covered in Chapter 22 (joint injuries and dislocations).

Non-accidental injury

Non-accidental injury is most commonly seen in children, inflicted by adults. Occasionally it may be seen in other dependent groups, e.g. those with 'learning difficulties' or the elderly. It is important to be aware of this possibility when examining children with any injury. Repeated attendance at

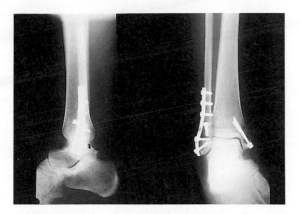

Figure 19.8 Internally fixed bimalleolar ankle fracture.

the A&E department, or an unsatisfactory or contradictory history, may lead to suspicion. Features to be sought include multiple bruises, burns or multiple fractures (especially of different ages). Some specific fractures (e.g. spiral femoral fractures in a child of less than walking age) are very frequently a result of non-accidental injury. Occasionally, a bone scan may reveal the presence of multiple fractures of different ages at various sites in the skeleton.

Non-accidental injury should be considered in many children attending A&E departments and orthopaedic clinics. For most, the possibility may be dismissed straight away, but if there is doubt a duty of care is owed to the child to take all necessary steps to protect him or her from further harm. Paediatricians are usually involved at an early stage in the management of such patients. It should be recognised that many children suffer fractures when not directly observed by a parent (so the lack of a perfect history is common), and that osteogenesis imperfecta (brittle bone disease) may present in a variety of forms, some of which are first detected in later childhood due to fractures with minimal trauma.

Neurological injuries

Complete neurological examination is obviously essential in patients with spinal injuries. However, limb injuries may also be associated with neurological damage. It may be simple and easily treated, such as the median nerve compression in the case history at the beginning of this chapter. The typical features are paraesthesiae or altered sensation in the radial three and a half fingers, caused by swelling or haematoma after distal radial fracture, and it is best treated by rapid decompression of the carpal tunnel. More extensive injuries, such as brachial plexus injuries, may be devastating, resulting in a useless ('flail') limb.

Dislocations are particularly likely to cause neurovascular problems. Sites often associated with such problems include the shoulder (brachial plexus injuries and circumflex humeral nerve injuries: usually transient), the hip (sciatic nerve injury) and the knee (vascular damage and peroneal nerve injury). Careful assessment is most important, both to identify the site and presence of injury and to provide an accurate prognosis.

Failures of normal union

The possibility of failure of the normal fracture-healing process has already been mentioned. Fractures at particular risk of delayed union or non-union are those occasioned by high-energy violence, which results in a great degree of soft tissue stripping from the bone, with consequent large areas of bone devascularisation. High-energy tibial fractures are particularly prone to this. Another type of fracture which may fail to unite is the displaced intra-articular fracture, such as that of the neck of the femur. Again, it is thought that these fractures are at risk because the blood supply of the fractured part of the bone is rather precarious.

Non-unions are traditionally classified into three types:

- Hypertrophic – there is a large amount of periosteal bone formation, but the fracture fails to unite. These fractures may be induced to unite by providing additional fracture site stability.
- Atrophic – there is very little sign of new periosteal bone formation. These fractures represent a failure of the fracture callus response. In addition to adequate mechanical stability, they require a biological stimulus such as a bone graft.

• Infected non-union. Infection in the area of the fracture healing response will usually result in the failure of the fracture to unite. Eradicating the infection and inducing union then present a considerable challenge. Thus, vigorous steps must be taken to prevent infection becoming established, including copious irrigation of any wound, removal of foreign material and debridement of devascularised material.

Another type of failure of normal union is *malunion*. Here, a fracture unites but does so in an anatomically or functionally unsatisfactory position. There may be gross angulation in the middle of a long bone shaft, a rotational deformity which leads to turning in or out of the foot, or loss of forearm rotation in the upper limb.

Algodystrophy

This condition, which is also termed reflex sympathetic dystrophy or (more recently) complex regional pain syndrome type I, can occur after any injury and is particularly common in the hand and foot. Patients develop abnormal amounts of pain, which is often of a disturbing burning quality with associated hyperaesthesia (see the description of neurogenic pain in Ch. 6, p. 91). There may be allodynia, which is an inappropriate sensation of pain on soft touch of the part. In addition they may have vascular instability (i.e. the limb is alternately hot and cold for no obvious reason) and swelling. The condition is frequent in a mild form especially after distal radial fractures, when it will often improve with time and physiotherapy. It may occasionally be very severe, in which case treatment is difficult and advice from a pain clinic may be helpful.

CLINICAL FEATURES
Clinical diagnosis of bony injury

Most fractures can be diagnosed clinically, and failure to examine patients adequately, in the belief that X-rays reveal all in fracture management, frequently leads to management errors. The principal presenting features for fractures are described below.

History of trauma. This would result from direct or indirect violence. Try to get an idea of the energy and mechanism of injury. (See the discussion of energy and mechanism of injury in Ch. 2, p. 6).

Pain. This is severe in most fractures, but the amount of pain does not accurately reflect the degree of displacement of the fracture. Pain is usually felt at the fracture site, but may be referred elsewhere (e.g. to the knee from hip fractures).

Loss of function. Loss of function is present after most fractures, but is not invariable. Patients occasionally appear having blithely used a fractured limb for several days; the failure to respond to the pain may be due to liberal intake of alcohol, or occasionally due to peripheral neuropathy (e.g. in diabetics). The function of joints adjacent to fractures is usually severely inhibited. This is due to reflex muscle spasm, which splints the affected part. Marked restriction of movement may be a good sign of a fracture; conversely, a joint permitting a full range of active and passive movement is unlikely to have a fracture in an associated bone. Thus, a patient with a suspicious line on an X-ray of the femoral neck may be (almost) exonerated of a fracture if found to have a full range of hip movement.

Deformity. This may be an obvious sign of fracture. Some injuries have characteristic clinical appearances, such as the dinner fork deformity in distal radial fractures (Fig. 19.1) or the appearance of anterior dislocation of the shoulder.

Tenderness. Fractures are generally tender; their distinguishing feature from sprains and soft tissue contusions is the presence of areas of maximum tenderness localised to bony surfaces. Thus, malleolar fractures can generally be most accurately distinguished from ankle sprains (usually of the anterior talofibular ligament) by determining the exact site of the maximum tenderness. In the case of a fracture, this will be over the fracture, while in the ligament sprain this will be accurately over the ligament.

Swelling. The amount of swelling after fractures varies, but may be considerable.

Radiological signs – definition of the fracture pattern

Fracture diagnosis was amongst the earliest clinical applications of Roentgen rays. Plain X-rays remain a principal tool for diagnosing fractures, for assessing fracture and implant position after treatment and for confirming fracture union. It is important that the whole bone, including the joints at each end, is seen in both anteroposterior and lateral views. The aim is twofold: to reliably detect the presence of fracture if there is one; and to define the pattern of the fracture to allow treatment planning.

Signs of fracture

The principal X-ray signs of fracture are described below.

Soft tissue swelling. This must be carefully assessed. In joint injuries, signs such as a lipohaemarthrosis may be observed; this strongly suggests the presence of an intra-articular fracture. Expansion of the prevertebral soft tissue shadow in the neck due to a haematoma may be the only sign of a vertebral fracture. Knowledge of the normal soft tissue appearance around joints is gained from observation of normal X-rays, but it is also useful to note that fat is usually very dark black on X-rays, while other soft tissues (including blood) are difficult to distinguish from each other.

Loss of continuity of the cortex on X-ray. This is the defining X-ray sign of a fracture; its detection is often easy, but sometimes may require a careful examination of all the cortical areas on two or more films of the injured area. Occasionally fractures are not visible on films on the day of injury, even in retrospect; generally these fractures become visible on repeat films taken 1 or 2 weeks later.

Angulation of bone. Angulation of bones is usually caused by fractures and is visible as a cortical break after a sufficient number of views. Occasionally bones undergo plastic deformation, where they bend without breaking. Far more common is the '*greenstick fracture*', where one cortex of the bone is bent or buckled while the other is frankly fractured. This fracture is characteristic of children before adolescence.

Changes in bone density. Osteoporosis is both a frequent cause and consequence of fractures. It may develop throughout the injured region (the so-called regional acceleratory phenomenon), or locally in the injured bone due to disuse. Pre-existing osteoporosis as a cause for fracture may be obvious on X-ray, but in general this is a poor method for identifying or quantitating

osteoporosis. However, other causes of pathological fractures (e.g. metastases) should be sought on the X-rays.

Fracture pattern

The principal aspects of the fracture pattern which the X-ray should define are those summarised in Figure 19.4:

- Is the bone broken in its diaphysis, metaphysis or epiphysis? This predicts the healing potential and is important for planning what sort of implant to use, if any.
- Does the fracture involve a joint surface; if so, is there displacement of the articular cartilage? Is the fracture actually a fracture-dislocation or fracture-subluxation? These predict the risk of secondary osteoarthritis and are important for deciding the necessity for open reduction and internal fixation.
- Is the fracture transverse, oblique or spiral? This indicates the stability of the fracture to axial loading after reduction and may determine whether operative treatment is required.
- Does the fracture involve a growth plate (in children) and, if so, does the fracture line actually cross it? This predicts the risk of growth disturbance and may also determine the need for operative treatment.

Additional imaging techniques

Some fractures may be difficult to diagnose on initial X-rays; a technetium bone scan to investigate the amount of osteoblastic activity may be useful in this situation. Some fractures are complex, and adequate planning of surgical approach and reconstruction require additional information. A CT scan is usually the most useful investigation for this.

Assessing the severity of the fracture

The more energy dissipated in the tissues at the time of fracture, the greater the degree of tissue damage and the lower the probability of swift, problem-free fracture union. Furthermore, certain components of the overall injury may have a big influence on the risk of the complications discussed earlier. Having detected the fracture and defined its pattern, it is vital also to assess its severity and modify the treatment plan accordingly. This requires attention to both the clinical examination and the radiological appearances.

The important clinical signs of fracture severity are:

- *Damage to the soft tissues overlying the fracture.* There may be an open wound in the skin, or there may be fatally crushed or devitalised, but intact, skin. There will be a very variable amount of devitalised muscle. Such devitalised tissue will have to be excised, and a significant extent of this constitutes a very severe injury. A rough grading of the severity of the open fracture is given by the Gustilo grading (1976).
- *Impairment of circulation to the limb beyond the fracture.* It is vital to check for the presence of pulses below the fracture, while keeping in mind the possibility that, even with palpable pulses, arterial damage may have occurred. Inordinate pain, excessive swelling and tension in the calf or forearm, and impaired sensation can all be signs of compartment syndrome. In high-risk cases of tibial fracture, compartment pressures should be monitored if equipment is available; in any case frequent clinical checks need to be carried out for 48 hours. There is usually marked swelling and local muscle tenderness. Remember: severe pain after fracture, persisting after immobilisation = compartment syndrome until proved otherwise.

The X-ray also contains clues as to the severity of injury. A high degree of comminution (multiple fragments), large distances between fragments, wide displacement between the main bone ends, and gross overlap with shortening of the limb are all signs that much energy was absorbed and the deep soft tissues nourishing the bone were badly damaged.

MANAGEMENT

First-aid management of fractures, before reaching hospital, includes immobilisation of the fracture using temporary external splintage, coverage of wounds with a clean (preferably sterile) dressing and administration of pain relief.

Management of fractures must be individualised. The optimum method of management of a particular fracture may change with the age and expectations of the patient, and other disease states present (including osteoporosis). The work and sporting requirements of the individual may require modification of treatment plans. Fractures in the elderly require a particular holistic approach, which is covered in detail in Chapter 21. A different approach is also needed for high-energy fractures with much surrounding soft tissue damage.

The principles of fracture treatment include:

- *reduction* (i.e. reduce the deformity and replace the bone fragments in their anatomical position)
- *maintenance of reduction* for as long as it takes for the fracture to unite
- Provision of *optimum conditions for healing*, for both the fracture and other damaged structures such as ligaments and joint capsules
- *early mobilisation* of adjacent joints to prevent stiffness; this is the first step in a phase of *rehabilitation* aimed at achieving sufficient function to allow early return of the patient to activities of daily living and to work
- *minimisation of complications*, including infection.

There are a wide variety of methods of fracture treatment, and none of them fulfils all of these conditions perfectly. All fracture treatment involves compromise, in order to minimise the risk of complications and the impact of any disadvantages of the particular method selected, while maximising its benefits. Broadly, there are six methods of fracture treatment:

- immediate or early mobilisation, essentially ignoring the fracture, providing minimal support (e.g. a sling).
- support/immobilisation in a plaster cast or plastic brace (Fig. 19.9)
- treatment by traction, which immobilises the fracture by applying a longitudinal force along the limb
- external fixation using a fixator applied with screws to the bone (Fig. 19.10)
- flexible internal fixation (usually with an intramedullary nail; Fig. 19.11)
- rigid internal fixation (usually with a stainless steel plate, which will minimise or prevent a callus response; (Fig. 19.7)

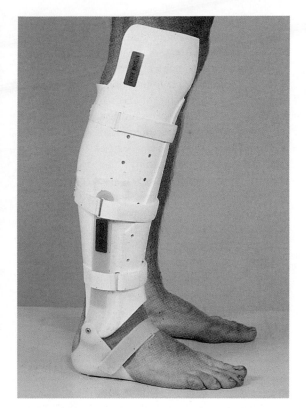

Figure 19.9 Functional tibial brace. It is closer fitting than a plaster cast and permits ankle and knee movement.

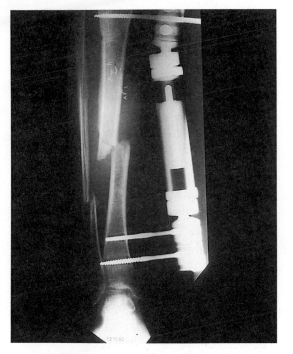

Figure 19.10 Externally fixed open (compound) tibial fracture. The position is poor, there is some evidence of the fixator pins coming loose and this fracture went on to heal very slowly.

This series of methods provides a progressive increase in rigidity of fixation, security of reduction and (usually) ability to mobilise adjacent joints. On the other hand, they have increasing risk of complications, including iatrogenic infections, because they are more invasive. In particular, rigid internal fixation increases the risk of failure of healing, and plating of shaft fractures increases the risk of infection due to the amount of soft tissue dissection required. Rigid fixation of articular fractures is, however, frequently carried out. The blood supply of cancellous bone is better than that of the cortical bone of the shaft (so healing is more assured and the risks of infection are somewhat less), and the importance of prevention of secondary osteoarthritis makes accurate reduction and early joint movement highly desirable. The essential logical step in planning treatment is thus to balance the risks of a given line of treatment against what is required to achieve a good functional result.

Because of the potentially devastating effects of compartment syndrome, many trauma units insert percutaneous pressure monitors into the anterior compartment of the leg after tibial fracture and take regular readings for the first 48 hours after fracture. Compartment syndrome is treated by division of the fascial wall of the affected compartments (fasciotomy). Undertreatment of this condition is commoner and more serious than overtreatment.

The approach to high-energy fractures

Extensive tissue damage has the potential not only to produce failure of fracture healing, but also to encourage infection of the open fracture by organisms. To prevent this serious complication, the following measures must be taken:

- Rigorous cleaning of the fracture wound and fracture site with large amounts of isotonic fluid. Excision of all severely contaminated and dead tissue.

- Fixation with devices which do not introduce implants directly into the fracture area, such as external fixators (Fig. 19.10).
- Early coverage of integument defects with skin grafts or larger areas of tissue transferred with a blood supply (flaps). Such surgery is generally carried out by plastic surgeons in collaboration with the orthopaedic team.
- Antibiotics. These are important, but will not be effective unless the other three factors described above are carried out meticulously. An appropriate agent should be used to cover for likely infecting organisms: Gram-positive cocci (i.e. staphylococci) and Gram-negative bacilli.

Treatment of late complications of fractures – including distraction osteogenesis

Detailed discussion of the treatment of non-unions, malunions and osteomyelitis complicating fractures is beyond the scope of this book. As described in the pathology section of this chapter, some non-unions can be induced to heal simply by the provision of mechanical stability, while others require a biological stimulus as well. Mechanical stability can be provided by intramedullary nailing, plating or external fixators of various designs.

The traditional biological stimulus is a bone graft – pieces of fresh cancellous bone harvested from the iliac crest. A more recent innovation, growing in popularity, is the Ilizarov technique, which is based on the discovery that distraction of non-union tissue induces osteogenesis – bone formation. A fresh bone cut (an osteotomy) also produces new bone under conditions of gradual distraction, provided the callus response is allowed a few days to start (usually 1 week) before distraction. This can be harnessed to regain length of a bone lost through fracture or to gradually correct a deformity resulting from malunion. This form of biological stimulus can obviate the need for taking bone graft, which is a good thing since there can be considerable donor site morbidity.

Fractures which have failed to heal because of uncontrolled infection present the greatest challenge. Some are so severe that amputation should be recommended. Others can be healed by excising infected bone and reconstituting the defect by massive bone graft or by distraction osteogenesis using the Ilizarov technique.

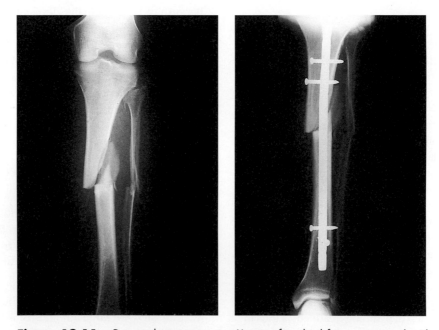

Figure 19.11   Pre- and post-operative X-rays of a tibial fracture treated with an intramedullary nail.

20 | An atlas of fractures

The practical treatment of fractures involves a great deal of pattern recognition. People tend to experience a variety of injury mechanisms which produce more or less constant patterns of injury. A great deal of time can be saved, and the risk of missing important complications reduced, by being aware of these patterns and learning how to recognise them. This is not to undermine the importance of the principles described in the previous chapter; they should also be constantly borne in mind and applied. It is simply a way of making use of the accumulated experience of generations of orthopaedic surgeons in the management of similar groups of injuries.

In the following pages, the common patterns of fracture will be listed, starting with the upper limb, and followed by the lower limb and the spine. For each, the classic pattern(s) of clinical and radiological presentation will be illustrated and the common injury mechanisms (to be listened for in the history) given. The common treatment(s) and complications will then be described.

An atlas of fractures

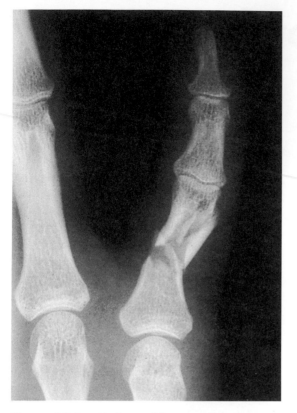

Figure 20.1   Phalangeal fracture of the little finger.

PHALANGEAL FRACTURES

Common mechanisms

Falls, fighting, industrial injuries.

Presenting features

Pain over site of fracture, deformity, poor hand movement. X-rays are required for adequate diagnosis, but clinical examination is the only reliable way to examine for rotational deformity.

Treatment

Most commonly splintage (e.g. to adjacent finger using adhesive tape ('neighbour strapping'). Occasional use of internal or external fixation.

Complications

Stiffness of hand or digit. Vigorous physiotherapy is often required. Malrotation or malunion occasionally leads to crossing of the fingers during flexion.

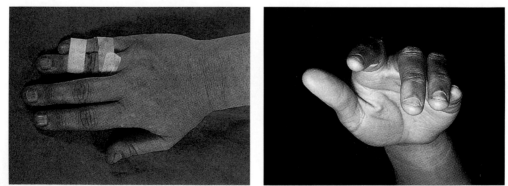

A   B

Figure 20.2   Neighbour strapping (A). This index finger shows malrotation (B); it is important to recognise and treat this problem in metacarpal or finger fractures.

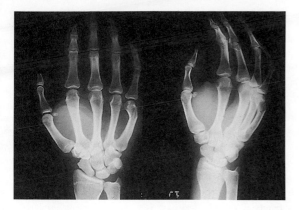

Figure 20.3   Fifth metacarpal neck fracture.

FIFTH METACARPAL NECK FRACTURES

Common mechanisms

Punching injury.

Presenting features

Pain and deformity of the knuckle of the little finger.

Treatment

Usually conservative (wool and crepe bandage).

Complications

Persistent mild deformity is usual, but normal function is almost invariable. Often there is temporary extensor lag of the little finger, recovering in a few months.

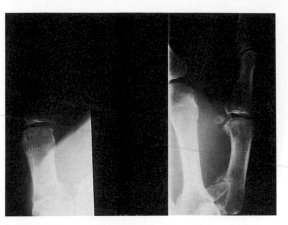

Figure 20.4 Bennett's fracture of base of thumb metacarpal.

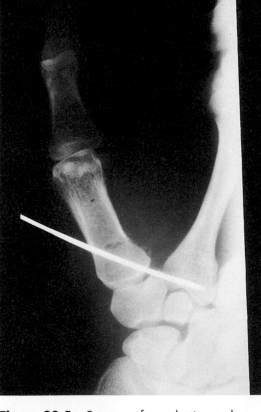

Figure 20.5 Fracture after reduction and Kirschner wire fixation.

FIRST METACARPAL BASE – BENNETT'S FRACTURE

Common mechanisms

Fall to thumb.

Presenting features

Pain in base of thumb; weak thumb. The Bennett's fracture is a fracture-subluxation of the carpometacarpal (CMC) joint – an intra-articular fracture.

Treatment

Controversial. Manipulation and plaster or internal fixation with K-wires are common methods.

Complications

Malunion is common. Arthritis in the CMC joint may result.

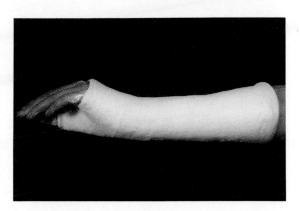

Figure 20.6 Scaphoid cast.

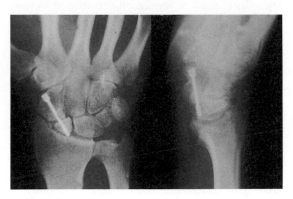

Figure 20.7 Herbert screw fixation of an ununited scaphoid fracture.

SCAPHOID FRACTURES

Common mechanisms

Falls to outstretched hand.

Presenting features

Pain and tenderness over radial side of wrist (anatomical snuff box). X-rays may not show a fracture initially – if clinical suspicion is high, repeat X-ray at 1 or 2 weeks (and leave in plaster during this period).

Treatment

Undisplaced fractures: scaphoid plaster 2–3 months. Displaced fractures: internal fixation.

Complications

Non-union of fracture, especially if displaced. Avascular necrosis of part of bone. Non-union may be followed by wrist osteoarthritis, even if the non-union is initially asymptomatic.

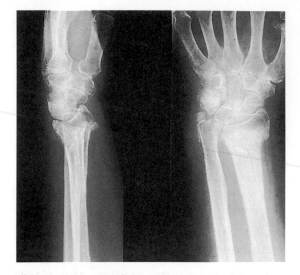

Figure 20.8 Distal radial fracture in patient with osteoporosis.

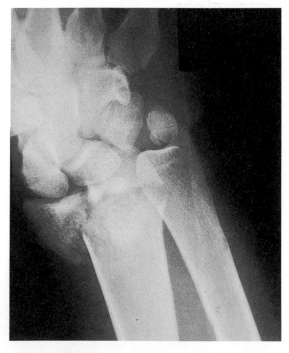

Figure 20.9 Severely displaced distal radial fracture in a young patient. There is often severe articular damage.

DISTAL RADIUS FRACTURES

Common mechanisms

Low-energy injury in elderly (major fracture of osteoporosis): fall to outstretched hand.
Higher energy injury in younger age groups: heavy fall, RTA etc.

Presenting features

Colles' fracture: dorsal angulation and dinner fork deformity.
Smith's fracture: palmar angulation deformity.
Ulna distal shaft or styloid often fractured as well as radius.

Treatment

Very variable. Treated with manipulation and plaster, internal fixation (especially with wires) or external fixation. Generally active (i.e. fixation) treatment with younger (less than 65) patients; more variable treatment in older patients.

Complications

Malunion may lead to persisting weak grip and poor range of motion of the wrist. There may be joint pain, especially in distal radio-ulnar joint. Algodystrophy is common after this fracture.

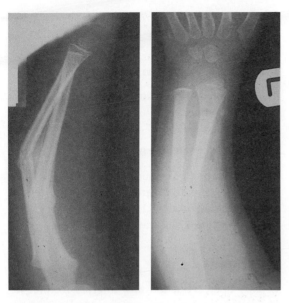

Figure 20.10   Greenstick radius and ulnar fracture in a child. These are nearly always treated with plaster fixation.

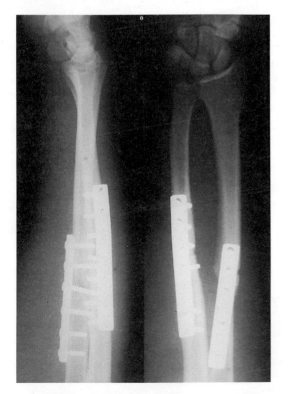

Figure 20.11   Internally fixed radius and ulnar fractures in an adult. There is a risk of loss of forearm rotation, so internal fixation is usual for adults.

RADIUS AND ULNA SHAFT FRACTURES

Common mechanisms

Falls, road traffic accidents. Common injury as a greenstick fracture in children.

Presenting features

Forearm deformity. There may be severe swelling (bad enough to require fasciotomy).

Treatment

Open reduction and internal fixation. In children (not adolescents), manipulation and plaster fixation with regular X-ray review on follow up.

Complications

Malunion may lead to gross restriction of forearm rotation. Now less common due to use of internal fixation.

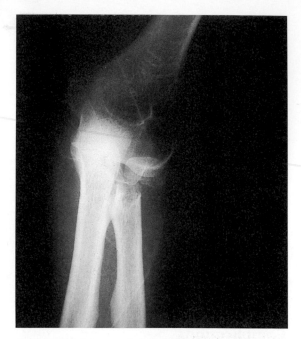

Figure 20.12 Radial head fracture. The head is completely detached from the shaft.

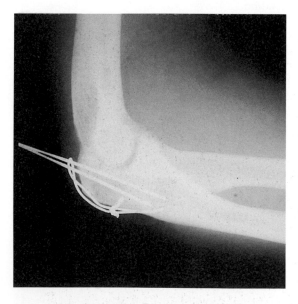

Figure 20.13 Internally fixed olecranon fracture. This is an intraoperative X-ray; the projecting wires will be cut and bent over before closing the skin. Taking an 'on-table' X-ray is usual practice during fixation.

RADIAL HEAD AND OLECRANON FRACTURES

Common mechanisms

Fall to outstretched hand (radial head) or tip of elbow (olecranon).

Presenting features

Pain and swelling at elbow. Markedly restricted elbow movement. Degree of comminution of fracture varies widely. High-energy injury may involve fracture-dislocation of elbow joint.

Treatment

Usually open reduction and internal fixation for olecranon. Radial head varies: simple ones left unfixed; severe ones treated by excision of the head – maybe at a later stage.

Complications

Stiffness. Characteristic problem is lack of full extension, which may be permanent. Requires early active movement and physiotherapy. Some risk of stiffness due to ectopic bone formation (myositis ossificans).

SUPRACONDYLAR HUMERAL FRACTURES

Common mechanisms

A child falling onto the outstretched hand.

Presenting features

Pain and swelling at elbow. Risk of damage or compression of brachial artery.

Treatment

Manipulation under anaesthetic, minimal internal fixation with K-wires, or traction in extension (if very swollen). Fracture is more stable when elbow is flexed, but too much flexion will occlude the artery.

Complications

Volkmann's ischaemic contracture: catastrophic ischaemia of forearm muscles.

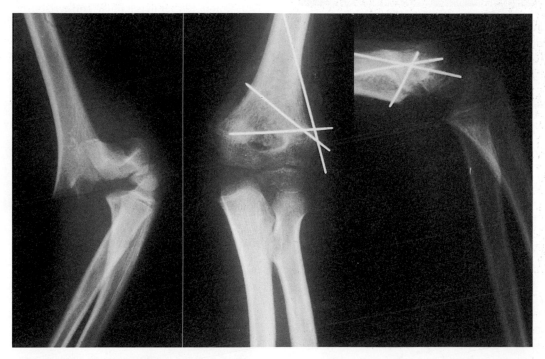

Figure 20.14   Severely displaced supracondylar fracture before and after wire fixation. Careful examination of forearm vascularity is required.

An atlas of fractures

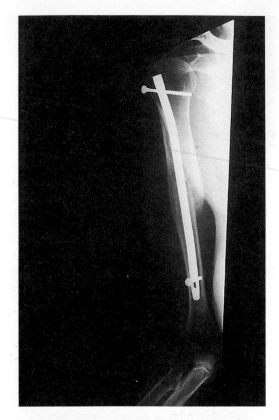

Figure 20.15   Humeral shaft fracture after nail fixation. Most such fractures can be treated conservatively.

HUMERAL SHAFT FRACTURES

Common mechanisms

Fall. Often a torsional injury, leading to a spiral fracture.

Presenting features

Pain in humerus. There may be spectacular bruising. Radial nerve at risk from injury at the spiral groove of the humerus (leads to wrist drop).

Treatment

Treated by traction (using 'hanging cast' as a weight) or with a fracture brace (or gaiter). If poor reduction or slow healing, consider intramedullary nail or plate.

Complications

Malunion (particularly varus), which may be obvious on X-ray but is rarely a clinical problem. Non-union. Radial nerve palsy and wrist drop.

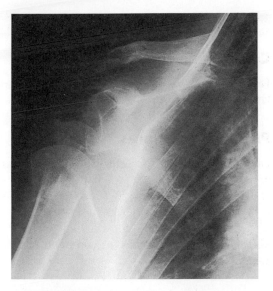

Figure 20.16   Humeral neck fracture.

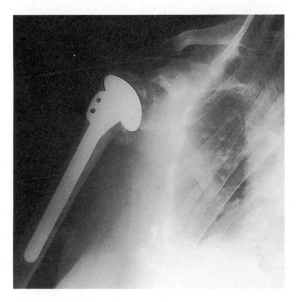

Figure 20.17   Fracture after Neer
hemiarthroplasty of the humeral head, undertaken
because of the very high risk of avascular necrosis
of the head in this particular fracture.

HUMERAL NECK FRACTURES

Common mechanisms

Fall. Very common in osteoporotic patients.

Presenting features

Pain and bruising (may be spectacular later). Very
variable degree of comminution – some have risk
of avascular necrosis of the humeral head.
Occasional fracture dislocation, or avulsion
fractures where rotator cuff is detached from
greater tuberosity.

Treatment

Humeral neck in elderly patients usually
conservative (sling). In younger patients,
occasionally operative fixation treatment is used.
Some humeral neck fractures with a risk of
avascular necrosis of humeral head are treated
with hemiarthroplasty.

Complications

Stiffness in shoulder. Weak shoulder (especially if
rotator cuff injured).

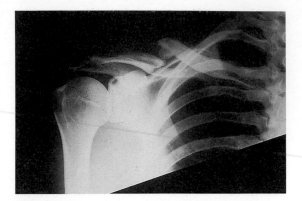

Figure 20.18   Clavicle fracture.

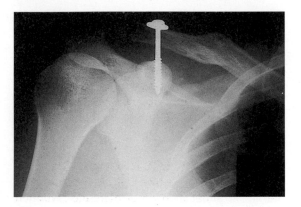

Figure 20.19   Distal clavicle fractures are often difficult to treat. This was treated with a screw to hold the clavicle down towards the coracoid.

CLAVICLE FRACTURES

Common mechanisms

Fall – usually to tip of shoulder. Common in children.

Presenting features

Obvious deformity, palpable in subcutaneous bone.

Treatment

Vast majority of fractures treated with simple sling.

Complications

Most patients have good functional result but obvious residual deformity at fracture site. This will remodel and diminish or disappear in children.

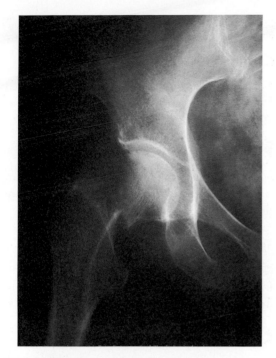

Figure 20.20   Displaced subcapital (intracapsular) femoral neck fracture.

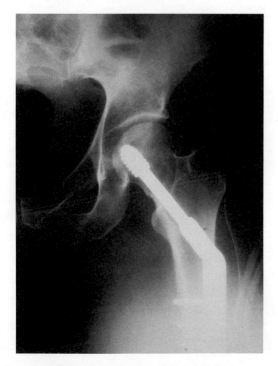

Figure 20.21   X-ray of an interochanteric fracture treated with a dynamic hip screw.

FEMORAL NECK FRACTURES

Common mechanisms

Fall. The classic osteoporotic fracture which forms a huge proportion of in-patient fracture work. Two quite different types: (1) transcervical or subcapital and (2) intertrochanteric.

Presenting features

Shortened, externally rotated leg (not in undisplaced fractures). Hip pain. Inability to bear weight.

Treatment

Internal fixation for intertrochanteric and undisplaced subcapital fractures. Displaced subcapital fractures – young patients: fixation; elderly patients: hemiarthroplasty.

Complications

High mortality rate in older patients. Subcapital fractures are intracapsular and the head therefore has a poor blood supply: risk of failure of fixation or avascular necrosis.

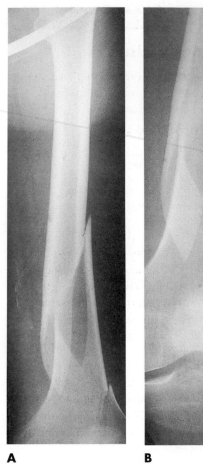

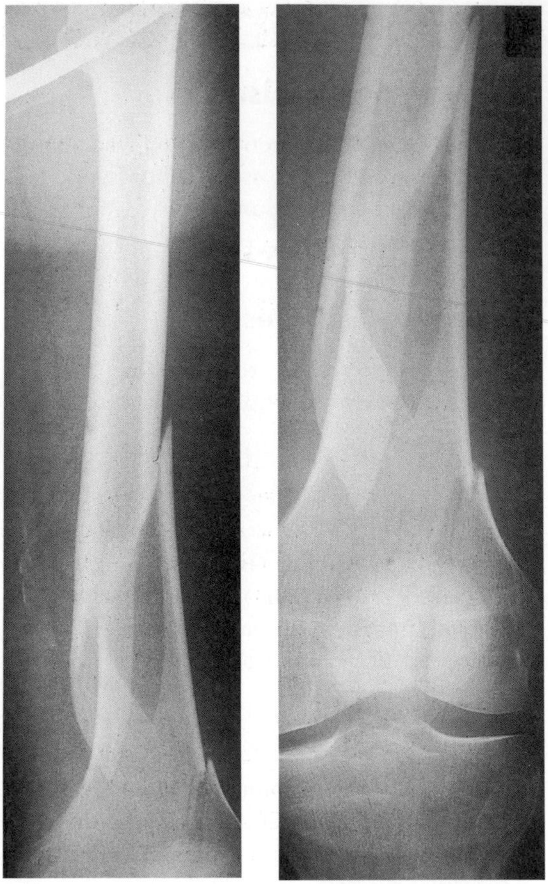

A   **B**

Figure 20.22   Femoral shaft fracture (A). The fracture extends into the knee joint (B).

FEMORAL SHAFT FRACTURES

Common mechanisms

Usually high-energy fracture (RTA, sporting etc.). Frequently associated with knee injuries such as cruciate ligament ruptures or meniscal tears.

Presenting features

Severe pain. Deformity and swelling at the fracture site. There may be substantial blood loss into the thigh.

Treatment

Conservative treatment (traction, possibly followed by a fracture brace) in children. Usually internal fixation with intramedullary nail in adults.

Complications

Risks of embolic phenomena during and after nailing. Knee stiffness. Occasional delayed union.

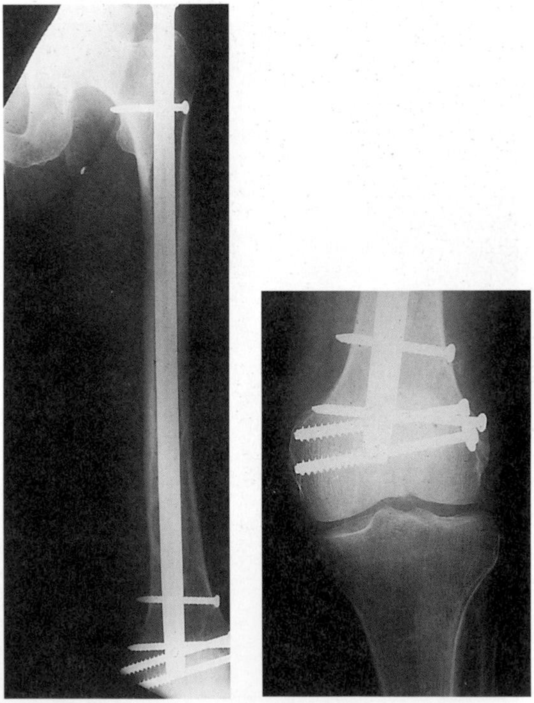

Figure 20.23   The femoral shaft fracture was fixed with a nail; two additional screws fix the lateral femoral condyle.

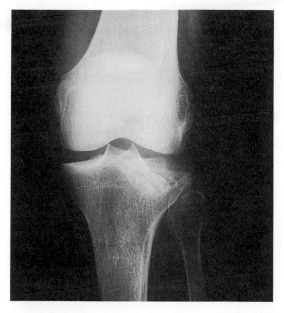

Figure 20.24 Depressed lateral tibial plateau fracture.

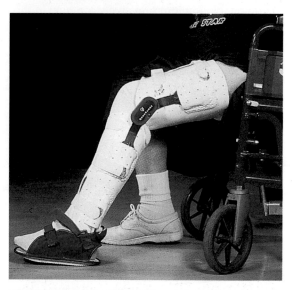

Figure 20.25 Hinged 'femoral' brace.

TIBIAL PLATEAU FRACTURES

Common mechanisms

Fall, sporting injury, 'bumper fracture', where a car strikes the knee from the side.

Presenting features

Pain around knee; loss of knee movement; haemarthrosis.

Treatment

Depends on degree of fracture displacement. Minimally displaced stable fractures: early movement, with or without a supporting brace, non-weight-bearing with crutches for 2–3 months. Displaced or unstable fractures: internal fixation and early movement.

Complications

Osteoarthritis of the knee is surprisingly uncommon. Knee stiffness. Concomitant ligament or meniscal injuries.

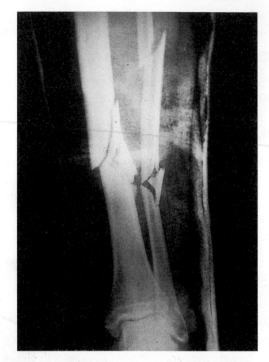

Figure 20.26   Tibial shaft fracture treated in plaster.

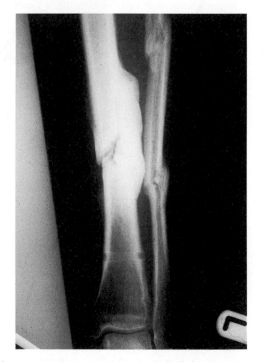

Figure 20.27   Healed tibial shaft fracture. Note after healing by external callus the fracture line is still visible.

TIBIAL SHAFT FRACTURES

Common mechanisms

Fall, road traffic accident, sports.

Presenting features

Pain, swelling, deformity at fracture site; unable to weight-bear. Often open fracture, due to subcutaneous position of bone.

Treatment

Closed fractures: plaster then brace, or intramedullary nail if good position of fracture unlikely in plaster. Open fracture: thorough wound toilet, external fixation, plastic surgery if necessary to achieve good quality soft tissue cover of bone.

Complications

Malunion. Non-union is relatively common in this bone, especially in high-energy open fractures. Compartment syndrome is a real risk – requires urgent fasciotomy.

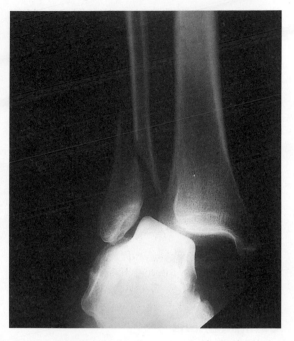

Figure 20.28 Ankle fracture. There is no medial fracture but the deltoid ligament has been ruptured. Ankle osteoarthritis is inevitable if not adequately treated.

ANKLE FRACTURES

Common mechanisms

Low- and high-energy injuries. Commonest is 'going over' on ankle on step or uneven ground.

Presenting features

Swelling, inability to weight-bear. Bony tenderness at medial or lateral malleolus. There may be obvious deformity, especially if ankle is subluxed.

Treatment

Undisplaced fractures – plaster immobilisation. Displaced fractures – internal fixation.

Complications

Ankle stiffness. Malunion in a proportion of displaced fractures treated conservatively – sometimes followed by osteoarthritis.

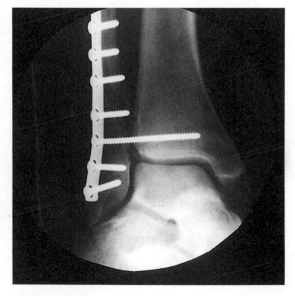

Figure 20.29 Ankle fracture after fixation with plates and screws.

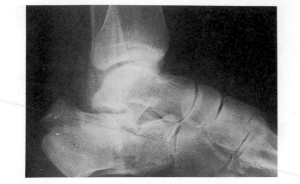

Figure 20.30   Calcaneal fracture.

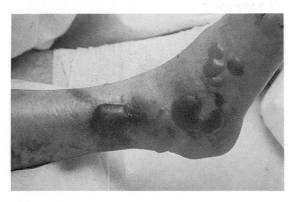

Figure 20.31   Calcaneal fracture. Marked swelling and blistering ('fracture blistering') are common after all fractures below the knee.

CALCANEAL FRACTURES

Common mechanisms

Fall from a height.

Presenting features

Swelling, may become gross over a few days. Bruising around hindfoot. Severe pain. Often associated with vertebral wedge fractures (cause back pain).

Treatment

Elevation, ice packs and early mobilisation. Increasing use of internal fixation for displaced fractures.

Complications

Frequently persisting pain. Stiff subtalar joint – causes difficulty on uneven ground due to lack of inversion/eversion.

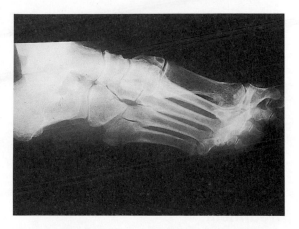

Figure 20.32   Fracture of fifth metatarsal base.

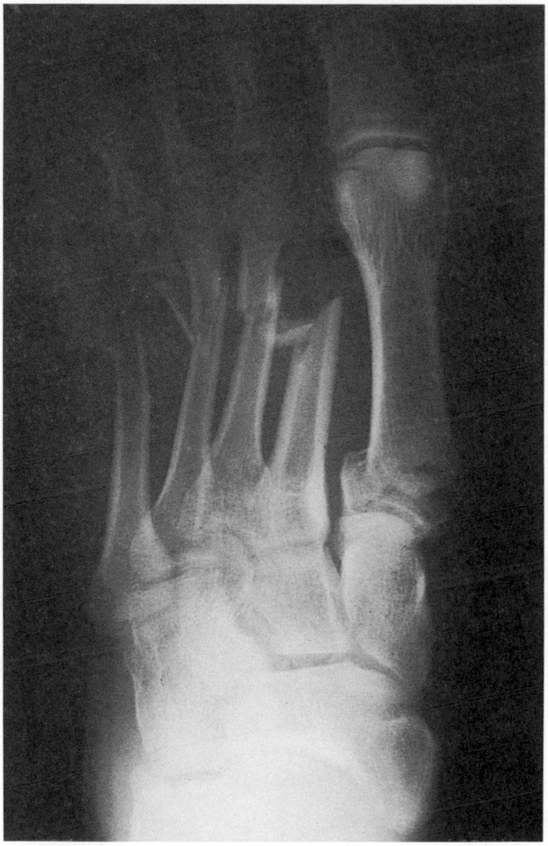

METATARSAL FRACTURES

Common mechanisms

Direct blow (e.g. dropping heavy weight on foot); inversion injury to foot (fifth metatarsal base fracture).

Presenting features

Swelling and local bony tenderness of foot. Obvious deformity only if multiple fractures.

Treatment

Plaster of Paris for single fractures. Internal fixation for multiple metatarsal fractures.

Complications

Occasional metatarsalgia. Non-union occurs occasionally in fifth metatarsal shaft fractures.

Figure 20.33   Fractures of metatarsal shafts. Metatarsalgia is likely unless these are reduced and fixed.

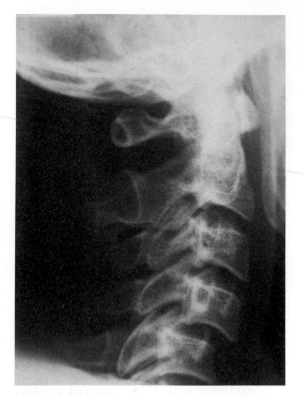

Figure 20.34 Cervical spine dislocation at C4/5. It is important to get views as far down as C7/T1 (not obtained in this example), as this is a common site of injury.

CERVICAL SPINE FRACTURES

Common mechanisms

Forced flexion, forced extension, lateral flexion.

Presenting features

Neck pain and tenderness. Pain radiating to arms or between scapulae. Weakness or paraesthesiae in arms or legs, or both.

Treatment

Immediate immobilisation of cervical spine. X-rays (and possible subsequent CT or MRI) to establish diagnosis. Treatment with traction, collar immobilisation or internal fixation.

Complications

Paraplegia, quadriplegia or more limited neurological damage. Persisting neck pain.

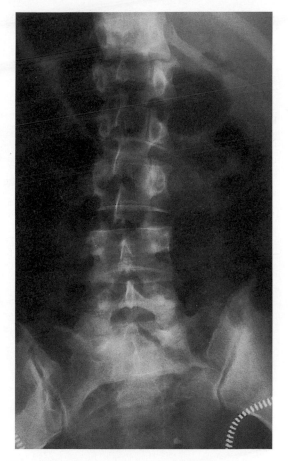

Figure 20.35   Lumbar spinal fracture. L1 is reduced in height and the distance between the two vetebral pedicles of L1 is increased (diastasis).

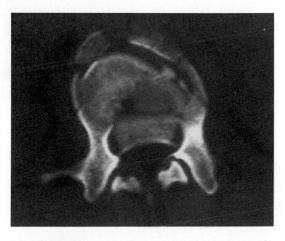

Figure 20.36   CT scan showing lumbar spinal canal compromise due to the fracture in Figure 20.35.

LUMBAR SPINE FRACTURES

Common mechanisms

Falls from height, road traffic accidents. Low-energy pathological fractures (osteoporosis, metastases).

Presenting features

Back pain. May be associated neurogenic pain. May be paraplegia; spinal cord ends at L1, so lower fractures will affect cauda equina (lower motor neurone). Examination of perineal area is mandatory.

Treatment

Immediate immobilisation of lumbar spine. X-rays (and possible CT or MRI) to establish diagnosis. Treatment with bedrest and pressure area care, or increasing use of internal fixation. Spine held to have four 'columns': anterior vertebral body and anterior ligament; posterior body and posterior interbody ligament; pedicles and facet joints; laminae and spinous processes and associated ligaments. Posterior two columns are probably most important for spinal stability.

Complications

Paraplegia or more limited neurological damage. Loss of urinary/bowel sphincter sensation or control in cauda equina injuries. Back pain.

21 | Fractures in the elderly

Case history

An 80-year-old woman was found on her kitchen floor by her home help. It appeared that she had been there all night, and on arrival in the A&E department she was noted to be extremely cold. She was confused and disorientated, insisting that she wanted to go home. Examination revealed that she was dehydrated, hypotensive and hypothermic, and appeared to be poorly nourished. She had a painful left hip, with tenderness in the groin and shortening and external rotation of the left leg. An X-ray confirmed a left subcapital femoral neck fracture (Garden grade 4, i.e. fully displaced), and after beginning to re-warm her and starting an intravenous infusion, she was transferred to the orthopaedic ward.

The woman's daughter said her mother had a history of angina which had been worsening recently, and had previously had a myocardial infarction. She took (unreliably) various medications including a calcium antagonist and a diuretic. Examination at the time of admission showed that she had widespread wheezes and coarse crepitations at the lung bases. In addition, she had an early sacral pressure sore which was thought to be related to the period of time she spent on the ground at home. ECG showed left axis deviation and ischaemic changes, together with evidence of an old infarct. Chest X-ray showed an enlarged heart and diffuse patchy pulmonary changes consistent with bronchopneumonia and pulmonary oedema. Her haemoglobin was 110 g/L. Urea and electrolytes showed sodium of 135 mmol/L (normal), potassium of 2.8 mmol/L (normal 3.5–5.0), urea of 13 mmol/L (normal 4.5–8.0) and creatinine of 200 mmol/L (normal max. 105).

The orthopaedic team asked their elderly care physician to advise on how best to prepare the woman for surgery. He recommended scheduling her operation for 48 hours later and set about correcting her fluid and electrolyte imbalance and prescribing antibiotic and physiotherapy treatment for her chest infection. On a scheduled trauma list, a partial hip replacement (hemiarthroplasty) was performed uneventfully under a spinal anaesthetic.

After her operation, the woman needed careful supervision by the orthogeriatric team. Her chest infection settled slowly on continued antibiotics and physiotherapy and, as her chest infection improved, her initial confusion subsided. Her early i.v. fluid therapy was carefully managed to avoid hyponatraemia and she was later encouraged to take a nourishing diet. To start with, she needed two people to assist her mobilising, but eventually she became independent with a frame. The occupational therapist visited her home and, after much discussion with her daughter, it was agreed that her ability to cope in her own home had become doubtful anyway, even before the fall. They decided to plan her discharge to an elderly person's home (EPH). Ten days after admission she was transferred to the elderly rehabilitation ward, where her cardiac drug therapy was fine-tuned. Two weeks later, she went to the EPH that her daughter had chosen.

Key points

- Elderly people with fractures usually have multiple problems – the fracture may merely be one incident in a long-term general failure of health

- A multidisciplinary approach, including both geriatricians and orthopaedic surgeons, is essential

- Falls occur for a variety of reasons, some of which may be treatable to prevent recurrence

- The key to treating elderly patients with fractures is early mobilisation

- Intravenous fluid therapy in the elderly is difficult

- The use of sedative drugs should be avoided if possible

PATHOLOGY

The fracture itself

The incidence of fractures in the elderly has increased sharply in the last 50 years and they now constitute a major public health problem, forming a large part of the work of orthopaedic units. This increase is occurring for at least two reasons:

- There is an increasing number of elderly patients in the population due to demographic changes. These changes have affected most developed countries and are likely to occur in other countries in the future as well.
- The age-specific incidence of fractures is increasing. This is certainly true for femoral neck fractures, but there is evidence of a similar increase in fractures at other sites. The most likely explanation for these changes is an increasing age-specific incidence of osteoporosis. There are several theories about why this may be occurring.

Although osteoporotic bone is more liable to fracture, the same bone is perfectly capable of mounting an adequate healing response. The mode of healing will depend on the method of treatment, as described in Chapter 19. Usually the method of fracture treatment will be dictated by the need to permit early mobilisation and rehabilitation. Osteomalacia is an occasional cause for low-velocity fractures in the elderly. The proportion of such fractures caused by osteomalacia is unclear, but it is important to check for the presence of this condition in elderly patients.

Metastatic disease is a common and important condition predisposing to low-velocity fractures. The incidence of bone metastases increases with age. Any of the common tumours which metastasise to bone may cause pathological fractures. Such fractures may be the presenting feature of patients with malignant disease. A history seeking the presence of pre-existing bone pain is important in all patients with these fractures. In addition, X-rays should be examined carefully for evidence of bone destruction at the site of the fracture and of metastases elsewhere on the X-rayed areas. Further management of metastatic bone disease is considered in Chapter 11.

The commonest fracture in the elderly which requires expensive in-patient treatment is described as a 'hip fracture' or a 'fractured neck of femur'. In fact, these terms cover two different types of fracture with different approaches to treatment.

Subcapital fractures of the femoral neck. These fractures are within the capsule of the hip joint and can damage the blood supply of the femoral head. This means that there is a risk of non-union and collapse of the head due to avascular necrosis. The degree of displacement is described by the Garden classification, which has grades 1 to 4. Undisplaced fractures (Garden 1 and 2), and displaced fractures in younger patients, are treated by screw fixation. In old people with displaced fractures, grades 3 and 4, the surgeon will often replace the head with a prosthesis – a hemiarthroplasty – rather than fix the fracture and aim for healing.

Intertrochanteric fractures. These fractures are extracapsular and not strictly in the neck of the femur at all. They run between the greater and lesser trochanters. Here the bone is much better vascularised, so internal fixation, with a view to obtaining fracture union, is the standard method of treatment.

Medical problems in elderly fracture patients at the time of presentation

It is vital to recognise that, in elderly patients, the fracture is frequently only one problem amid a more generalised medical deterioration. Thus the fracture may arise due to a fall caused by some other current medical condition. Frequent causes for falls (Box 21.1) include visual impairment, cerebrovascular accidents and cardiac problems, including dysrhythmias and myocardial infarction, as well as treatment with drugs which depress consciousness or cause postural hypotension. Other causes of unsteadiness include musculoskeletal diseases such as arthritis. Environmental causes for falls are also important in elderly patients, many of whom are sufficiently infirm to have to struggle to walk. These causes include loose flooring materials (e.g. rugs), steps in the home and builders' insistence on placing electrical sockets at floor level.

Several conditions at the time of presentation may influence the overall outcome in patients with osteoporotic fractures. These comorbidities are particularly important in patients who require surgery. Careful medical assessment of these patients at the time of admission is vital. Problems include the presence of pulmonary disease, diabetes and vascular disease. The nutrition of many elderly patients at the time of presentation is poor and, regrettably, is frequently even worse at the time of their discharge from hospital.

The mental condition of the patient is an important prognostic factor for outcome after fractures in the elderly. Confused patients have a more difficult rehabilitation and poorer prognosis after operation. Confusion frequently occurs due to the injury and treatment. An episode of confusion is a frequent complication of admission of an elderly patient with a fracture. Areas worth checking in such patients include the chest (hypoxia is a common cause of confusion: check the blood gases if necessary), hyponatraemia (check the electrolytes: see below) and drug-related problems. Many elderly patients respond poorly to sedative drugs and analgesics; thus confusion may require a trial of withdrawal of medication to make sure that the medication is not the cause. Treatment of confusion in the elderly with sedatives may make things worse; administration of oxygen is far more likely to be helpful.

MANAGEMENT OF ELDERLY FRACTURE PATIENTS

It is clear from the above that the management of elderly fracture patients requires a combination of physicians' and surgeons' skills, as well as those of nurses and many others. Medical problems, which may not have been known about before, must now be addressed if the patient is to do well following the acute incident of trauma. In addition, the particular responses of the elderly to fracture must be taken into account.

Medical problems arising from the injury

Most elderly patients have only undergone low-energy trauma when sustaining their injury; nonetheless the metabolic effects of the trauma

---

Box 21.1 Common medical conditions in elderly fracture patients

- Cardiovascular
  - CVA
  - dysrhythmias
  - myocardial infarction
  - cardiac failure

- Neurological
  - dementia and confusion
  - Parkinsonism

- Poor nutrition

- Respiratory
  - bronchopneumonia
  - pulmonary oedema

- Endocrine
  - diabetes
  - exaggerated metabolic response to trauma

- Drug-induced
  - sedation
  - postural hypotension

may be marked. There is evidence of an altered physiological response to trauma in the elderly; in particular, there are abnormal and prolonged hormonal responses. An enhanced glucocorticoid response to trauma is common. Prolonged and inappropriate secretion of antidiuretic hormone (ADH) may result in severe difficulties in controlling fluid and electrolyte balance. Most patients are fluid-depleted at the time of presentation to hospital – from blood loss, and having been unable to drink between sustaining the fracture and attending hospital – and require fluid resuscitation. It is best to avoid excessive amounts of non-electrolyte based fluids (e.g. 5% dextrose) in these patients. The abnormal ADH secretion, which is part of the injury response, may then lead to fluid overloading, with concentrated urine being excreted and blood biochemistry showing a low sodium, a normal potassium and a low urea and creatinine. This condition is generally managed by restriction of fluids. Thus, there may be a difficult balancing act between adequate fluid resuscitation and overloading, compounded by the precarious cardiac reserves of some of these patients. Inappropriate ADH secretion occurs most commonly in the postoperative phase, and dehydration is much commoner than overloading in pre-operative patients.

Elderly patients with fractures are at severe risk if placed on prolonged bed rest. Careful nursing will minimise complications, but these patients risk developing broncho-pneumonia, thrombo-embolic disease (the risk of which is dramatically increased in the elderly) and pressure sores. The decision to undertake surgical treatment in an elderly patient depends on balancing the risks of conservative treatment against those of operative treatment. Improvements in anaesthesia and surgical technique have resulted in a marked increase in such surgery in the elderly over the past 25 years. In particular, almost all femoral neck fractures are now treated by surgical intervention.

Surgery

Surgical treatment of fractures in the elderly poses particular technical problems. These patients are frequently unfit for prolonged anaesthesia. Further, failed surgery is likely to have disastrously poor results, and frequently the demise of the patient. It is therefore important that surgery be technically reasonably simple and deliver robust results. The technical problems of surgery in the elderly include the difficulty of achieving sound fixation of fractures in weakened or osteoporotic bone, and failure of fixation is unfortunately not rare. A meticulous surgical technique is required to minimise these difficulties. If there is a choice, intramedullary devices (nails) are generally better than plates which are held in place by screws that can easily pull out. General complications of surgery are more frequent in elderly patients, including wound infection. There are also several specific complications of osteoporotic fractures which may be troublesome. Thus, fixation of displaced subcapital femoral neck fractures (Garden 3 and 4) may be followed by avascular necrosis of the femoral head and osteoarthritis of the hip.

Rehabilitation

The problems facing elderly fracture patients are not complete after operation, as rehabilitation in such patients poses particular problems. This is reflected by the very poor outcomes after some fractures in the elderly. Thus, mortality rates of 30% are common at 6 months after femoral neck fracture. Rehabilitation is frequently complicated by dementia (present at the time of accident) or by postoperative confusion. Such symptoms may be difficult to diagnose, but assessment should include investigation of possible hypoxia and drug-related confusion. Rehabilitation is also complicated by the significant muscular weakness present in elderly patients. In a patient of 80, the simple exercise of standing from a chair without using the arms is likely to require close to 100% of available muscular effort from the quadriceps muscles. This weakness severely hampers and prolongs efforts at rehabilitation.

Rehabilitation of elderly patients includes addressing the cause of their initial fall and fracture. Patients should be assessed for cardiac and neurological causes of falling; this is best done in consultation with a physician with an interest in the elderly. Many of these patients are clinically malnourished at the time of presentation, and efforts (which must continue after discharge) should be made to correct this. Many fractures in this age group are related to osteoporosis, and consideration should be given to bone mineral density measurement and appropriate treatment.

Because of the many medical and social factors which have to be addressed in elderly fracture patients, the provision of an effective service requires a team approach (Box 21.2). Most orthopaedic units are developing collaborative care plans, patient pathways and the like, which

---

Box 21.2   The team approach to fractures in the elderly

- Doctors
  — orthopaedic surgeon
  — elderly care physician
  — ward-based doctors
  — general practitioner

- Nurses
  — orthopaedic
  — elderly care
  — community

- Rehabilitationists:
  — physiotherapy
  — occupational therapy

- Social worker (if local authority residence needed)

- Relatives and carers

---

aim to integrate the activities of the various professional groups in a patient-centred system. Considerable thought has to be given to the maintenance of continuity of care, especially when the patient is transferred from the acute orthopaedic ward to an elderly rehabilitation ward.

Great improvements have occurred recently as a consequence of the introduction of named nurses, who are best placed to integrate all the information and the efforts of other members. Another helpful innovation has been the discipline of discharge planning, which can begin almost as soon as the patient is admitted. The large volume of hip fractures has driven considerable clinical audit efforts, including a major initiative by the Royal College of Surgeons, to investigate which improvements in practice affect the outcome significantly.

CONCLUSION

It is worth repeating that, in the elderly patient, a fracture is usually only one feature of gradual physical deterioration. This renders management of elderly patients with fractures a challenge which is presented daily in most hospital orthopaedic departments. The management strategy for such patients must emphasise the importance of concurrent medical problems, in the interests of both the efficiency of the process of managing such patients while in hospital and the quality of the eventual outcome.

22 | Joint injuries

Case history

An 18-year-old student injured his right shoulder whilst playing rugby. He fell heavily during a tackle, and felt severe pain in the right shoulder. He was unable to move his shoulder subsequently. He was taken to the A&E department where he was noted to have an obvious shoulder deformity. A clinical diagnosis of a right anterior shoulder dislocation was made. Further, it was noted that he had an area of numbness over his right deltoid. There did not appear to be any other neurovascular signs in the right arm. X-ray confirmed the shoulder dislocation, and this was reduced under general anaesthetic.

After his shoulder dislocation, he wore a sling for 6 weeks and then mobilised his right shoulder with physiotherapy. The area of numbness over his deltoid resolved within about 2 months of the injury. He did not notice any particular weakness, but the orthopaedic surgeons examined the muscles in his shoulder at regular intervals to ensure recovery. He regained a full range of shoulder movement over the next 2 months. However, when he returned to playing rugby, he sustained a further right shoulder dislocation within a couple of weeks, and subsequently had four further dislocations over the following 2 years. Each of these was reduced in hospital, initially under general anaesthetic, but with the last one being reduced in the A&E department with analgesia. He had further physiotherapy to his shoulder which did not seem to improve the situation appreciably.

The student attended the orthopaedic outpatients, where he was noted to have some apprehension on external rotation of his right arm. Further X-rays were taken which demonstrated a Hill Sacks lesion – a notch in the bone of the humeral head. In view of the many dislocations of his shoulder and the severe effect this was having on his sporting activities, surgery was advised. Under general anaesthetic, the shoulder joint was exposed from the front and the detached glenoid labrum was reattached to the glenoid rim, thus reconnecting the anterior glenohumeral ligament to its correct insertion at the edge of the glenoid. The torn joint capsule was also tightened. Postoperatively, he was allowed to mobilise his shoulder after 6 weeks in a sling. He initially had some restriction of external rotation of his arm, but otherwise he recovered full movements quickly. He has not had any further dislocation.

Key points

- Joint injuries can result in long-standing problems:
  — stiffness
  — instability
  — arthritis

- Dislocations require reduction

- Following surgical treatment, injured joints should be moved as early as possible, to encourage nourishment of injured cartilage by synovial fluid

- Recurrence of instability is common and sometimes requires surgery

Dislocations and other joint injuries are second only to fractures in their prevalence as injuries presenting to orthopaedic departments. Because normal function in the major joints is essential for the use of the limbs, it is important to take joint injuries very seriously. Inadequate treatment will lead to long-term problems due to:

- stiffness
- instability
- secondary osteoarthritis

Joints can be injured in several ways (Box 22.1). *Dislocation* is defined as complete loss of contact between normally congruent surfaces; *subluxation* means partial loss of contact. These may occur with or without an associated fracture, and intra-articular fracture will damage joint surfaces with or without associated dislocation. *Ligament ruptures* may present even without subluxation/dislocation – although some loss of joint congruency must have occurred at the moment of injury. *Ligament sprain* means that the ligament was stressed sufficiently to cause some damage of collagen fibres, but complete structural failure did not occur. *Meniscal injuries* are common in the knee.

Box 22.1   Joint injuries

- **Dislocations (and subluxations)**
- **Fracture-dislocations (and fracture-subluxations)**
- **Intra-articular fractures**
- **Ligament ruptures (and sprains)**
- **Meniscal tears**

In this chapter, there is first a general discussion of the pathology, clinical features and management of joint injuries, and then an atlas of the commonly encountered joint injuries.

PATHOLOGY

Articular cartilage is a complex structure consisting of cells and extracellular matrix. The principal cell type is the chondrocyte, and the extra-cellular matrix which these cells produce consists of collagens and proteoglycans. The cartilage matrix is capable of absorbing a relatively large amount of water, which is expelled under pressure. Thus joint movement, with changing pressures on different areas of articular cartilage, results in a circulation of the fluid between the articular cartilage and the surrounding synovial fluid in the joint, which nourishes the cells in this avascular tissue. It also encourages the development of a thin fluid layer at the surface of the area of contact between two articular surfaces, which promotes lubrication of the joint.

The dependence of articular cartilage on movement to obtain synovial fluid circulation in this way means that early movement of joints after injury is likely to improve results. It both improves the nutrition of chondrocytes, which may be marginally viable after injury, and decreases the risk of adhesion formation. It is now possible to provide such early movement on a prolonged basis using continuous passive motion machines which move the affected joint through a desired range of movement.

Articular cartilage only exhibits a weak ability to repair itself after injury. When full-thickness defects develop in hyaline cartilage, subsequent repair is generally by fibrocartilage in adults. This cartilage tends to be mechanically unsatisfactory and deteriorates at a relatively early stage. Injuries to articular cartilage may include intra-articular fractures, such as osteochondral fractures where a piece of underlying bone and its attached cartilage lie free in the joint. Articular fractures may result in an abnormal contour, such as a step, in the articular surface. This produces abnormally high loads passing through localised areas of the joint surface, causing cartilage breakdown and eventual osteoarthritis.

The other structures frequently damaged in joint injuries are menisci and ligaments.

Menisci are composed of fibrocartilage, where in addition to collagen type II there is collagen type I. They are present in the wrist (in the distal radio-ulnar joint), the temperomandibular joint, the acromioclavicular joint and the knee. Damage to knee menisci are common causes for persisting symptoms after injury and a good deal is now known about their physiology. They are important in load-bearing, equalising the pressure distribution across the articular cartilage of the tibiofemoral joint. Thus, removal of a whole meniscus results in localised high pressure on the articular cartilage of the knee, rather than evenly spread moderate pressures. Total meniscectomy therefore predisposes to articular cartilage breakdown and osteoarthritis. The central portion of the meniscus is avascular, but the peripheral part adjacent to the synovium does have a blood supply and therefore the potential to heal after injury.

Ligaments. These are responsible for controlling the stability of joints, together with the bony architecture of the joint and the surrounding muscles. They may be separate from the fibrous tissue of the joint capsule, but more commonly exist as named thickenings in it. The principal ligaments of the knee and ankle are shown in Figure 22.1.

CLINICAL FEATURES OF JOINT INJURIES

Most patients with primary joint injuries will give a history of an episode of trauma. However, joint injuries may characteristically be the causes of recurrent problems, and when patients present with such recurrences there is frequently no recent history of trauma, or only very minimal violence. Such conditions include recurrent shoulder dislocation and recurrent mechanical instability of the knee following previous meniscal injuries.

Acute dislocations

Patients generally give a history of specific trauma. In the upper limb this is frequently a fall to the outstretched hand. Such a mechanism can cause a wide variety of relatively common injuries, such as glenohumeral dislocations in the shoulder and dislocations of the elbow. In addition, this may cause less common injuries such as dislocations of carpal bones. In the lower limb, substantial force is required to cause dislocations due to the strong ligaments. Thus the characteristic cause of hip dislocation is a longitudinal force applied along the

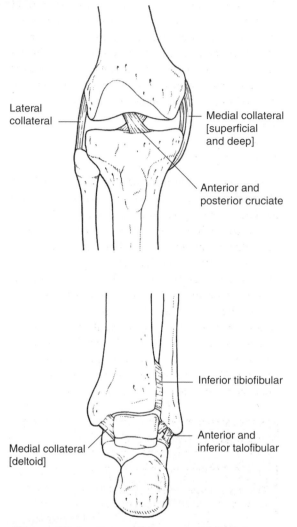

Figure 22.1 Principal ligaments of the knee and ankle.

femur due to dashboard injury in a high-velocity road traffic accident. Knee dislocations also characteristically require substantial force, although dislocations of the patellofemoral joint can occur with relatively little violence.

Examination

Examination of dislocated joints is frequently all that is required to establish the diagnosis. However, it is sometimes difficult to distinguish between fractures close to a joint and dislocations.

X-rays are important in ensuring accuracy of diagnosis. Inspection of a dislocated joint will frequently reveal characteristic deformities, which may in some circumstances be easier to discern than the abnormalities on the X-ray. These are described for individual joints in the atlas section (p. 317). One situation where X-rays are difficult to interpret is the posterior dislocation of the shoulder. The loss of the normal prominence of the shoulder tip, combined with the obvious and abnormal posterior prominence of the humeral head makes this clinically almost unmistakable. In contrast, the anteroposterior (AP) X-ray in particular may frequently be passed as normal.

Significant swelling is often present as well as deformity. Discerning the degree of the swelling may be difficult if the joint is deeply placed (e.g. hip joint). The dislocation is frequently associated with extensive bruising. Substantial haemarthrosis after such injuries is unusual since dislocations, almost by definition, result in capsular rupture; this results in any haemarthrosis being allowed to escape. As with fractures, there is substantial loss of functional ability with dislocation. Usually it is impossible to achieve even a few degrees of movement in any direction in the affected joint because of the protective spasm which arises in the surrounding muscles.

Investigations

X-rays are useful to diagnose dislocations, and it is important to obtain adequate views in two orthogonal planes. The anatomical AP and lateral views may not be the most useful, as some joints do not lie parallel to the conventional anatomical axes. For example, the glenohumeral joint lies approximately 30° internally rotated from the sagittal plane and an ordinary lateral view would be unhelpful because the thorax is in the way. So, in order to obtain orthogonal views of the glenohumeral joint, the AP X-ray must be taken at 30° from the sagittal plane; the lateral is replaced by the so-called axial view where the X-rays are directed from above the shoulder into the axilla.

It should be emphasised that the fact that a joint is no longer dislocated at the time of X-ray does not mean that the joint has not been dislocated during the injury and then reduced. Useful signs may still be present on X-ray suggesting substantial joint injury. These include evidence of lipohaemarthosis (the fat is detected as a very dark area with a fluid level due to the blood). Soft tissue swelling may be obvious on the X-ray. In addition, avulsion fractures from the margins of the joint indicate a high degree of likelihood of avulsion injuries of ligamentous origins or insertion.

Sometimes it is desirable to investigate the anatomy of the dislocation in more detail. The best choice of investigation varies, but computed tomography is frequently employed. This is of particular value if there are associated fractures (fracture-dislocation).

Problems associated with dislocations

Dislocations cause neurovascular problems rather more commonly than do fractures. This may be because of the persisting stretching caused by a joint which remains dislocated for any significant period of time. Nerves which are particularly at risk include the axillary nerve at the shoulder, the ulnar nerve at the elbow and the sciatic nerve at the hip. Similarly, blood vessels are sometimes at substantial risk. In particular, knee dislocations are attended by frequent damage to the popliteal artery. This may result in severe distal ischaemia, and it is vital to double check both distal pulses and capillary circulation. Some surgeons would recommend angiography as a routine investigation in this circumstance. A vascular problem which may arise more insidiously after dislocation is that of avascular necrosis. Some areas of bone have relatively precarious blood supplies which may be interrupted by dislocation. These areas include the femoral head. The two large feeder arteries in the dorsal capsule of the femoral neck are frequently damaged by posterior dislocation of the hip. This means that reduction of a dislocated hip is a surgical emergency. Early reduction minimises the risk of avascular necrosis of the femoral head which would lead to osteoarthrosis of the hip due to bony collapse of the femoral head.

Acute dislocations may lead to severe joint stiffness if they are managed by reduction and then prolonged immobilisation. The healing response following soft tissue trauma of dislocation includes substantial scarring, and tissues allowed to organise around the joint may result in 'arthrofibrosis'. Thus early mobilisation of the affected joint, possibly achieved by use of a continuous passive motion machine, is best. Physiotherapy at this stage after the dislocation is principally employed to ensure an adequate range of movement, thus minimising the risk of important adhesion formation. Once severe arthrofibrosis has developed it usually proves very difficult to treat.

A further complication of joint dislocation is recurrent instability. Once ligaments have been substantially damaged, they may not resume their normal strength. This is particularly the case if the affected joint has relatively poor bony stability and relies heavily on soft tissues for stability. For example, in young sporting males, recurrent dislocation may occur in up to 50% of those who sustain acute shoulder dislocation. In contrast, recurrence is far less common after this injury in the older age groups. This appears to reflect the differing degree of violence acquired to achieve the original dislocation in the two different groups. Recurrent dislocations may arise with relatively minor trauma after the initial injury; the mechanism of injury in the first few dislocations may be similar to the original injury, but eventually even trivial disturbances of the joint may result in dislocation. In addition to the pain that this causes, a substantial loss of confidence results such that the joint cannot be relied upon to function normally in any critical situation. The anatomical basis of this recurrent instability includes the development of a notch in the humeral head (the Hill Sacks lesion) and detachment of the glenoid labrum and anterior glenohumeral ligament, which normally limits external rotation and anterior translation of the humeral head. Patients may also report sensations of the joint 'coming out' when complete dislocation has manifestly not occurred; this is common if subluxation occurs (e.g. at the shoulder or knee) and should not be dismissed.

Acute ligament injuries

These injuries may occur without frank dislocation, but usually require a definite history of trauma. Occasionally, patients present with deficient ligaments of long standing, but no history

of trauma is recalled. It is generally held that such patients have had a previous injury which they have forgotten.

The principal feature of joints with a ligament injury is the presence of abnormal mobility. The direction and magnitude of the abnormal mobility is determined by the normal function of the ligament affected, and the presence of any secondary restraints. Thus, in a complete disruption of the lateral ligament complex of the ankle, abnormal mobility may be detected on forced inversion of the heel (the talus tilts into varus due to the lack of restraining forces). However, the action of the peroneal tendons will resist varus tilt. Therefore, detection of the abnormal mobility may be difficult in the unanaesthetised patient due to (often involuntary) muscle forces.

The abnormal joint mobility leads to clinical symptoms, characteristically of two types:

- *Instability and giving way of the joint.* This is true both of upper limb and lower limb joints. The characteristic movement required to elicit instability varies from joint to joint; in the knee, twisting on a partially flexed loaded knee (such as when changing direction while running) will frequently result in transient subluxation of the ACL deficient knee
- *The joint is often painful.* The pain may be principally associated with episodes of instability or subluxation, where tissues are stretched abnormally. Later, recurrent instability may lead to degenerative changes (osteoarthritis) in the joint, so it may be painful even without additional episodes of subluxation or instability.

Instability of the joint may also lead to secondary damage to other structures, such as menisci. For example, subluxation of the knee due to ACL laxity often leads to subsequent meniscal damage.

Meniscal injuries

In contrast to ligament injuries, it is now clear that degenerative changes in knee menisci (including some tears) can occur due to ageing processes, without abnormal loading or trauma being applied. These become commoner with increasing age, while trauma is overwhelmingly the commonest cause of fibrocartilage problems in young patients.

There are three principal features of fibrocartilage damage in a joint, exemplified by the features of meniscal tears in the knee:

- the joint may be painful, with the area of pain usually well localised to the damaged area of cartilage on the tibiofemoral joint line
- the joint may be unreliable, with recurrent giving way under load
- the joint may lock and become stuck due to a mechanical block to movement caused by a fragment of the fibrocartilage becoming trapped between the opposing joint surfaces.

In the case of the knee, the standard terminology is that a 'locked knee' is one with a block to extension, rather than flexion. This is frequently caused by a meniscal tear but can also be caused by a loose body – a fragment from an old osteochondral fracture – within the knee. A block to flexion is not commonly caused by meniscal tears. A history of the joint becoming temporarily completely immovable because of severe pain is known as 'pseudolocking'. This is generally caused by pain around or within the joint rather than a mechanical problem.

Differentiating between cartilage and ligament injuries is frequently difficult, and is of increasing importance as meniscal repair is now undertaken for some cartilage injuries. One useful pointer is whether a haemarthrosis is present. A haemarthrosis occurs rapidly, taking only an hour or so to develop after the traumatic incident. Haemarthrosis occurs in ligament injuries (especially cruciate ligament injuries) and some (peripheral) meniscal injuries. In contrast, an effusion of synovial fluid comes up over a period of about 12 hours, often overnight. Effusions occur in most isolated meniscal injuries.

Investigations
Adequate diagnosis may be difficult in these injuries. There is often nothing to see on plain X-ray. Eliciting abnormal mobility of the joint, especially in the first stage after the causative injury, may be impossible without examination under anaesthesia (EUA), possibly with an arthroscopic examination of the affected joint. If such an EUA is not undertaken, subsequent diagnosis may remain difficult, requiring stress X-rays, arthroscopy or MRI to reach a firm diagnosis.

MRI permits imaging of soft tissue structures. The use of this technique in the diagnosis of meniscal injuries is now widespread. There is some concern about the difficulty of interpretation of MR images, and the role of this investigation in joint injuries is still evolving.

Problems associated with ligament and fibrocartilage injuries
Although ligament and fibrocartilage injuries tend to require significant *initial* precipitating trauma, subsequently they may cause recurrent symptoms of pain, instability or locking with minimal precipitating cause. These symptoms may be very disabling, particularly for sports players and manual workers. An unreliable limb may result in some patients, e.g. those who work at a height such as painters or roofers, losing their job.

Diagnosis may be difficult, and some patterns of such injuries may still be unrecognised. Thus the recognition that anterior cruciate ligament laxity permits recurrent subluxation of the tibiofemoral joint is only relatively recent, but very large numbers of patients are now clearly seen to be suffering from problems of ACL laxity. Presumably, these symptoms were previously undiagnosed. Similarly, symptoms due to acetabular labral tears are only now beginning to be recognised.

MANAGEMENT OF JOINT INJURIES
Acute dislocations

Dislocations almost invariably require reduction. The only common exception to this rule is the acromioclavicular joint, which is often left unreduced, as the difficulty of obtaining and maintaining a reduction means that operative reduction and fixation with a screw provides the only really effective method of treatment. Some authors feel that the risks of this procedure outweigh the possible benefits. However, other dislocations should be reduced as promptly as possible under an appropriate degree of anaesthesia.

Manipulative reduction is possible for most dislocations. Occasionally the reduction of a dislocation may be blocked by an avulsed tissue component or a bony fragment. Under these circumstances, an *open reduction* may be necessary to ensure adequate reconstitution of the joint. After dislocation, the joint is generally rested for a few days either in a cast or a bulky plaster wool and crepe bandage in the lower limb, or in a sling in the upper limb. A plaster slab may be applied across the joint if severe pain and swelling appear likely.

There is debate about how long to immobilise some joints after injury. On the one hand, it may be that immobilisation will allow ligaments to heal in a more nearly physiological configuration. On the other hand, joint surfaces are thought to benefit from early movement, as described above. This debate is not fully settled, but there is an increasing trend towards early mobilisation, not necessarily combined with weight-bearing, of all joint injuries.

Acute ligament injuries

Ligament injuries may require examination under anaesthetic to establish an adequate diagnosis. Many patients can compensate for the abnormal mobility of their joint by adequate muscular strength and control, which may develop following physiotherapy regimes. If these are insufficient, ligament reconstruction can be undertaken. Generally this is performed using a piece of tendon as a graft (e.g. middle third of patellar tendon for an anterior cruciate ligament reconstruction). Such a graft will eventually reform a satisfactory ligament. Synthetic ligament substitutes have also been employed.

Meniscal injuries

Fibrocartilage injuries may be treated by either repair or excision. Repair is difficult as the periphery is the only part with any significant vascular supply. Tears in the substance of the fibrocartilage (rather than around the rim) are unlikely to heal and partial excision is generally the treatment of choice. The fibrocartilages may have an important role in load distribution across the joint surface. Meniscectomy in the knee markedly increases loading on the central cartilage of the femoral and tibial condyles and may ultimately lead to osteoarthrosis. It is therefore now common policy to minimise the amount of cartilage resected during a meniscectomy, so that only the markedly unstable tissue is removed.

Recurrent joint instability

Recurrent instability of joints particularly affects the shoulder, where either subluxation or dislocation may occur, and the knee and ankle, where subluxation is common after ligament injuries. Recurrent dislocation is fairly common after total hip replacement, but is very rare in the hip otherwise. It is important to realise that patients may describe a variety of symptoms from subluxation, including the joint 'coming out', giving way, pain and clicking. X-rays are often normal, at least initially, and there may be little to find on simple clinical examination, but patients' complaints should not be dismissed without considering instability as a possible cause of their symptoms.

Recurrent shoulder instability most commonly follows an initial shoulder dislocation, especially in young men (below 25 years). Subsequently, multiple episodes of dislocation or subluxation may occur, with each episode being precipitated by progressively smaller amounts of trauma. This instability is associated with damage to the anterior glenohumeral ligament and glenoid labrum (Bankart lesion) or an impression defect on the posterior surface of the humeral head (Hill Sacks lesion; this tends to cause subluxation with the humerus in external rotation). Physiotherapy may be of some value; however, many patients come to surgery. Various operations are used, the principles being to limit external rotation (e.g. by reefing subscapularis and the anterior shoulder capsule, as in the Putti–Platt procedure) or to reconstruct the labrum and glenohumeral ligament (as in the Bankart procedure). Operation is usually successful, providing the diagnosis is correct (which includes the direction in which instability is occurring).

Knee and ankle instability usually follow ligament injuries (cruciate and anterior talofibular, respectively). Many patients can be managed adequately with physiotherapy, or occasionally with braces or supports; if surgery is required, the commonly employed procedures involve using a section of tendon as a ligament subsitute, usually aiming for a replacement of the ligament in an anatomical position.

AN ATLAS OF JOINT INJURIES AND DISLOCATIONS

In a similar fashion to fractures, joint injuries and dislocations frequently occur in characteristic patterns. The following pages present an outline of mechanisms, presenting features, treatment and consequent problems for the commoner joint injuries. Although ligament damage is common in spinal injuries, the issues of their management and diagnosis have been addressed in the atlas of fractures, as ligament injuries and fractures often coexist in the spine. Ligament sprains of the spine are common as a component of back injuries, but are not well characterised.

Joint injuries

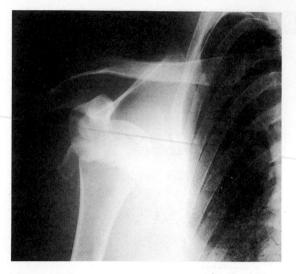

Figure 22.2   Anterior dislocation of the anterior shoulder.

ANTERIOR SHOULDER DISLOCATION (GLENOHUMERAL JOINT)

Common mechanisms

Fall to outstretched hand. Often recurrent (sometimes with minimal trauma).

Presenting features

Loss of shoulder contour. There may be loss of sensation in axillary nerve area (i.e. skin overlying deltoid).

Treatment

Manipulative reduction, under GA preferably, but can be done with analgesia and sedation.

Special problems

Check axillary nerve before manipulation. Palsy leaves deltoid paralysed. May need surgical stabilisation if dislocations are recurrent.

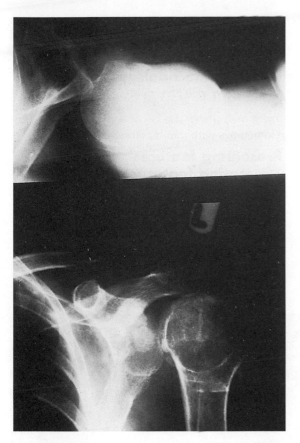

Figure 22.3 Axial and AP views of posterior shoulder dislocation. The AP view shows the 'light bulb' sign where a lateral view of the humeral head is seen on the AP film.

POSTERIOR SHOULDER DISLOCATION (GLENOHUMERAL JOINT)

Common mechanisms

Fall to outstretched hand. Fits. Electric shocks.

Presenting features

Loss of shoulder contour. Humeral head prominent posteriorly, but 'empty' glenoid anteriorly. AP X-ray can be deceptive, but axial view shows it well.

Treatment

Manipulative reduction.

Special problems

Diagnosis often missed. Always get an axial view if there is any possibility of dislocation.

ACROMIOCLAVICULAR DISLOCATION

Common mechanisms

Fall to point of shoulder; blow due to sporting injury.

Presenting features

Obvious prominence of tip of clavicle (which may tent the skin).

Treatment

Controversial. Either ignore *or* carry out surgical maintenance of reduction.

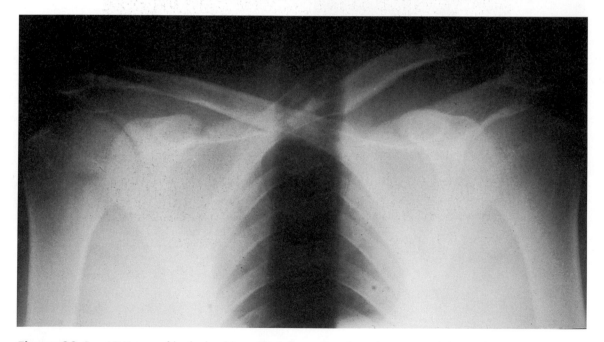

Figure 22.4   AP X-rays of both shoulders. The left acromioclavicular joint is dislocated.

INTERPHALANGEAL JOINT DISLOCATION (FINGER)

Common mechanisms

Direct blow to fingertip.

Presenting features

Obvious deformity of finger.

Treatment

Manipulative reduction and early mobilisation.

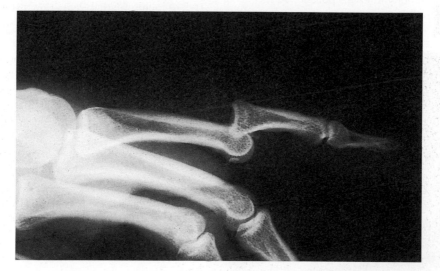

Figure 22.5 Interphalangeal joint dislocation in index finger.

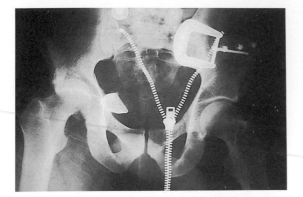

Figure 22.6   Right hip dislocation. The acetabulum overlies the femoral head. The hip had dislocated posteriorly, and this patient had a sciatic nerve palsy.

HIP DISLOCATION

Common mechanisms

Often after road traffic accident (dashboard injury to front of knee).

Presenting features

Flexed, slighty adducted and internally rotated hip (posterior dislocation). There may be associated acetabular rim fracture.

Treatment

Urgent manipulative reduction. May need open reduction and internal fixation of associated acetabular fracture.

Special problems

Risk of avascular necrosis of the femoral head and sciatic nerve palsy.

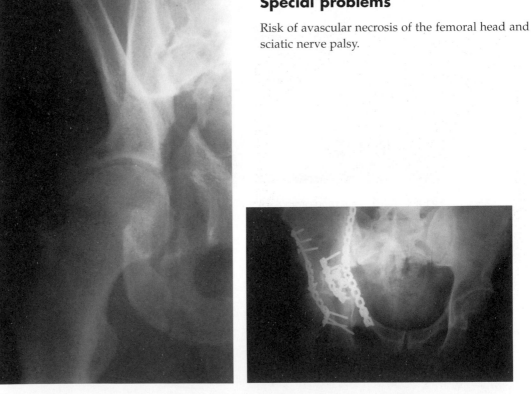

Figure 22.7   X-rays after a severe acetabular fracture and subsequent fixation.

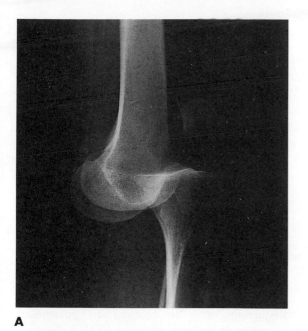

A

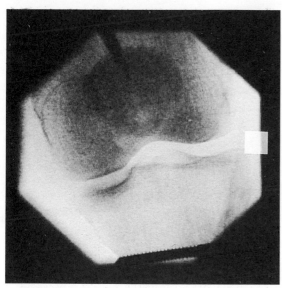

B

KNEE DISLOCATION

Common mechanisms

RTA or other high-energy injury. Often forced varus/valgus stress, or anteroposterior force.

Presenting features

Obvious swelling and deformity. Major risk to neurovascular structures. There may be vascular damage even if pulses are normal.

Treatment

Urgent reduction. Knee ligaments not usually readily repairable. Vascular consultation and/or angiography.

Figure 22.8   Lateral X-ray of knee dislocation (**A**). As well as complete ligament disruption, vascular damage is common. An intra-operative angiogram (**B**) shows a block of the femoral artery at the popliteal fossa. The dye has shown the femoral artery proximally (behind the upper pole of the patella), but it has not filled distally.

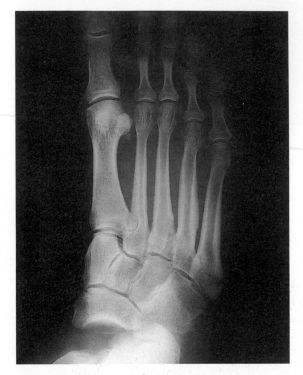

Figure 22.9 X-ray of subtalar/talonavicular dislocation. The medial skin was rented over the talar head and required urgent reduction.

SUBTALAR DISLOCATION

Common mechanisms

Forced inversion injury.

Presenting features

Talar head appears prominent on medial side of foot. There may be marked tenting of skin, leading to ischaemic damage.

Treatment

Urgent manipulative reduction.

Special problems

Reduction may be blocked by interposed ligaments or tendons.

ANTERIOR CRUCIATE LIGAMENT INJURY

Common mechanisms

History of twisting injury on flexed knee, or hyperextension injury. Often history of 'popping' sound. After first injury, recurrent giving way when twisting on flexed knee.

Presenting features

Haemarthrosis (acute injury). Positive anterior drawer sign, Lachmann sign or pivot shift (see Ch. 3).

Treatment

Initially, physiotherapy. Cruciate ligament reconstruction if recurrent symptoms.

Special problems

Long-term risk of osteoarthritis; effect of treatment on preventing this is unclear. Also risk of meniscal injury.

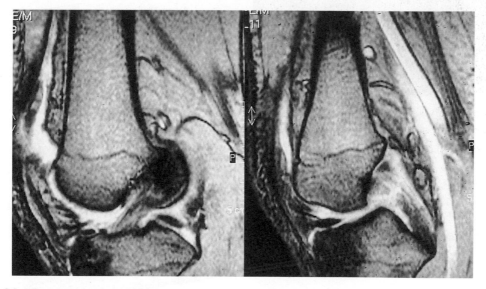

Figure 22.10 Anterior cruciate ligament injury. MRI scans are useful in assessing the cruciate ligaments. This image shows the knee of a patient with recurrent giving way; the anterior cruciate is intact in this patient (left), the posterior cruciate ligament is difficult to see and is ruptured (right). There was a posterior 'sag' sign (or false anterior drawer sign (Fig. 3.23)), which enabled the clinician to tell that the posterior rather than the anterior cruciate was ruptured.

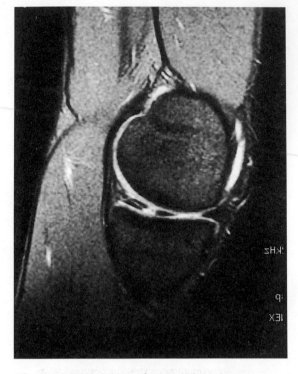

Figure 22.11 MRI of meniscal tear. It is possible to see a white (fluid) line in the posterior horn of the medial meniscus. This represents a tear in the substance of the meniscus.

MENISCAL INJURY (KNEE)

Common mechanisms

Twisting injury or forced varus/valgus. Often recurrent locking, giving way or joint line pain.

Presenting features

Block to extension; effusion; joint line tenderness.

Treatment

Investigation by MRI scan or arthroscopy. Treatment by meniscal repair (occasionally) or partial meniscectomy (usually).

ANKLE LIGAMENT INJURY (ANTERIOR TALOFIBULAR LIGAMENT)

Common mechanisms

Inversion strain. There may be recurrent instability of the ankle, with tendency to 'go over' on uneven ground.

Presenting features

Tenderness and swelling over anterior talofibular ligament. There may be evidence of tibiotalar instability on examination.

Treatment

Investigation with strain views of ankle. Physiotherapy. If still unsatisfactory, consider reconstruction of ankle ligaments.

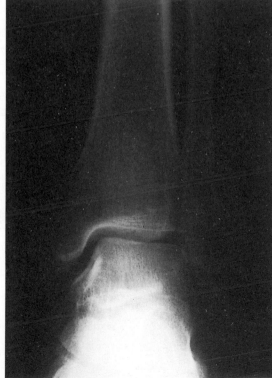 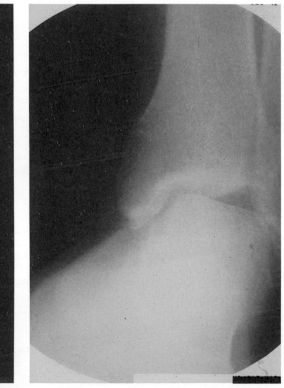

A   B

Figure 22.12   X-rays of unstable ankle at rest (**A**) and with varus stress applied under general anaesthetic (**B**).

23 | Soft tissue injuries (in the limbs)

Case history

Following an episode of heavy drinking a 19-year-old man presented to the A&E department. He had got into an argument with a man as he was leaving the pub and, in his own words: 'I became so angry, I stuck my hand through the window'. On examination he was noted to have several lacerations on the palmar surface of his forearm and wrist. The most substantial one was a laceration crossing most of his forearm from the ulnar side about 2 inches proximal to the wrist. This was bleeding copiously. He was rather uncooperative, and asserted that sensation in his hand was entirely normal. He was unable to actively move the little or ring finger at all. It was difficult to assess intrinsic muscle function at this stage. Vascularity of the hand appeared normal. The other lacerations were extensive but appeared superficial. An X-ray of his forearm and hand clearly demonstrated the presence of a substantial piece of glass in the deep laceration. His wound was covered with an antiseptic pressure dressing, which controlled the bleeding, and he was booked for the next day's trauma list.

By the next morning, having sobered up, the young man realised that in fact he had a completely numb little finger. At surgery the piece of glass was removed and the wounds were thoroughly explored. He was found to have a complete division of both ulnar nerve and ulnar artery, and several flexor tendons. The median nerve was explored and appeared to be intact. The tendons were all repaired. The ulnar nerve was repaired using an *epineural repair*, and the ends of the ulnar artery were tied together to take the tension off the nerve

repair. Postoperatively, he was managed in a *back slab* for a period of 4 weeks to ensure that the nerve repair was not disrupted by wrist movement. During this time he was started with active and passive finger stretching exercises to guard against the development of an ulnar claw hand.

On removal of his back slab, more active physiotherapy was undertaken and he was provided with a splint to wear at night, again to guard against the development of an ulnar claw hand. He regained active finger flexion quite quickly over a period of approximately 3 months, but many of the fine movements in his hand were unsatisfactory. He found writing

Key points

- Penetrating limb wounds form a large part of the work of A&E, orthopaedic and plastic surgery departments

- Wounds may involve damage to:
  — skin and muscle
  — peripheral nerves
  — arteries and veins
  — tendons

- The healing of a soft tissue wound depends on the vascularity of the tissues at the wound edges

- It is essential to be aware of the deep structures that could be damaged by any given wound and to know how to test their function

- If in doubt, assume that deep structures at risk have been damaged and arrange to have them surgically explored

difficult (which didn't bother him much). He also found himself completely outclassed in the darts team whereas previously he had been an excellent darts player. More mundane things such as tying shoelaces were also difficult. Over a period of approximately 18 months there was some improvement in the fine movements in his hand, and sensation on the ulnar side of his hand did slowly improve. However, when he was eventually discharged from follow-up 2 years after the accident, use of his hand was still somewhat restricted for tasks involving fine movement.

PATHOLOGY

This chapter is mainly concerned with penetrating wounds in the limbs. Soft tissues can of course be damaged by blunt injury as well but, with the exception of ligament injuries (see Ch. 22), their management is mainly supportive. The incidence of soft tissue injuries is unknown, but their management forms an important part of the work of A&E, orthopaedic and plastic surgery departments. Such injuries may be divided into skin and muscle injuries, nerve injuries, vascular injuries and tendon injuries.

Skin and muscle injuries

Skin injuries can be classified as contusions or abrasions, where there is partial-thickness damage to the skin, and lacerations, where there is full-thickness damage to the skin. However, closed injuries can involve full-thickness damage when the perforating blood supply to the skin from the underlying fascia is sheared – this is known as *degloving* and its diagnosis is both difficult and important. Common causes for lacerations include knife injuries and injuries on glass. However, in old people with fragile skin, lacerations can also be caused by shearing of the skin; this often happens over the front of the tibia. In younger people, lacerations can also be caused by crushing injuries – the 'burst laceration'.

The repair process seen following such injuries is in many ways the paradigm of wound repair, which may be by primary or secondary intention.

Primary intention

An excellent example of wound repair by primary intention is that which occurs after a clean incised surgical wound is subsequently neatly sutured. The amount of tissue necrosis will be minimal, and because of the wound edge apposition and lack of dead space in the wound, the distances which must be traversed by the epidermis (on the surface) and by the granulation tissue and scar tissue (deep to the surface) are minimal. The wound is therefore sealed to bacteria after a very short period of time and attains a functional level of wound strength within 3–4 weeks.

Secondary intention

Wound repair by secondary intention occurs in a ragged or contaminated wound which is left open. Even if contaminated material is thoroughly excised and removed, the amount of damaged tissue and consequent necrosis will be greater than in the clean wound. Additionally, because the wound edges have not been brought together the distances which both scar tissue and epidermis have to traverse to seal and then heal the wound will be greater. Initially, there is bleeding and a clot forms. This will turn into a scab which forms a protective layer over the underlying repair process. The defect will be partly filled by granulation tissue which will be gradually covered by migrating epidermis to recover the wound. Cicatrisation (wound contracture) will reduce the size of the wound, making epithelialisation faster. Secondary wound healing takes longer than primary wound healing, is less predictable and may give very unsatisfactory cosmetic results. If the wound contracture is over a joint, the range of movement at this joint may be markedly diminished, leaving a permanent contracture.

Peripheral nerve injuries

Nerve injuries may occur due to all of the mechanisms described under soft tissue injuries. A further mechanism of injury is when an acute traction force is applied to a nerve; this will often result in substantial internal disruption. Such injuries are not generally amenable to operative repair, and the prognosis for their spontaneous improvement is unfortunately poor. These injuries often affect the brachial plexus, typically in motorcyclists who fall from their machines at high speeds, when loading on the shoulder drives the shoulder distally, causing a massive distraction force on the brachial plexus and serious injury. However, the majority of severe peripheral nerve injuries are caused by lacerations, most often on broken glass.

In general, repair in the central nervous system is considered to occur only by formation of scar (glial) tissue, with no attempt at nerve regeneration. In contrast, nerve regeneration does occur in the peripheral nervous system, albeit to a rather meagre extent. Much research and development work is currently underway to increase the vigour of nerve regeneration after injury, using molecular biological methods.

Each peripheral 'nerve fibre' consists of the nerve axon, the protracted process of the nerve cell whose cell body is in the spinal cord. The axons may be myelinated or unmyelinated, depending on whether they have Schwann cells forming a tube of myelin insulation around them. The Schwann cells with non-myelinated fibres provide a purely supportive function. In either case, each axon runs in its own thin connective tissue tube, formed by the *endoneurium*. Fascicles (bundles) of nerve fibres are each covered in a *perineurial* sheath. There are several such fascicles in most named peripheral nerves, and the fascicles are held together to form the complete peripheral nerve by the *epineurium*.

Maintenance of normal nerve function depends on distal transport of protein manufactured in the cell body. The cell body, being in the central nervous system, is remote from the more peripheral parts of the nerve and therefore a specialised axoplasmic transport system exists. However, a nerve injury (such as a laceration) will inevitably interrupt transport processes, and subsequent to this the part of the nerve distal to the laceration will die. This, together with the scavenging of the consequent debris, is known as Wallerian degeneration.

Nerve injuries have classically been graded into three types, depending on two crucial issues of severity:

- whether there has been death of the axon distal to the lesion, or just a temporary conduction block
- whether there has been physical disruption of the connective tissue tubes in which the axons run.

Neurapraxia, axonotmesis and neurotmesis

Neurapraxia describes a recoverable conduction block due to crushing of the nerve. Good return of function can be expected and regeneration does not need to take place. *Axonotmesis* results from a more severe crush, or traction injury, where Wallerian degeneration takes place, but the endoneurial tubes remain intact. Here nerve regeneration is required but, since the new axons have intact conduits to guide them to their correct destinations, reasonable function will eventually return. Exploration or attempted repair is most unlikely to be beneficial.

In contrast, *neurotmesis* describes the situation where the nerve is actually divided. Under these circumstances, after a lag period, neural sprouts grow out of the proximal cut end of the nerve and can cross the gap and enter the empty endoneurial tubes of the distal stump. Suturing the cut ends together aids this process, but the problem is getting the appropriate sensory and motor end organs joined to the appropriate central cells, to allow full functional recovery. Unfortunately, it is currently impossible to achieve accurate guidance of such neural sprouts to their correct endoneurial tubes. The best that can be done is to place the nerve ends in as macroscopically close and accurate apposition as possible. Young patients are much better able to adapt to the scrambled information carried by nerves after injury and repair; functional results are usually poor in adults.

In between axonotmesis and neurotmesis are degrees of disruption of the fascicles within an intact epineurium. This is the common pattern after severe traction injuries and the potential for healing is very poor. Usually there is quite a lengthy segment disrupted and the only hope for recovery is to excise this and replace it with a *nerve graft*, usually from the sural nerve.

Vascular injuries

Vascular injuries may arise due to lacerations or to blunt trauma. An example of closed injury is popliteal artery damage due to a knee dislocation; although the artery is not totally disrupted, intimal damage leads to the arterial lumen being blocked. With skilled surgical technique, the cut ends of an artery or vein can be anastomosed. The walls heal by fibrosis and the lumen can be preserved. Sometimes extra tissue needs to be imported, in the shape of a patch graft of harvested vein to prevent constriction at the site of suture. However, there is always a risk of thrombosis and, in practice, the question is whether a particular severed vessel needs to be repaired. In the example case history above, the ulnar artery was not repaired because the radial artery is able to compensate for its absence.

Tendon injuries

Tendon injuries may occur due to direct injury (generally lacerations) or degenerative change. Degenerative change is common in mid-to-late adult life and results in dramatic weakening of the tendon substance. The pathogenesis of this process is not entirely clear, but it appears to be related to vascular changes in the tendons. The result is a weakening of the tendons so that rupture may occur with relatively minor trauma.

Following division, the cut tendon ends can be surgically repaired and will heal by a process consisting principally of fibrosis. The problem is that the scar which forms, as well as joining the tendon ends together, will also tend to join the tendon to its surrounding sheath. In the case of finger tendons, especially flexors, this scarring can limit movement of the digit so much that the functional result is poor to useless.

CLINICAL FEATURES OF SOFT TISSUE INJURIES IN THE LIMBS

Skin and muscle injuries

Penetrating wounds by definition involve disruption of skin, and the most obvious way to describe a laceration is to quantify the size of the

hole that has been created. However, the state of health of the edges of the wound is often the more crucial factor, as should be obvious from the discussion of the healing process above. Furthermore, infection is a potent inhibitor of healing. It is important, therefore, to note the quality of the wound edges and the degree of contamination of the wound, as well as its size.

Incised, torn or crushed muscle has good capacity for repair, provided it has an adequate blood supply. On the other hand, muscle that has been rendered ischaemic by the injury is not only unable to heal, but also constitutes a great danger to the patient because dead muscle is such an excellent culture medium for bacteria.

The essence of clinical assessment of wounds in skin and muscle is, therefore, in addition to describing the structural damage, to estimate the condition, especially the vascularity, of the remaining tissue.

Peripheral nerve injury

Following peripheral nerve injury, many patients are initially unaware of any sensory deficit. The main reason for this is the fact that their body image is so firmly set, and they are so absorbed in the pain of the laceration itself, that they are initially unable to accept that there has been a change in sensibility beyond the laceration. It is also just possible that some crude nerve conduction may be able to 'jump the gap' and give rise to spurious sensibility in the early period before the distal nerve has degenerated. Whatever the reason, there is a great danger of missing significant injury if clinical testing, particularly sensory testing, is done casually.

Adequate knowledge of the motor and sensory function of individual nerves, and the anatomical paths taken by them, is required to predict likely damage from a particular injury. Mild weakness may be explained by pain inhibition, but severe weakness or paralysis not explained by muscle or tendon laceration must be presumed to be due to nerve division until proved otherwise. Sensory testing must be rigorous, otherwise the patient, believing sensibility to be intact, will falsely reassure the examiner. It is important to shield the area being tested from sight of the patient so that they cannot use visual cues. Do not ask 'can you feel me touch you?', but instead set a discriminatory task which can only be achieved if sensibility is present. The simplest is to see if the patient can reliably distinguish the sharp and blunt ends of a safety pin on a series of several random applications. Remember that peripheral nerves may be partially damaged, so test several areas in the territory of a nerve under suspicion.

Vascular injuries

Vascular injuries may affect arteries or veins, or both. Blood loss is an obvious complication of such injuries, and associated nerve injuries are frequent. In general, injury to a single artery is more critical than injury to a single vein as there is usually a more adequate collateral venous circulation. Some arteries also have adequate collateral circulation, but it is imperative to ensure that there is adequate supply before a decision to tie off a vessel, rather than reconstruct or repair it, is taken.

The classical features of arterial insufficiency are:

- pallor
- pulselessness
- paraesthesia (and weakness).

It should be noted, however, that the presence of distal pulses does not rule out arterial injury and associated ischaemia, especially following an intimal injury where a pulse may be present initially, only to disappear later.

Tendon injuries

Any tendon may theoretically be affected by an incised injury, but those at the wrist and in the hand are most frequently involved. The exact site of injury of a particular tendon is important. Thus, laceration of finger flexor tendons at the wrist may be followed by almost normal function after repair. However, laceration in the synovial flexor sheath between the distal palmar crease and the proximal interphalangeal joint presents a very difficult problem of surgical management because of the problem of adhesions forming between the

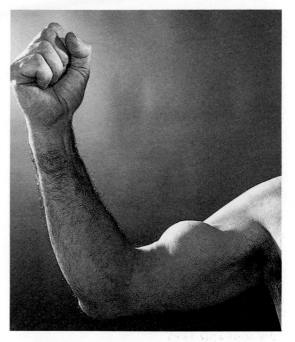

Figure 23.1 Biceps tendon rupture. The tendon of the long head ruptures, often spontaneously. The cosmetic effect is often more marked than the functional effect.

repaired tendon and the flexor sheath, resulting in very poor or even absent finger flexion.

The characteristic feature of any tendon injury is lack of movement at the joint to which the tendon provides motive power. This is sought by examination of the joint for appropriate active movement. The incised wound is usually obvious, but the size of wound may bear little relationship to the degree of underlying damage.

Degenerative tears

Degenerative tears in tendons usually present as a result of mild trauma. The tendons characteristically affected are the Achilles tendon, the quadriceps and patellar tendons of the knee, and the rotator cuff, particularly the supraspinatus. Because of the lack of incised injury, and the history of minimal (usually indirect) trauma, diagnosis is often difficult. The patient complains of pain and some weakness. The weakness complained of frequently appears disproportionate to the injury involved, and there is an unfortunate risk of these patients being dismissed without adequate examination. Examination will reveal a rather boggy and indistinct gap in the tendon. Such a gap is not generally palpable in the muscles of the rotator cuff, which are covered by the acromion. There will be a reduction in power of movement of the affected joint, but this is often incomplete as the tear in the tendon frequently does not extend to the extreme medial and lateral edges.

Several classic sites of degenerative tendon rupture have well-defined clinical tests associated with them:

- The appropriate test for the *Achilles tendon* is Simmond's test, which is performed with the patient kneeling up on the couch, facing away from the examiner. Gently squeezing the calf muscle will normally cause plantarflexion of the ankle; if the Achilles tendon is ruptured, the foot remains flaccidly still.
- The appropriate test for the tendons of the *knee extensor apparatus*, above and below the patella, is to ask the recumbent patient to perform a straight-leg raise.
- The appropriate test for the *rotator cuff* is to look for loss of the ability to *initiate* abduction or to externally rotate the arm against resistance (see shoulder examination, Ch. 3).

MANAGEMENT OF SOFT TISSUE INJURIES

Management of soft tissue lacerations starts with an adequate history to determine the cause of the laceration, the symptoms which have developed since the injury and any other factors such as fitness for anaesthetic. A careful examination must then be undertaken to define the probable extent of damage to deep structures and the vascularity of the wound edges. This requires an adequate knowledge of anatomy and of the techniques of functional examination, particularly of the limbs, as described above.

Skin and muscle injuries

Closure of many incised wounds may be under-taken in the A&E department under local anaesthetic. This only applies to wounds which are adequately clean and where the doctor is satisfied that no deep structures could possibly be involved. Otherwise the wound should be referred for exploration under general or regional anaesthesia, so that structures which might be damaged by the injury can be directly visualised and either confirmed as undamaged or repaired. Ideally, open wounds should be taken to theatre as soon as possible, to reduce the risk of colonisation by hospital organisms. However, little harm comes from a few hours delay, provided the wound is kept covered with an antiseptic dressing, and it is often better to wait until the patient is in a better state for anaesthesia and until the surgical and theatre staff can be present in greater numbers and are more mentally alert.

If there is to be a delay, it is essential to elevate the damaged limb, using a roller towel for the upper limb, and pillows or a frame for the lower limb. This apparently minor and 'low-tech' detail makes a huge difference to outcome because it reduces the development of oedema, which is good for infection and bad for healing.

At surgery, contaminated wounds must be thoroughly cleaned, and all devitalised tissue and foreign material removed. Damaged deep structures should be repaired. Contaminated wounds which are capable of being sutured should not be closed at the same time as they are cleaned but rather 2 or 3 days later at a 'second look' procedure — '*delayed primary closure*'. Prophylactic antibiotics are given, but adequate cleaning and wound excision are more important in preventing wound infection than the use of antibiotics.

Wound repair by secondary intention is often a protracted process. Accordingly, referral to a plastic surgery unit should be considered for patients who have wounds which cannot easily be treated, so they wound heal by primary intention. De-gloving injuries, where a shearing force has been applied to the skin and removed it from all its underlying blood supply, may be extremely difficult to assess, and in general the damage may be much more extensive than is first appreciated. Where this is suspected, the injury should also be assessed by plastic surgeons.

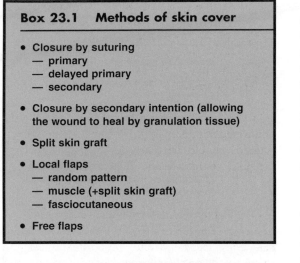

Box 23.1   Methods of skin cover

- Closure by suturing
  — primary
  — delayed primary
  — secondary

- Closure by secondary intention (allowing the wound to heal by granulation tissue)

- Split skin graft

- Local flaps
  — random pattern
  — muscle (+split skin graft)
  — fasciocutaneous

- Free flaps

There are a plethora of methods available for achieving skin cover in traumatic wounds (see Box 23.1). In addition to immediate or delayed suturing, these include skin grafting, local flaps and free flaps. The latter two categories are usually the province of plastic surgeons.

Skin grafting. This procedure takes skin from elsewhere in the body, transferring it to the area of need. *Split-thickness skin grafting* is commonest; the epidermis and part of the dermal layer are removed, leaving the remainder of the dermis and dermal appendages (e.g. hair follicles) to permit skin regeneration at the donor site. The recipient site must be clean, not infected, and have an adequate blood supply to permit the graft to 'take'. Some tissues (e.g. bare cortical bone, tendon) will not accept a skin graft.

Local flaps. Achieving skin cover with local flaps involves rotating an area of full-thickness, vascularised tissue so that it covers the defect while remaining attached to its origin. The rotated tissue may be muscle or skin. An example of a *muscle flap* is use of a medial gastrocnemius-based flap to cover a skin defect over the medial border of the tibia after a fracture. The distal part of medial gastrocnemius is mobilised subcutaneously, leaving the proximal part of the muscle attached to its origin and hence its blood supply. The muscle flap is moved to cover the defect over the fracture and then a split skin graft is placed on it to provide skin cover.

When skin is rotated to cover a defect, the flap may be supplied with blood via a defined pedicle with a known vascular supply or may rely simply on having a wide base. The latter is known as a *random pattern flap*, the name being a description of the vascular supply. Flaps with a defined pedicle include *fasciocutaneous* flaps, where the deep fascia that is moved with the skin carries the artery providing the blood supply. The rotation manoeuvre uncovers an area of (uninjured) muscle, which is itself covered by a split skin graft – this is known as the 'secondary defect'.

Free flaps involve the movement of a remote area of tissue with its own feeder vessels. The vessels are divided and reattached using microsurgical techniques to appropriate arteries and veins at the recipient site. There are now many described flaps of this nature; one of the earliest was the Chinese forearm flap, which moved skin from the radial border of the forearm based on the radial artery and veins. Venous drainage is often more of a problem to maintain than arterial inflow. Similar microsurgical techniques are used in replantation surgery after traumatic amputations.

Peripheral nerve injuries

Management of nerve injuries largely depends on whether they are closed or open. Closed nerve injuries have a variable prognosis. Compression injuries, frequently causing neurapraxia, have a relatively favourable prognosis and surgery is unlikely to be necessary. Conversely, traction injuries have a poor prognosis. Surgery should be reserved for specialised units, where a decision for or against exploration (possibly with nerve grafting of the damaged areas) will be made.

Most peripheral nerve injuries are the result of lacerations. Such wounds should be explored, the only exceptions being lacerations on the digit distal to the proximal interphalangeal (IP) joint, where the nerve is generally held to be too small to be readily repairable. At exploration, the nerve is generally repaired using magnification to ensure coaptation is as accurate as possible. Every effort is made to ensure that the repair is not under tension. The most common suturing method is *epineural repair*, where the outer coverings of cut ends of the whole nerve are coapted. Many hand surgeons use the operating microscope and very fine sutures to carry out a *perineural repair*, coapting individual fascicles, but as yet there is little evidence that this makes much difference.

Postoperative care

Postoperative care of patients with nerve injuries is extremely important. All patients are likely to require physiotherapy to guard against joint contractures which may occur. These may happen as a result of splintage, associated injuries to muscles and tendons, or muscle imbalance following nerve injury. A nerve frequently involved in the latter is the ulnar nerve, injury of which below the elbow results in the so-called *ulnar claw hand*, where there is muscle imbalance due to the loss of action of intrinsic muscles of the hand. The deformity consists of hyperextension at the MTP joint and marked flexion at the DIP and PIP joints of the ulnar two fingers (see Ch. 3). Management of ulnar nerve injuries needs to ensure that permanent joint contracture of the affected joints does not take place during the time that nerve regeneration is occurring. If the intrinsic muscles are to have any chance of effective function, normal joint movement must be maintained by passive physiotherapy and appropriate splinting while re-innervation is awaited.

Nerve regeneration is generally considered to proceed at a rate of 1 mm/day, so a lesion which is proximal in a limb may easily take a year to recover, and further motor recovery may be anticipated for 2 years. Sensory function can go on improving even longer, perhaps for 4 years, as the new axons mature and the brain learns to interpret the new pattern of signals. As a consequence of the many peripheral nerve injuries sustained in World War II, the Medical Research Council developed scales of recovery of sensory and motor function after nerve suture (Boxes 23.2 and 23.3). These scales are subtly different from the MRC scales of sensory and motor function presented in Chapter 3: they deal specifically with nerve recovery after injury.

The progress of the regenerating axons can be followed by the 'Tinel sign', which consists of parasthesiae felt in the denervated territory when

---

Box 23.2   The MRC scale of sensory recovery

S0 – absence of sensibility

S1 – recovery of deep cutaneous pain sensibility

S2 – return of some degree of superficial cutaneous pain and tactile sensibility

S3 – return of superficial cutaneous pain and tactile sensibility throughout the autonomous area with disappearance of overreaction

S3+ – return of sensibility as in stage 3 with the addition that there is some recovery of two-point discrimination

S4 – complete recovery

Box 23.3   The MRC scale of motor recovery

M0 – no contraction

M1 – return of perceptible contraction in the proximal muscles

M2 – return of perceptible contraction in the proximal and distal muscles

M3 – return of function in both proximal and distal muscles of such degree that all important muscles can act against resistance

M4 – return of function as in stage 3 with the addition that all synergic and independent movements are possible

M5 – complete recovery

---

the nerve is tapped at the level the new axon tips have reached. Once a given area of skin has been reached, sensibility will begin to reappear there. At first the sensation produced by stimulating the skin is highly unpleasant; hopefully it improves with time as more new fibres arrive and then mature.

Nerves recover poorly in all adult patients, and nerve injuries may be devastating, particularly for hand function. It is important to give early advice about the length of time over which recovery may be expected and about the prognosis. Unfortunately, recovery is extremely unpredictable. Patients may have to accept that they have had very substantial acute loss of limb function as a result of a nerve injury, and appropriate social and psychological support is required. Occasionally, palliative surgery such as muscle transfers may be helpful in the long term.

Vascular injury

Vascular injuries should be managed, as a matter of urgency, together with a vascular surgeon or plastic surgeon. Generally, a large artery is best operated on by a vascular surgeon, but small ones such as the digital arteries are more the province of the plastic surgeon. Arteriography may be needed to define the lesion before surgical exploration. The main decision is whether repair of the vessel is needed. If one digital artery is destroyed, the other will probably be adequate; one of the radial or ulnar arteries can usually be lost. Loss of a major artery below the knee may or may not be sustainable, depending on the individual patient's vascular anatomy.

The orthopaedic surgeon gets involved with vascular injuries because they are often part of a composite injury involving many tissues and structures in a limb. Trauma is no respecter of anatomical or interdisciplinary boundaries. The key to good management, as with so many things in musculoskeletal medicine and trauma, is teamwork.

Tendon injuries

Management of open tendon injuries involves exploration of the wound and appropriate repair. Injuries to the flexor tendons within the flexor sheaths in the palm of the hand require particular attention, and demand meticulous postoperative care with early active or passive movement of the tendon to ensure that adhesion formation is minimised. The technical challenge of achieving strong healing of the tendon, without adhesion formation between the tendon and its surrounding structures, has been one of the main reasons for the emergence of hand surgery as a subspeciality. Close collaboration between the surgeon and the physiotherapist is essential for success. The patient has to work hard to regain finger flexion, otherwise there is a real risk that the stiff digit will become so much of a liability that late amputation has to be advised.

The treatment of closed degenerative tendon ruptures varies according to site. Tears of the patella and quadriceps tendon should be repaired surgically as soon as they are recognised. The management of Achilles tendon ruptures is controversial. Some surgeons also treat these by surgical means and this can lead to excellent results. Unfortunately, the skin over the Achilles tendon has a precarious blood supply, and if wound infection occurs this can lead to rather extensive tendon necrosis and very delayed healing. Accordingly, other surgeons will treat such injuries in casts in plantarflexion, initially having the ankle fully plantarflexed for a period of approximately 4 weeks, and subsequently with decreasing plantarflexion for a further 4 weeks. Injuries to the supraspinatus are generally treated conservatively initially, but the results following such treatment are very variable and subsequent repair of the defect in supraspinatus is sometimes required. This may be due to persistent pain in the subacromial region or to weakness, or both.

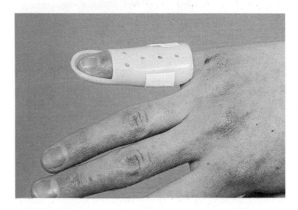

Figure 23.2 Mallet finger splint. A mallet finger occurs with rupture of the extensor tendon close to its insertion, leading to a lag at the DIPJ. Splintage is usually adequate treatment.

Index

Index

Index